Introduction to Phonetics and Phonology

Introduction to Phonetics and Phonology

FROM CONCEPTS TO TRANSCRIPTION

Jacqueline Bauman-Waengler

Boston ▪ New York ▪ San Francisco
Mexico City ▪ Montreal ▪ Toronto ▪ London ▪ Madrid ▪ Munich ▪ Paris
Hong Kong ▪ Singapore ▪ Tokyo ▪ Cape Town ▪ Sydney

Executive Editor and Publisher: Stephen D. Dragin
Series Editorial Assistant: Christina Certo
Marketing Manager: Kris Ellis-Levy
Production Editor: Paula Carroll
Editorial Production Service: Publishers' Design and Production Services, Inc.
Composition Buyer: Linda Cox
Manufacturing Buyer: Linda Morris
Electronic Composition: Publishers' Design and Production Services, Inc.
Interior Design: Publishers' Design and Production Services, Inc.
Cover Administrator: Kristina Mose-Libon

For related titles and support materials, visit our online catalog at
www.pearsonhighered.com.

Between the time website information is gathered and then published, it is not
unusual for some sites to have closed. Also, the transcription of URLs can result in
typographical errors. The publisher would appreciate notification where these errors
occur so that they may be corrected in subsequent editions.

ISBN-13: 978-0-205-40287-8
ISBN-10:   0-205-40287-9

Library of Congress Cataloging-in-Publication Data was not available at the time of
publication.

Printed in the United States of America

10 9 8 7 6 5 4 3   EDW   11

Allyn & Bacon
is an imprint of

www.pearsonhighered.com

Jacqueline Bauman-Waengler has been a university professor for over thirty years. Her main teaching and clinical emphases have been in the areas of phonetics and phonology, including disorders of articulation and phonology in children. She has published and presented widely in these areas both nationally and internationally. In addition to this book, the third edition of *Articulatory and Phonological Impairments: A Clinical Focus* was recently published by Pearson/Allyn and Bacon.

CONTENTS

Transcription Workbook   *317*

The concept for this book developed from two perceived necessities: to connect phonetics and phonology into a conceptual unity and to demonstrate the clinical relevance of phonetics, phonology, and phonetic transcription for beginning students within communication disorders. Although there are many excellent textbooks that deal with both phonetics and phonology, they are typically more linguistically oriented, and, therefore, their application to communication disorders falls short. This textbook attempts to tie phonetics and phonology into a framework that can be utilized by readers as they begin to learn about the assessment and treatment of individuals with articulation and phonological disorders. This relates directly to demonstrating the clinical relevance of these concepts. First, phonetics and phonology as practical, usable notions are demonstrated by many clinical examples. These examples draw from several sources, including not just speech-language pathology but audiology, linguistics, communication, teaching English as a second language, and teaching within a classroom. A clinical case study is developed at the beginning of each chapter and followed throughout the chapter to demonstrate that particular subject area. In addition, clinical examples and applications are a portion of each chapter.

Integrated into this textbook is the gradual yet systematic development of phonetic transcription. There is a phonetic transcription workbook at the end of this text, which offers many transcription exercises. These exercises allow the reader to learn transcription skills in a comprehensive manner while targeting specific problems that beginners may have when learning these skills. For example, word stress and vowel variations are an integral portion of the workbook. At the same time the text attempts to demonstrate how transcription skills can be used and why they are important. Too often our students exit the beginning transcription course with some basic skills but no understanding of the relevance and importance of their utilization within the clinical process. This book demonstrates in various scenarios the practical application of phonetic transcription. The end result will hopefully be a more user-friendly text that introduces students to concepts within communication, linguistics, and teaching as well as speech-language pathology and audiology.

The textbook has nine chapters. Each chapter begins with chapter highlights and typically one case study that is followed and unfolds throughout the chapter. Each of the chapters includes a separate case study at the end of the chapter, followed by a chapter summary, which briefly discusses the chapter highlights. Key terms for the chapter are also located at the end of each chapter, along with additional readings and exercises labeled "Think Critically." The last portion of each chapter is a group of multiple-choice questions that the reader can work through independently.

The first chapter introduces the concepts of phonetics and phonology with basic core definitions. However, the end of the chapter ties the two concepts together while introducing articulation and phonological disorders to exemplify two facets of these concepts. The second chapter is an overview of the respiratory, phonatory, resonatory, and articulatory systems. In addition, a brief review outlines acoustic phonetics and resonance properties. Chapter 3 introduces phonetic transcription and the International Phonetic Alphabet, while Chapters 4 and 5 define and classify the vowels and consonants of American English. Chapter 6 is an extensive chapter on dialect. It defines core terms and discusses in depth regional and ethnical dialectal variations within the United States. In addition, the definition of the limited English proficient student is presented within the context of English as a second language. The vowel and consonant systems of six prevalent foreign languages within the United States are presented, along with typical pronunciation problems for individuals learning English as a second language relative to each of these languages. Chapter 7 contains the concepts of coarticulation and assimilation, the suprasegmentals, and finally, the diacritics—narrow transcription markers—are introduced and practical examples given. Chapter 8 covers normal phonological development and relates this acquisition to three theoretical models: distinctive feature, natural phonology, and nonlinear phonology. Chapter 9 is a practical application chapter that demonstrates how phonetics and phonology can function together when analyzing the speech of children and adults.

The final portion of this text includes a transcription workbook, an extensive glossary, and a reference list. Key concepts are outlined and definitions provided. The reference list includes updated references for a wide variety of topics. It is hoped that this text will be easy to read and provide enough applications to the real world that the reader will be able to easily apply these concepts to an array of situations.

Acknowledgments

A project of this size always has a great number of people who are responsible for guiding and helping throughout the process. First, I would like to acknowledge all my students who demonstrated the evolution of phonetic transcription skills in my classes. Those who struggled with transcription taught me a great deal about which basic skills are necessary and which ones are difficult. I have used this knowledge many times in the book and in the phonetic transcription workbook.

The person who has been instrumental in keeping me motivated and pushing me along, maybe dragging me at times, is Steve Dragin, Allyn and Bacon's executive editor and publisher. He did not lose sight of the project when I almost did at certain times. He is patient and understanding in a world that is extremely busy for him. I also gratefully acknowledge Katie Heimsoth, former editorial assistant at Allyn and Bacon. She prepared multiple "to do" lists, which did keep me on track, especially in the final stages of this project. Special gratitude goes to my research assistants Cassie Hall and Traci Davenport, who helped with references and proofreading, and to ZestNet producers Duane Eells and Ric Ruffinelli, who are responsible for editing and creating the phonetic transcription DVD. Thanks to Lorraine Storm, an art student at the University of Redlands, who is responsible for the illustrations. Special thanks to two dear friends, Dee and John Lockwood, who helped coordinate and video the children and adults on the DVD. I would also like to thank Castaway Seven Studios Ventura, CA, for their help with this production. A special thank you to my companion and technical guide Les Beears. His patience and help throughout the project has meant so much. I also would like to acknowledge all the reviewers who gave their time and beneficial suggestions: Michael Blomgren, University of Utah; Carolyn Chaney, San Francisco State University; Gayle H. Daly, Longwood University; Patricia Lohman-Hawk, California State University–East Bay; Lauren K. Nelson, University of Northern Iowa; Horabail S. Venkatagiri, Iowa State University; and Roberta Wacker-Mundy, State University of New York, Plattsburgh.

CHAPTER 1

Introducing Phonetics and Phonology

Chapter Highlights

- What is phonetics?
- What three areas of study are emphasized in phonetics?
- What is phonology?
- What is the difference between a phoneme and an allophone?
- What is the difference between free variation and complementary distribution?
- How are form and function related to phonetics and phonology?

Chapter Application: Case Studies

This is Andrea's first year of graduate school, where she is studying communication disorders. Although she feels that she has a good background in speech development and language disorders, she has never been in a clinical setting. Suddenly she is in the clinic and planning therapy for several children who have speech sound problems. For example, Megan seems to be having trouble with her s-sounds—they sound more like "th," while Jess is clearly saying "wabbit" for "rabbit." Frank seems to have quite a different problem: He leaves off the ends of the words, which makes him hard to understand at times. He will say "toe" for "toad" or "bow" for "boat." Andrea wonders about the differences in their problems. Some children seem not quite ready to say their sounds correctly; however, Frank can say the sounds, but not at the end of words. Is there a difference in the speech sound problems of these children? Her supervisor suggests that she review her notes for the basic definitions of phonetics and phonology. Andrea wonders how this will help her in understanding the speech sound problems of these children.

Lynda has always been interested in languages. Her family lived for several years in Thailand when she was a child, and she learned Thai in school as well as being exposed to other languages that were spoken in the small towns where she was living. Lynda is now at the university studying linguistics, which is the study of language and languages. For Lynda's senior project she would like to compare the speech sounds of Thai to American English. Her instructor tells her that she should think about the phonetic and phonological differences in the two languages. How would Lynda analyze the two languages based on phonetic versus phonological principles?

Communication, the exchange of information, is central to all human beings. We communicate in many different ways, by waving to someone we know, by smiling to a companion, by writing a note to our roommate, and by e-mailing our friends and family. However, our primary means of communication is speech. We talk about the weather, what we did over the weekend, as well as our hopes and aspirations. Speech is by far the most widely used means of exchanging information.

If we examine the use of the term **speech**, we find we are referring to oral, verbal communication. Speech, as a communication mode, is the exchange of information through speaking or talking. This term can be used in a number of ways. First, *speech* is often used together with the term *language* to imply the mental faculty of verbal communication. For example, speech and language distinguish man from other species of animals. In this context speech refers to the cognitive ability of *Homo sapiens* to use oral language.

The term *speech* can be used to denote a more formal spoken communication to an audience: for example, "She gave a *speech* on the development of computer technology in the last ten years," or "He was required to give a *speech* for his introductory philosophy course."

In addition, *speech* can be used to indicate the manner of speaking or the actual way in which the verbalization is delivered. Examples of the term *speech* used in this way would include "His *speech* was marked by a foreign accent" and "Her *speech* was hard to understand because she mispronounced certain sounds."

The slightly different definitions of the term *speech* are also helpful when establishing the importance of speech for various interests and professions. Within the field of communications, which encompasses radio and television broadcasting, speech delivery plays an important role. Thus, for individuals interested in broadcasting, the ability to effectively use speech—referring not only to the delivery of an oral message but also to the manner of speaking and pronunciation—is an important variable. Oral communication skills will also be important for anyone involved in theater, acting, or public speaking, as well as specific aspects of business and education.

In a narrower sense, specific aspects of speech are the primary focus within linguistics, teaching English as a second language, and communication disorders, which encompasses speech-language pathology and audiology. For each of these professions, the study of speech and **speech sounds**, i.e., the individual units of speech, are fundamental.

To understand speech, there is no better starting point than basic knowledge in phonetics. Generally speaking, **phonetics** is the study of speech emphasizing the description of speech sounds according to their production, transmission, and perceptual features (Bauman-Waengler, 2008). This study encompasses an objective description of how speech units are produced and tries to measure speech characteristics as accurately as possible.

The next section of this beginning chapter will discuss this definition of phonetics in more detail by elaborating on the three specific branches of study within this discipline. Throughout the chapter, the relevance of phonetics and its application will be highlighted by referring back to the case studies at the beginning of the chapter and by further examples.

Defining Phonetics

The discipline of phonetics involves studying speech sounds. Although there are countless sounds we humans can produce—whistles, cries, groans, and moans, for example—only those sounds that make up a "word" are considered speech sounds. If we say the word "lip," for example, three distinctly ordered speech sounds "l-i-p" have been uttered to convey an explicit meaning.

These segment-sized units known as speech sounds are the basic unit of phonetics. A phone is another term for these phonetic sound units. A **phone** is any particular occurrence of a sound segment that is used by a speaker saying words, regardless of whether the target language uses them (Velleman, 1998). In a phonetic analysis, they are described using phonetic transcription and are placed in brackets. Thus, [t] would exemplify the first speech sound in the word "tooth." Phonetic transcription is the use of a specific written notation to record utterances, specifically to describe speech sounds. Phonetic transcription will be further defined and examples given in Chapter 3.

Acoustics is a subfield of physics that deals with the generation and transmission of sound (Shriberg & Kent, 2003).

There are many different ways to examine speech sounds as a portion of the total speech communication process. Speech sounds could be analyzed according to their *production* characteristics. For example, we could examine how sounds are actually articulated: the physical structures that are used and the oral movements necessary to say the sound. Or speech sounds could be viewed in relationship to their acoustic *transmission* properties, which include specific characteristics relative to the frequency, intensity, and duration of a specific sound. Finally, we could study speech sounds according to how they are *perceived*, how speech sounds are recognized and distinguished from one another. These three areas are labeled (1) articulatory phonetics, the branch of phonetics that examines production features of speech sounds, (2) acoustic phonetics, the branch that documents the transmission properties of speech sounds, and (3) auditory phonetics, which studies the perception of speech sounds. The following section will expand upon each of these areas of phonetics, providing examples for each.

FOCUS 1: *What is phonetics?*

Phonetics as Production, Transmission, and Perception of Speech Sounds

The first area of phonetics, **articulatory phonetics**, examines how the different speech sounds are generated; it describes and classifies speech sounds according to parameters of their actual production. One basic type of classification is derived from the specific structures that are used to produce the various speech sounds: the lips, tongue, alveolar ridge, mandible

Concept Exercise ARTICULATORS

Say the first sound in "<u>f</u>oot." Note how the bottom lip and the top teeth come close to one another, as air is passing between the two. Now say the first sound in "<u>b</u>oy." Which articulators are involved in the production of this sound?

The alveolar ridge is the ridge directly behind the upper front teeth. The palate is the hard, bony roof of the mouth. The velum or soft palate is the soft, muscular rear portion of the roof of the mouth.

(lower jaw), teeth, hard palate, and velum. Those <u>anatomical structures</u> <u>directly involved</u> in the generation of speech sounds are referred to as **articulators**. One aspect of articulatory phonetics is the classification of speech sounds according to these articulators. The first sound in "far," "f," involves the integrated action of the lower lip and upper teeth. These two articulators would classify "f" as a labio- (=lip) dental (=upper teeth) sound.

Another categorization divides speech sounds into two general groups: vowels and consonants. **Vowels** are relatively open productions, without articulatory constriction, whereas **consonants** are relatively closed productions, typically with significant articulatory constriction (Small, 2005). Examples of vowels include the first sound in "<u>i</u>t" and the last sound in "m<u>e</u>." Consonants are exemplified by the first sounds in "<u>t</u>oe," "<u>s</u>o," and "<u>r</u>ow."

Reflect on This: Clinical Application

How does our knowledge in articulatory phonetics help us in our work with individuals demonstrating speech difficulties? The following scenario can possibly show this: An 8-year-old child is brought to you by her parents. They are concerned because Sandy cannot say her s-sounds correctly. She does not have a hearing loss or any structural problems that might hamper her production, but every time she says her name, for example, she produces a sound that is clearly not a normal "s." First, you would probably want to know how she is making her particular off-target sound. By closely observing her mouth and by listening carefully as she says a word with "s," you should be able to get a fair impression of how her articulators are positioned during the production. You would then compare her articulation to what is considered to be the typical articulation of "s." After this, you can effectively help Sandy by providing specific directions and using certain techniques to adjust her articulators so that a normal "s" results.

What role did articulatory phonetics play in this process? First, you had to know in detail what the articulators should be doing and where they should be placed for a regular "s" production. This information is gained

Concept Exercise VARIATIONS OF "S" PRODUCTION

Prolong the s-sound, the first sound in the word "saw." During this "s" production move the tongue slightly forward in your mouth, toward the front teeth. Do you hear the way the "s" changes its quality? Go back to your typical s-production and glide the tongue slightly back in your mouth. Now how does the "s" sound? These two variations in [s] can be noted in children with s-problems.

from sound descriptions articulatory phonetics has to offer. Second, based on your knowledge of the typical "s" articulation, you then had to judge how Sandy's sound was productionally different. Similarities and differences between speech sound productions are main issues in articulatory phonetics. These principles could be applied to children or adults with speech sound disorders. Because of its decisive clinical role, the major emphasis of this book will be articulatory phonetics. Knowledge gained in studying aspects of articulatory phonetics will provide the cornerstone for assessment and treatment of these problems.

The second portion of our definition of phonetics examines the physical properties of speech sounds as they are transmitted through the air. This branch is referred to as **acoustic phonetics**. Professionals specializing in acoustic phonetics study speech sounds in the form of sound waves that travel through the air from a speaker to a listener (Lyons, 1981). Acoustic phonetics deals with the properties of speech sound waves such as their frequency, intensity, and duration.

For example, certain speech sounds, such as "s" and "z," contain high-frequency components (from approximately 4000 to 12,000 Hz) that are relatively intense (Ohde & Sharf, 1992). This gives them their characteristic quality. Vowels, on the other hand, contain more intense frequency areas, clearly below 4000 Hz. Principles of **resonance**, another area of study within acoustic phonetics, are important to our understanding of how specific speech sounds are generated.

The third portion of our definition of phonetics examines the *perception* of speech. This subdivision is called **auditory** (Lyons, 1981) or **perceptual phonetics** (Edwards, 2003). As sound waves are received by the hearing mechanism, they must be identified and interpreted. Auditory (perceptual) phonetics is the study of how speech sound waves are identified and perceived by the listener (Edwards, 2003).

In order to delineate acoustic from auditory phonetics, let's look at how each of the branches might approach the study of speech events. As previously stated, professionals specializing in acoustic phonetics examine the frequency, intensity, and duration of speech sounds. They could do this by using instrumentation to analyze the physical parameters of speech sounds and arrive at a relatively objective determination of their frequency and intensity components, for example. On the other hand, in auditory phonetics the terms *pitch* and *loudness* are used instead of *frequency* and *intensity* to underline speech sound perception. Is that just splitting hairs again? Surely frequency and pitch or intensity and loudness are identical. Are we just using different labels to identify the same thing? A wide variety of studies, many dating back for over seventy years (e.g., Nordmark, 1968; Riesz, 1928; Shower & Biddulph, 1931; Stevens, 1935; Stevens & Volkmann, 1940), found that the parameters of frequency-pitch and intensity-loudness do not have a one-to-one correspondence. That means that the objective physical properties of a given sound, intensity, for example, and the perceived subjective interpretation of that sound as loudness are not identical. Assume that you are asked to match the perceived *loudness* levels of two tones, one tone that is 100 Hz, a low hum, and one that is 1000 Hz, a fairly high-pitched tone for a female voice. Your task is to make the two tones perceptually of equal loudness. You have a dial that increases or decreases the objective intensity of each tone, and you can switch back and forth from one tone to the other to compare the two loudness levels.

Reflect on This: Clinical Application

How does our knowledge in acoustic phonetics help us in our work with clients with speech impairments? Examine the following clinical example: Jeff's wife urged him to come to the Speech and Hearing Clinic. She noticed that he frequently misunderstood words and that some of his sound productions, such as "s" and "z," were often imprecise. Jeff was a 35-year-old operator of heavy machines who worked primarily on large construction jobs with very loud equipment. He has never worn any ear protection against the noise. A hearing evaluation revealed that Jeff had a substantial high-frequency hearing loss (4000 Hz and above) in both ears. From knowledge gained in studying acoustic phonetics, we know that certain sounds, such as "s" and "z," contain high-frequency components that are above 4000 Hz. In fact, it is these high-frequency components that determine the characteristic quality of these sounds. In order to understand and discriminate "s" and "z" from other sounds, Jeff must not only be able to hear these high frequencies, he must also be able to distinguish various intensity levels of these frequencies. For example, if an individual cannot hear specific intensity differences above 4000 Hz, there is a good chance that "s," "f," and "th" will be confused (Ohde & Sharf, 1992). The knowledge gained in acoustic phonetics would allow us to conclude that both Jeff's discrimination and, therefore, his production of certain sounds could be affected by the acoustic characteristics of his hearing loss.

Although the two tones are different frequencies, you will find that it is not difficult to reach a setting that will make the two tones sound as if they are equally loud. However, when you arrive at this subjective interpretation of equal loudness, you will find that the two tones have very different objective intensities. For example, if the 1,000 Hz tone is at 40 dB, the 100 Hz tone will be adjusted to over 60 dB (Ohde & Sharf, 1992). Differences will also be found between objective measurements and subjective perceptions if we try a comparable experiment with frequency and pitch. These results demonstrate the careful distinction we should make between the objective physical properties of sounds (frequency, intensity) and the subjective perception of these sounds (pitch, loudness).

How does the information learned in auditory (perceptual) phonetics help us in our work with clients with communication disorders? Adult speakers learning English as a second language are often interested in intervention to reduce their foreign accent. One of the problems that they demonstrate is confusing sounds used in their own native language for somewhat comparable sounds of General American English. A prominent example is the mix-up of "l" and "r" by Japanese speakers learning English. In Japanese these are not two distinct sounds but rather productions of similar sounds that can be used interchangeably. For the Japanese speaker, it is not a matter of objectively hearing the physical acoustic properties that differentiate "l" and "r"; we can verify that their hearing is within normal limits. For these Japanese speakers of American English, it is a question of perceiving the contrasts between "l" and "r." In spite of repeated exposure to speakers of American English, native speakers of Japanese have difficulty perceiving these differences.

Reflect on This: Clinical Application

Leila, an executive at a computer firm, came to the Speech and Hearing Clinic with a problem. Her hearing was normal, and her written English demonstrated competency in differentiating "l" and "r." However, she would often mix up these two sounds in her spoken conversation. She had difficulty perceiving the distinctions between "l" and "r" in her own speech as well as in the speech of others. The knowledge gained in auditory phonetics emphasizing the subjective perception of these sounds applies directly to Leila's situation. In order to help Leila, we needed to develop her perceptual abilities. By pairing the perceptual and production differences for "l" and "r" (also using our knowledge from articulatory phonetics), Leila became better at perceiving and articulating the two different sounds.

To summarize, production aspects of speech sounds are reflected in articulatory phonetics, and transmission properties in acoustic phonetics, while perception of speech sounds is correlated with the branch known as auditory (perceptual) phonetics.

FOCUS 2: *What three areas of study are emphasized in phonetics?*

The next section examines a completely different aspect of speech sounds: their *function* or use within a language system. In this new section, the focus will be not on how speech sounds are produced, transmitted, or perceived but rather on how they are used within a language, i.e., what kind of system and organization can be documented as these units are put together to form meaningful words.

Defining Phonology

Phonology studies the structure and systematic patterning of sounds in a particular language (Akmajian, Demers, Farmer, & Harnish, 2001). Therefore, phonology includes the description of the sounds a language uses and the rules governing how these sounds are organized. In other words, phonology is concerned with *which* speech sounds a language uses and how they are *arranged* and *function* within that language (Poole, 1999).

Phonology is considered a branch of linguistics. Linguistics is an area of study that remains rather unclear to most. Some think of a linguist as a person who speaks several languages fluently, while others postulate that linguistics has to do with using correct grammar. In actuality, **linguistics** is a field that is concerned with the nature of language and communication (Akmajian et al. 2001). Linguists are interested in the principles that govern languages, the systematic rules that determine pronunciation, word formation, and grammatical constructions. However, when linguists talk about "rules," they are not talking about how you *should* pronounce something, or, for example, that you should not say "ain't," but about rules that describe the actual language of a particular group of speakers.

At the present time, programs and courses in phonetics are also housed within the department of linguistics. However, historically, phonetics owes its development to physicians and scientists (see Moses, 1964; Ohala, 1991; Panconcelli-Calzia, 1957), and at different points in time the two disciplines were separated (Ohala, 2004). There is a movement, continuing today, to reintegrate phonetics and phonology.

Linguists assume that human language is at all levels rule-governed. In this sense, "rule-governed" indicates that there are certain generalizations and regularities in the structure and function of a particular language, not that, for example, you need to follow certain rules of grammar.

Going back to our original definition, the study of phonology examines how speech sounds function within a language. Here we are referring to their *linguistic* function. Although speech sounds can be described according to their phonetic production features, such as vocal fold vibration during the production of the sound and the articulators involved during the production of the sound, these sounds also have a linguistic function. When arranged in certain ways, these sound units make up words with a specific meaning. Two words can be very different in their sound structure. For example, words such as "map" and "potato" vary considerably in the arrangement of sounds and in the number of syllables. However, other words are different by only one unit: "bee" and "beet," for example. Here the presence (or absence) of "t" is the distinguishing factor resulting in two distinct words with very different meanings. The words "hit" and "him" also demonstrate this principle. In this case, "t" and "m" differentiate between the two words, each with their characteristic sound structure that signals to us two different words with two different meanings. The smallest linguistic unit that is able, when combined with other such units, to establish word meanings and distinguish between them is referred to as a **phoneme**.

Phonemes, then, are sound units with a special, language-dependent function: the linguistic function to establish and distinguish between word meanings. The phoneme is the central unit of phonology. The term *phoneme* references a particular language. Therefore, one speaks about the phonemes of American English or Spanish, for example. In addition, when phonemes of a particular language are represented, they are placed between slanted lines, or virgules. For example, /t/ signifies the phoneme "t." Using our previous example, the phoneme /t/ distinguishes between "bee" and "beet." Words that differ in only one phoneme value, such as the examples given previously of "bee" and "beet" or "hit" and "him," are called **minimal pairs**.

The distinction between phonetics and phonology can be exemplified in the following example. The human vocal mechanism can produce a very wide range of sounds; however, only a small number of these are used in a language to construct all of its words. Phonetics is the study of all possible speech sounds, while phonology studies the way in which the speakers of a particular language use a selection of these sounds in order to express meaning.

In phonology, first we look at which sounds a language uses. If we choose American English as our language to be examined, we would first note the sound units that are used in American English, thus, all the vowels and consonants that establish words. When we attempt to do this, we find that there are quite a few different vowels and consonants.

Second, phonology looks at how these sound units are arranged within a particular language. Arrangement pertains to the rule-governed ordering or patterning of speech sounds within that language, such as which consonants can begin or which ones can end a word or syllable. *Rule-governed* also pertains to which speech sounds can or cannot be combined to create words. Using American English, we could examine the list of vowels and consonants and see which rules might be operating within the word inventory. We might notice, for example, that "ng," the last sound in "ring," cannot be at the beginning of any words in American English; it exists only at the end of words or syllables such as "sing" or "singing." This, then, would be one characteristic of the phonological system of American English. On the other hand, the phonemes "h" and "w" can appear only at the beginnings of words or syllables, such as in "house," "a-hoy," "wagon," and "a-way." But what about words such as "how" and "borrow"—they have "w" at the end of the word? Remember that we are talking about sound units, not letters. Although "how" and "borrow" are spelled with a "w" letter at the end of the word, there is not a w-sound at the end of the words. If you say "how" you will notice that the last sound is the one in "<u>ou</u>t" or "<u>ou</u>ch," while the last sound in "borrow" is the "o" as in "<u>oat</u>" or "<u>oak</u>." Also, when looking at the arrangement of speech sounds, we would find that certain consonants can be combined together in words while others cannot. If a word begins with "f," we know that a combination of f + r, as in "<u>fr</u>ee," is acceptable, f + l, as in "<u>fl</u>y," works as well, but f + t is not a sound combination that is found at the beginning of an American English word. However, if we analyze a bit further, we will find that the f + t combination of sounds is acceptable at the ends of words, as in "li<u>ft</u>" and "le<u>ft</u>." Phonology describes how the speech sounds can and cannot be arranged to form meaningful words. **Phonotactics** is the <u>specific branch of phonology that deals with restrictions in a language on the permissible combinations of phonemes.</u> Phonotactics identifies permissible syllable structure, consonant clusters, and vowel sequences within a particular language.

 FOCUS 3: *What is phonology?*

 ## Reflect on This: Clinical Application

Imagine Larry, the linguist, who has learned that a group of people speaking an unknown language has just been discovered in the depths of the jungle. Larry has traveled to these people and would like to record and document the language they speak. What would he probably do? First, he would have several people name objects, say words, and describe pictures and try to document, using phonetic transcription, the speech sounds that these individuals use. By observing how the various speech sounds are produced, Larry would be using phonetics, specifically, articulatory phonetics. Second, he would probably examine the way these sound units are arranged to form meaningful words; thus, he would be examining the phonology of the language. Which sounds can occur at the beginning and which ones at the end of words and syllables, for example, is one aspect of the phonology of a particular language. Also, which consonants can be acceptably combined to form words and which ones cannot is a portion of the phonological analysis of this new language. Larry the linguist would also try to discover rules about the phonology of this new language. How many consonants can be combined at the beginning and at the end of a syllable would exemplify one type of phonological rule. Thus, Larry would use information from phonetics, specifically articulatory phonetics, and phonology to document this new language.

Phonemes and Allophones

The phoneme concept at first appears to be simple and straightforward. If we look at a previous definition we find that the phoneme is the smallest linguistic unit that is able, when combined with other such units, to establish word meanings and distinguish between them. To demonstrate this, we could take a word, such as "bat," replace one sound with another, and see whether a difference in meaning results. If so, we would know that those two sounds are phonemes within that particular language. Given this concept, if we replace the /b/ in "bat" with an /r/, then a different word emerges, namely "rat." We know then that /b/ and /r/ are different phonemes of American English. Using this same technique we find /s/ (sat), /m/ (mat), /f/ (fat) and /h/ (hat) are further examples of phonemes in American English. The idea of the phoneme is considered to be an abstraction, as phonemes are not single, concrete, unchanging entities. A phoneme is an abstraction from the many different variations that occur for a particular sound as it is heard in differing contexts of conversational speech. This does not necessarily make the phoneme concept complex or difficult to understand. We constantly deal with abstractions. Take, for example, the concept "car." A car is not a single, unchanging entity. There are big cars and small cars, cars with solid roofs and those that are convertibles, and cars of various colors and designs. However, there are certain characteristics that we accept as being typical to the concept of "car." We could say that the car concept embraces a whole family of units that are related yet somehow distinct. Even two cars of the same model, color, and year will have slight variations that can be detected. If we apply this to the phoneme concept, we find a similar abstraction. So, when we speak of a particular phoneme, /t/ for example, we are referring to the typical "t," but we also take into consideration the varieties of "t" that are used in various contexts and by different speakers. The term **allophone** is used to refer to the variations of the phoneme used by various speakers in differing contexts. While a phoneme belongs to a basic group of sounds that can distinguish word meaning, i.e., changing one phoneme in a word can produce a different word, an allophone is a variation in phoneme realization that does not change the meaning of a word. An allophone is one of several similar phones that belong to the same phoneme family; it represents a slight variation of the basic sound unit. Speakers of a particular language perceive a phoneme as a single distinctive sound in that language, while an allophone is considered to be a variation, but not a meaning-distinguishing production difference. Within the phonological system of American English, there are many examples of allophones.

Several allophonic variations can occur with the /p/ phoneme in various contexts. At the beginning of a word, as a single sound unit, /p/ is typically aspirated. Aspiration is that slight puff of air that you hear if you pronounce the word "pie" or "pot." This is transcribed as [pʰ], the small raised ʰ representing the puff of air or aspiration in phonetic transcription. However, /p/ is typically unaspirated following "s," as in "spy" or "spot." These allophonic variations, exemplified by aspiration or lack of aspiration, do not have phonemic value within the phonological system of American English—they do not change the meaning of the word. In other words, we can hear these differences, but both aspirated and unaspirated *p*-sounds are considered one phoneme, /p/.

Let's consider one other allophonic variation of /p/. At the end of a word, /p/ can be unreleased. In this case, *unreleased* means that the lips come together but there is no releasing movement of the lips. The lips, therefore, remain closed; there is no movement to separate the lips again. If the unreleased [p] is substituted for the typical [p] that occurs at the end of a word, the meaning of the word will not change. These two production variations are allophones of the /p/ phoneme. Say the word "mop," bringing the lips together for the final "p" and then opening them slightly after the production. This is a released [p]. Now try the same word, but this time leave your lips together at the end of the word. This is an unreleased [p]. You can probably feel and hear the difference between the two p-sounds; however, if you say one or the other (released or unreleased), we would still understand the word to be "mop." These two allophonic variations do not change the word meaning.

Beginning Case Study

LYNDA STUDYING LINGUISTICS

Lynda was presented at the beginning of the chapter. She is studying linguistics and would like to compare the speech sounds of Thai to those of American English. How would phonetics and phonology help this analysis? First, when comparing the production aspects of the speech sounds, their phonetic characteristics, Lynda could note that there are many similar vowels, such as "ee" and "oo." However, there is also a vowel in Thai that is similar in production to "oo" but without the characteristic lip rounding noted in the American English "oo" vowel. These two vowels—"oo" with lip rounding and "oo" without lip rounding—are two different phonemes in Thai: They signal meaning differences in Thai. In addition, "p," "t," and "k," when produced with aspiration (that characteristic puff of air that can be heard after these consonants in words such as "pie," "toe," and "key") versus without aspiration (the lack of this puff of air in words such as "spoon," "stove," and "ski"), also have phonemic value. Thus a word produced with an aspirated "p" and one produced without aspiration in Thai will have two different meanings; "p" with aspiration and "p" without aspiration are two different phonemes in Thai. To go one step further, the aspirated and unaspirated "p" are allophonic variations of the /p/ phoneme in American English. In Thai, they are not; the aspirated and unaspirated /p/ represent two distinct phonemes of this language.

While other differences exist between the phonetic production features and the phonological system of Thai, these examples demonstrate to Lynda the value of both phonetic and phonological analysis in her studies.

FOCUS 4: *What is the difference between a phoneme and an allophone?*

Free Variation or Complementary Distribution

In the preceding section, different allophones of /p/ were introduced. For example, depending on the context and the position in the word, /p/ can be aspirated or unaspirated and released or unreleased. The term **free variation** is used to indicate two allophones of one phoneme that could be exchanged for one another in similar contexts. Therefore, it is optional and unpredictable whether one or the other is produced in that context for that particular phoneme (Akmajian et al., 2001; Grunwell, 1987). Free variation can be a matter of personal habit or possibly regional pronunciation. Given our previous examples, we could say that the released or unreleased variation of the /p/ at the end of a word is in free variation. A particular speaker in a given context may choose to release the /p/ while in a different context may demonstrate an unreleased /p/. Given the context this allophonic variation is not predictable and it is optional. On the other hand there are other allophonic variants that are context conditioned, and their occurrence is predictable. **Complementary distribution** is used to indicate the mutually exclusive relationship between two phonetically similar segments. A mutually exclusive relationship means that one segment occurs in an environment where the other segment never occurs. Mutually exclusive refers to linguistic environments that do not overlap.

Think about a baseball team: Each player standing on the field has his own "environment" where he waits for the ball to be hit. This environment is the territory where he launches an offensive strategy, the territory that he covers when the opposite team hits the ball into the field. He may be the center fielder, the right fielder, or the first baseman. His position or territory is defined relative to the bases and whether it is inside or outside the base lines, for example. (Hopefully you have never seen two players collide because they have lost sight of their territories.) Any single player with any of these territories is not the team—the team is the whole collection of players with their territories. Think of the phoneme like the team and the allophones like the players. Allophones also have their "territories" or linguistic environments that they cover, and no allophones of a phoneme in complementary distribution will have overlapping territories. When one sound enters the territory of another, you know they are on opposing teams, i.e., members of different phoneme groups. When you define the territory of an allophone, you are defining its distribution, the set of places within words in a language where the allophone appears.

Here is an example: "spin" versus "pʰin," "spool" versus "pʰool," "spot" versus "pʰot." The aspirated "p" (pʰ) and the unaspirated "p" are in complementary distribution. At the beginning of a word "p" is aspirated while following "s" the p-sound is not aspirated. An English speaker hears these sounds as the same sound; thus, these two variations in pronunciation will not be heard as different words with different meanings.

Another example might be helpful. In American English there are two distinct allophones of "l." The first one, which is called the light "l," is produced typically at the beginning of a word, when "l" precedes a vowel or follows an initial consonant. Thus, the light "l" is used in words such as

The light and dark "l" allophones demonstrate distinct production differences. The front portion of the tongue has a convex shape for the light "l," while the dark "l" changes qualitatively due to the elevation of the tongue's posterior portion (Heffner, 1975; Shriberg & Kent, 2003). To demonstrate the different tongue shapes, say the word "little," noting the differences between the beginning "l" and the "l" at the end of the word.

"lip" and "slip." The second variation of "l," called the dark "l," is found, for example, in word-final positions and when it precedes a consonant. Word examples for the dark "l" include "full" and "told." These two types of /l/ allophones are in complementary distribution; they are predictable, dependent on the context, and they occur in mutually exclusive contexts. You would not typically substitute the dark "l" in a context where the light "l" occurs.

FOCUS 5: *What is the difference between free variation and complementary distribution?*

Interrelationships Between Phonetics and Phonology

Although closely related, phonetics and phonology represent two distinct areas of study. The concepts *form* and *function* have been used to characterize this distinction. Phonetics emphasizes the form of speech sounds by describing and categorizing their physical attributes, that is, their articulatory and acoustic components and their auditory effects. Phonology stresses their function as meaning-establishing and meaning-differentiating phonemes within a language system. Adequate form and function of all sound segments are basic requirements for meaningful utterances in any language. Adequate form is established by the way the sound in question is produced, that is, by articulatory events. If the end product of these events is qualitatively acceptable to the speakers of a specific language, they perceive it as being a speech sound of their system. Adequate function relates to the observance of language-specific rules regarding the use and arrangement of these sound segments. The end product is the establishment of words that convey a particular meaning within that specific language.

Every utterance has two facets: an audible sequence of speech sounds and the specific meaning conveyed through this sequence. For example, if someone says, "Look at that bee," there is an audible sequence of sounds that conveys a meaning. If you are not particularly fond of bees, this sequence of sounds could convey a warning, at least an alert that a bee is in the vicinity. If, however, someone says, "Look at that beet," the production has changed, there is the addition of an extra sound—a "t"—and, in addition, the meaning has changed. This statement would not send a warning to you but would just direct your attention to a harmless form of vegetable. Both the form, i.e., the production of the sound units, and their function, the arrangement of these units into a meaningful word, are important in our understanding of speech.

Close interrelationships exist between form and function; they are largely dependent on one another. Without acceptable production features, without the acceptable form, sound segments cannot fulfill their linguistic function. A child might produce a sound in words, for example, that is perceived as not quite "s" and not quite "sh" but somewhere between the two speech sounds, an s-sh-type production; in other words, speech sound form is inadequate. This child now turns to Mom and says, "I want a s-ship." Does the child want a sip or a ship? Due to the child's aberrant form, we are not sure what is meant. The language function of this particular segment cannot be fulfilled, and communication is affected. On the other hand, if the form is acceptable but the function is aberrant, communication will also be problematic. A child, for example, can produce an acceptable "t" (adequate form) but may leave off that sound at the end of all words (inadequate function). Therefore, words such as "toe" and "tea" will be understood, but words such as "boat" and "bow" will be confused, since the linguistic function of /t/ as a final consonant signaling the differences in meaning between the two words, "bow" and "boat," is not being realized. For the purpose of effective verbal communication, both regular segment form and function are indispensable.

 FOCUS 6: *How are form and function related to phonetics and phonology?*

Understandably, in clinical assessment the interrelationship between form and function is very important as well. When analyzing segment form, a clinician will examine the production features that are normally associated with the articulation of the speech sound in question. Perhaps the tongue is positioned too far forward in the mouth or too far back. Or maybe this particular sound should be a voiced sound, such as [b], but is perceived as being a voiceless one, such as [p]. Phonetic analysis of speech sounds examines the production form, the adequacy of the production features. If the individual's speech sound form deviates significantly from the norm, this may be diagnosed as an articulation disorder. An **articulation disorder** refers to difficulties with the motor production aspects of speech, or an inability to produce certain speech sounds (Elbert & Gierut, 1986). An articulation disorder is a phonetic production problem; it represents difficulties with speech sound form.

On the other hand, when analyzing segment function, the clinician needs to examine the rule-governed distribution, places within a language where the phoneme appears, and the organization of these sound units within this language. The clinician examines which phonemes are used and how they are arranged and function within that language. Therefore, the clinician will see if the phonemes the child uses are comparable to those normally used, in other words, assess the adequacy of the child's *inventory* of phonemes. In addition, their arrangement will be assessed to determine if these phonemes are actually being used to establish and distinguish between word meanings. A **phonological disorder** refers to an impaired system of phonemes and phoneme patterns (Grunwell, 1986).

Children with phonological disorders have difficulties with the function of phonemes within a language. For clinicians, both areas, speech sound form and phoneme function, are equally significant for the evaluation of speech disorders.

Beginning Case Study

ANDREA IN COMMUNICATIVE DISORDERS

From the beginning of the chapter, Andrea was concerned about planning therapy for several children who have speech sound problems. Two of the children, Megan and Jess, seem to be having trouble with the actual production of specific sounds. Megan's "s" sounds more like "th," while Jess says "wabbit" for "rabbit." For these two children, the speech sound form is clearly not acceptable: They have phonetic difficulties. The positioning of the articulators may need to be changed somewhat to achieve an adequate sounding "s" and "r." However, Frank does seem to have quite a different problem: He can say the sounds in question but he leaves them off the end of the words. He will say "toe" for "toad" but can produce the "d" in "do" or "day." Frank does not have difficulty with the actual speech sound production but with the systematic organization of these phonemes; he has phonemic difficulties. Frank's therapy will need to focus on the function of these phonemes within the language system. In this example, knowledge of both phonetics and phonology would be important for understanding the problems that these three children demonstrate.

Summary

FOCUS 1: *What is phonetics?*

Phonetics is the study of speech and speech sounds. It was defined broadly as the science and study of speech emphasizing the description of speech sounds according to their production, transmission, and perceptual features. The basic unit of phonetics is the speech sound.

FOCUS 2: *What three areas of study are emphasized in phonetics?*

The three areas of phonetics consist of (1) articulatory phonetics, (2) acoustic phonetics, and (3) auditory (perceptual) phonetics. Articulatory phonetics is that branch that is concerned with how the different speech sounds are generated; actual parameters of speech sound production are described and classified. The articulators are those anatomical structures directly involved in the generation of speech sounds. One aspect of articulatory phonetics is the classification of speech sounds according to these articulators. For example "m" is considered to be a bilabial sound (bilabial = two lips), as the upper and lower lips come together to produce the sound.

The second area noted is acoustic phonetics. This branch of phonetics studies speech sounds in the form of sound waves that travel through the air from a speaker to a listener. Acoustic phonetics deals with the objective, physical properties of speech sound waves such as their frequency, intensity, and duration. Frequency was exemplified by noting that certain sounds, such as the fricatives "f" and "s," contain high-frequency sounds.

The third area of phonetics, auditory (perceptual) phonetics, is the study of how speech sound waves are perceived by the listener. In auditory phonetics, the terms *pitch* and *loudness* are used instead of *frequency* and *intensity* to underline speech sound perception. Examples were given to demonstrate the differences that occur when we compare the objective measurements of amplitude and frequency to the subjective measurements of loudness and pitch.

FOCUS 3: *What is phonology?*

Phonology is the study of how speech sounds are put together to form words that convey meaning within a specific language system. Phonology emphasizes the linguistic function of these speech sounds within a particular language. Therefore, which sounds can occur at the beginning of a word, which sounds can end words, and the type of sound combinations that can exist within a particular language are all a portion of phonology. Phonology studies the structure and systematic patterning of sounds in a particular language and includes the description of the sounds a language uses and the rules governing how these sounds are distributed or organized. In other words, phonology is concerned with *which* speech sounds a language uses and how they are *arranged* and *function* within that language.

FOCUS 4: *What is the difference between a phoneme and an allophone?*

The phoneme is the basic unit of phonology. It is defined as the smallest linguistic unit that is able, when combined with other such units, to establish word meanings and distinguish between them. Phonemes, then, are sound units with a special, language-dependent function, the linguistic function to establish and distinguish between word meanings. The idea of the phoneme is considered to be an abstraction, as phonemes are not single, concrete, unchanging entities. A phoneme is an abstraction from the many different variations that occur for a particular sound as it is heard in differing contexts of conversational speech. When we speak of a particular phoneme, /t/ for example, we are referring to the typical "t," but we also take into consideration all the varieties of "t" that are used in various contexts and by different speakers. These realizations of the phonemes have often been labeled *allophones*. Allophones are production differences that occur as phonemes are realized in certain contexts. Allophones are variations in phoneme realization that do not change the meaning of a word. An allophone is one of several similar phones that belong to the same phoneme family; it represents slight variations of the basic sound unit. Speakers of a particular language perceive a phoneme as a single distinctive sound in that language, while an allophone is considered to be a variation, but not a meaning-distinguishing production difference.

FOCUS 5: *What is the difference between free variation and complementary distribution?*

The term *free variation* is used to indicate two allophones of one phoneme that might occur within similar contexts. Therefore, it is optional whether one or the other is produced in that context for that particular phoneme. An example was given in the chapter in which either a released [p] or an unreleased [p] could occur at the end of a word. The term *complementary distribution* is used to indicate two allophones of the same phoneme that have no environment or contexts in common. At the beginning of a word, "p" is always aspirated, while following /s/ the unaspirated [p] is always used; other allophonic variations are not produced in that particular context. Therefore, in this context the unaspirated [p] is in complementary distribution with the aspirated [p].

FOCUS 6: *How are form and function related to phonetics and phonology?*

The concepts form and function were used to characterize the differences between phonetics and phonology. Phonetics emphasizes the form of speech sounds by describing and categorizing their physical attributes, that is, their articulatory and acoustic components and their auditory effects. Phonology stresses their function as meaning-establishing and meaning-differentiating phonemes within a language system. Adequate form and function of all sound segments are basic requirements for meaningful utterances in any language. Adequate form is established by the way the sound in question is produced, by articulatory events. If the end product of these events is qualitatively acceptable to the speakers of a specific language, it is perceived as being a speech sound of their system. Adequate function relates to the observance of language-specific rules regarding the use and arrangement of these sound segments. The end product is the establishment of words that convey a particular meaning within that specific language.

Further Readings

Akmajian, A., Demers, R., Farmer, A., & Harnish, R. (2001). *Linguistics: An introduction to language and communication* (5th ed.). Cambridge, MA: MIT Press.

Grunwell, P. (1987). *Clinical phonology* (2nd ed.). Baltimore: Williams & Wilkins.

Parker, F., & Riley, K. (2005). *Linguistics for non-linguists: A primer with exercises* (4th ed.). Boston: Allyn and Bacon.

Key Terms

acoustic phonetics p. 5
allophones p. 10
articulation disorder p. 14
articulators p. 4
articulatory phonetics p. 3
auditory phonetics p. 5
complementary distribution p. 12
consonants p. 4
free variation p. 12
linguistics p. 7
minimal pairs p. 8

perceptual phonetics p. 5
phone p. 3
phoneme p. 8
phonetics p. 2
phonological disorder p. 14
phonology p. 7
phonotactics p. 9
resonance p. 5
speech p. 2
speech sounds p. 2
vowels p. 4

Think Critically

1. You are working with a preschool child who has difficulties producing [f]. This sound is described as a labio-dental sound. What does the term *labio-dental* mean? How would you instruct the child to put the articulators for the correct placement?

2. How could you use minimal pairs to test a child's knowledge of phonology? Which minimal pairs could you construct that would test an understanding of [f] versus [s]?

3. What are some sound combinations in American English that do not occur at the beginning of words or syllables but can occur at the end of a word or syllable? List two sound combinations that do not occur at all in American English.

4. Explain in your own words how the area of phonetics relates to speech sound form while phonology encompasses the function of phonemes within a language.

5. Based on one of the case studies presented in this chapter, explain the importance of phonetics and/or phonology.

Test Yourself

1. Any particular occurrence of a sound segment that is used by a speaker in words may be referred to as a
    a. phone.
    b. minimal pair.
    c. phonotactic.
    d. phoneme.

2. Auditory phonetics may also be referred to as
    a. articulatory phonetics.

b. acoustic phonetics.

c. perceptual phonetics.

3. How speech sounds are produced and classified would be studied in which area of phonetics?

a. articulatory phonetics

b. acoustic phonetics

c. auditory phonetics

4. If we were looking at how different sounds are perceived and interpreted by a listener, we would be studying which area of phonetics?

a. articulatory phonetics

b. acoustic phonetics

c. auditory phonetics

5. If we were using equipment to analyze the frequency and intensity components of speech sounds, we would be studying which area of phonetics?

a. articulatory phonetics

b. acoustic phonetics

c. auditory phonetics

6. The study of the structure and systematic patterning of sounds in a particular language is referred to as

a. phonetics.

b. linguistics.

c. phonology.

d. phonotactics.

7. Variations in phoneme realizations that do not change the meaning of a word when they are produced in various contexts are referred to as

a. allophonic variations.

b. consonants.

c. vowels.

d. all of the above.

8. The terms *form* and *function* are related to

a. free variation and complementary distribution.

b. phonotactics and minimal pairs.

c. phonetics and phonology.

d. speech sounds and articulators.

9. The concept that two allophones of one phoneme might unpredictably occur within similar contexts is known as

a. phonotactics.

b. free variation.

c. complementary distribution.

d. minimal pairs.

10. The concept that two allophones of one phoneme have no environments or contexts in common is known as

a. phonotactics.

b. free variation.

c. complementary distribution.

d. minimal pairs.

Answers: 1. a 2. c 3. a 4. c 5. b 6. c 7. a 8. c 9. b 10. c

For additional information, go to www.phonologicaldisorders.com

CHAPTER 2

An Overview of Speech Production

Chapter Highlights

- What are the structures and general functions of each of the four subsystems of the speech mechanism?
- How do the inspiratory and expiratory muscles regulate the pressure needed for speech?
- What is the mechanism involved in vocal fold vibration?
- Why is the velopharyngeal mechanism important for resonance?
- What are the specific articulators?
- What role does resonance play in the production of vowels?

Chapter Application: Case Study

Julie would like to be an audiologist. She enjoys learning about and using the instrumentation associated with hearing testing. During the summer, she had an opportunity to visit an aural rehabilitation clinic. Julie learned that aural rehabilitation is accomplished through an educational and clinical program. It is implemented primarily by audiologists but may also include other team members such as speech-language pathologists or educators of the deaf. The program is designed to help those children with hearing impairments reach their full potential. Julie was extremely interested in the program and became rather attached to the children in the program. She noticed that the children with more severe hearing impairments were far more difficult to understand, and the vowel and consonant quality of their speech was affected, while those with milder hearing impairments were easier to understand but often had trouble with sounds such as "s," "sh," and "f." She also noticed that children with more severe hearing impairments often had a different quality to their voice. Julie began to wonder about how the children's specific hearing losses impacted their speech. The audiologist at the aural rehabilitation clinic told Julie that it had to do with the degree of hearing loss and the frequencies that were affected. Julie couldn't quite connect the testing she had done that assessed the various frequencies and intensities and the resulting impact on speech sounds. She remembered that it had something to do with the acoustics of speech.

The purpose of this chapter is, first, to give an overview of the anatomical-physiological mechanisms and processes that are the foundation for speech production. *Physiological phonetics* will be used as a broad term to encompass this discussion. Therefore, those structures and processes involved in breathing, producing voice, and creating certain speech sound qualities will be summarized. Second, this chapter will examine a specific aspect of acoustic phonetics, resonance. Basic principles of resonance are important as we attempt to understand how specific adjustments to the articulators result in varying sound qualities. Thus, changes within the vocal mechanism create and form specific sound qualities due to resonance properties. Clinical examples will be used throughout the chapter to exemplify and apply the topics and information.

Physiological Phonetics: The Anatomical-Physiological Foundation of Speech Production

Physiological phonetics examines the anatomical-physiological prerequisites for speech and hearing, in particular the functional adequacy of all structures that are a portion of the speech process. We will be looking at one portion of this area of study, those elements involved in the speech process. The structures that are involved in producing speech are cumulatively labeled the **speech mechanism**. The speech mechanism is further subdivided into the following systems:

1. Respiratory
2. Phonatory
3. Resonatory
4. Articulatory (e.g., Creaghead & Newman, 1989; Zemlin, 1998)

The **respiratory system** consists primarily of the lungs and airways, including the trachea, rib cage, abdomen, and diaphragm (Ferrand, 2007). These are the structures directly related to respiration, the exchange of gases necessary for sustaining life. In addition, these structures are necessary to generate the airflow, which makes voice and speech possible. The **phonatory system** consists of the larynx and is responsible for **phonation**, the production of tones resulting from vibration of the vocal folds. The **resonatory system** is composed of a series of cavities: the oral, nasal, and pharyngeal cavities. This system plays a vital role in **resonance**, the selective absorption and reinforcement of sound energies, which create the characteristic quality of certain speech sounds. Finally, the **articulatory system** contains the mandible, tongue, lips, teeth, alveolar ridge, hard palate, and velum. These articulators are important in forming the individual speech sounds. The articulatory system fine-tunes the production, resulting in speech sounds that are distinct and qualitatively acceptable. An overview of the resonatory, phonatory, and respiratory systems is shown in Figure 2.1, while Figure 2.2 represents most structures of the articulatory system.

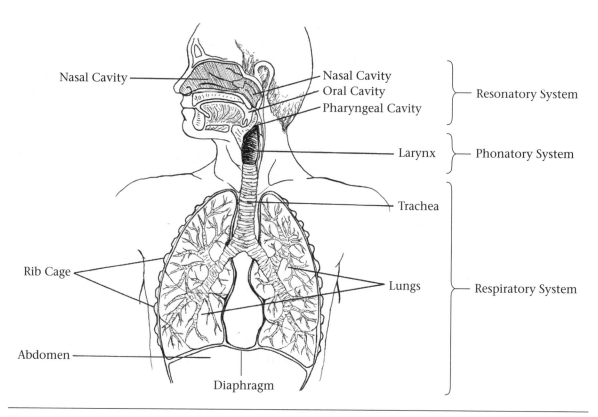

Figure 2.1 Overview of the Respiratory, Phonatory, and Resonatory Systems

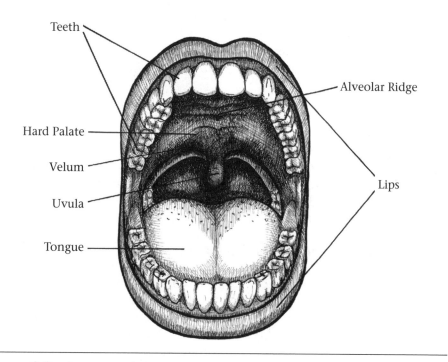

Figure 2.2 Overview of the Articulatory System

Thus, physiological phonetics encompasses breathing and its adequacy for speech (respiratory system), the function of the vocal folds, which are the sound source for speech (phonatory system), the way the various cavities of the head and neck modify this sound source (resonatory system), and the structure and function of the articulators as they form the various speech sounds (articulatory system).

 FOCUS 1: *What are the structures and general functions of each of the four subsystems of the speech mechanism?*

The articulatory system, as one portion of the speech mechanism, has a good deal of overlap with the previously mentioned phonetic branch labeled articulatory phonetics. Physiological phonetics provides us with the totality of anatomical structures and physiological processes that are the foundation for speech production, while articulatory phonetics emphasizes the specific production characteristics of the speech sounds. The fine-tuning of the articulators to produce various speech sounds remains a central feature of articulatory phonetics.

Areas of interest within physiological phonetics might include the differences in breathing patterns that occur when breathing without speech (quiet breathing) versus speech breathing. Or physiological phonetics could include vocal fold activity during speaking as opposed to singing, for example. Articulatory phonetics, on the other hand, encompasses how the articulators are positioned during the production of speech sounds, giving them their characteristic qualities. Vocal fold vibration (or lack thereof on certain sounds) and the use of certain resonating cavities are used as descriptors, further delineating the production features. So, while physiological phonetics examines the totality of the anatomical and physiological necessities for speech and hearing, articulatory phonetics emphasizes only one specific area, the classification and production characteristics of individual speech sounds.

How does physiological phonetics differ from general anatomy and physiology of these respiratory, phonatory, resonatory, and articulatory structures? Physiological phonetics translates data from anatomy and physiology to their special prerequisites for the speech process. One could also say that general courses in anatomy and physiology would concentrate on the primary functions of the speech mechanism. In physiological phonetics, the emphasis remains on anatomical and physiological factors related to the secondary functions the speech mechanism serves in speech production.

A **primary function** depicts the life-supporting tasks of the speech mechanism. The primary function of the respiratory system, for instance, is the life-preserving exchange of gases, while the laryngeal system's primary function is to prohibit foreign matter from getting into the respiratory airway. Primary functions are also referred to as **vital functions**. **Secondary functions** are called **overlaid functions**, indicating functions that are merely placed onto the original functions. However, the term *overlaid* is somewhat misleading, as the structure of the speech mechanism has undergone considerable evolutionary development that has increased its functional efficiency for the act of speaking (Lieberman, 1998).

The Respiratory System

The respiratory system consists of the lungs, rib cage, thorax, abdomen, trachea, and those muscles associated with breathing. The primary function of the respiratory system is to provide the vital exchange of gases that is necessary for life. The secondary function of this system is generating a source of energy in the form of a stream of air for the production of speech. Without this pressurized air flow, voice is not possible and speech sounds remain inaudible. A brief review of the basic structures and their function during one cycle of breathing will be used to illustrate this process.

The principal muscle of inhalation is the diaphragm, which divides the torso of the body into the thoracic and abdominal cavities. The thoracic cavity, which is primarily filled with the lungs and heart, is bounded by the sternum (breast bone) and the rib cage in the front and by the spinal cord and vertebrae in the back. The abdominal cavity, or abdomen, contains the digestive tract, glands, and other organs. The diaphragm consists of a strong fibrous central portion, known as the central tendon, as well as peripheral muscular portions. The muscular portion of the diaphragm is connected anteriorly (at the front) and laterally (on the sides) to the lower edges of the ribs. Its posterior connection is the upper lumbar vertebrae. (The upper lumbar vertebrae are located toward the lower back area.) There are several other thoracic muscles that are also considered muscles of inhalation. These muscles may aid in the elevation of the ribs during inhalation. In this respect, two sets of muscles are very important: the external and internal intercostals. The fibers of the external intercostals are attached at the lower edges of the ribs, coursing downward at an angle to the upper edges of the ribs below. The internal intercostals are under the externals, and the fibers again run from the lower edges to the upper edges of the ribs below, but the angle of the fibers is in an opposite direction.

The diaphragm during its rest phase, i.e., between respiratory activities, resembles the shape of an inverted bowl. However, it should be kept in mind that the shape of the diaphragm is affected by the organs of the abdominal cavity upon which it rests, primarily the liver. In addition, the posterior muscular attachments of the diaphragm are much lower than those in the front of the body. Therefore, it is a rather asymmetrical inverted bowl shape. See Figure 2.3 for the positioning of the diaphragm and the intercostal muscles.

As inhalation begins, the muscular portion of the diaphragm contracts. This contraction, shortening the muscular fibers, pulls the central tendon down and somewhat forward. As the diaphragm moves downward, the vertical up-and-down dimensions of the thoracic cavity increase; thus, the contents of the abdominal cavity are compressed. At the same time contractions of the external and internal intercostals and other so-called accessory muscles elevate the entire rib cage, the ribs swing up and outward. This increases the front-to-back and side-to-side dimensions of the thoracic cavity (see Figure 2.4).

For respiration to occur, the lungs must increase and decrease their volume through expansion and contraction. Since the lungs contain very little muscle, this process must be mediated by external forces. This external force is created through the structure and connections of the lungs to the thorax, known as pleural linkage.

Adhering to each of the lungs is a membrane, known as the pleura (plural form = pleurae). Covering the outer surface of the lungs is the visceral, or what is also called the pulmonary pleura. The outermost membrane, which covers the inner surface of the thorax and the top portion of the diaphragm, is known as the costal or parietal pleura. The two membranes are airtight and fused together, producing a small amount of fluid that provides smooth, lubricated movement of the lungs during respiration. There is a powerful negative pressure between the two pleural membranes. This pressure links the costal and visceral membranes so closely that the lungs cohere to (stick to) the thoracic walls. Thus, any movement of the thoracic cavity results in a movement of the lungs. As the dimensions of the thoracic cavity increase, these airtight membranes cause the lungs to follow the thoracic walls as they enlarge. Therefore, as the diaphragm

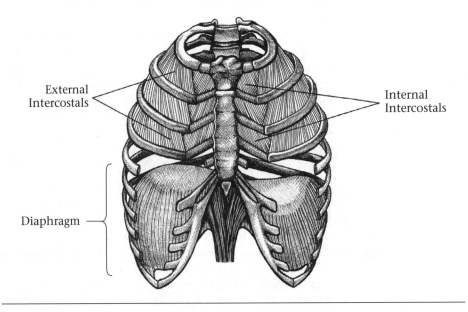

External Intercostals

Internal Intercostals

Diaphragm

Figure 2.3 The Diaphragm and Intercostal Muscles

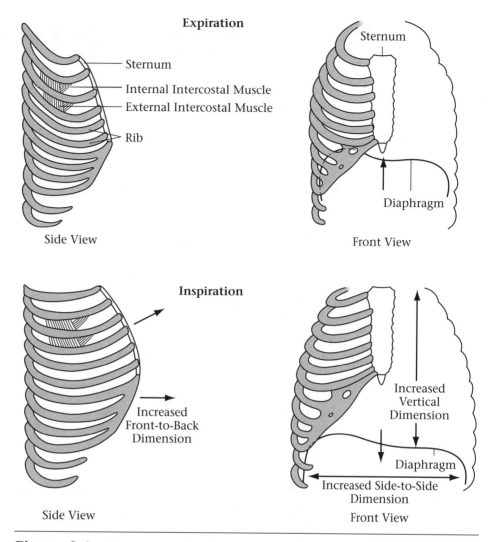

Expiration

Sternum

Internal Intercostal Muscle

External Intercostal Muscle

Rib

Side View

Sternum

Diaphragm

Front View

Inspiration

Increased Front-to-Back Dimension

Side View

Increased Vertical Dimension

Diaphragm

Increased Side-to-Side Dimension

Front View

Figure 2.4 Changes in the Dimensions of the Thoracic Cavity During Inhalation

Source: From *Human Anatomy and Physiology* (2nd ed., p. 562), by J. E. Crouch and J. R. McClintic, 1976, New York: John Wiley and Sons. Copyright 1976 by John Wiley and Sons. Reproduced with permission.

descends and the dimensions of the rib cage increase, the lungs are forced into expanding. During rest, the pressure within the lungs, the so-called **alveolar pressure**, is equal to the outside air, the **atmospheric pressure.** However, as inspiration begins, the increase in the thoracic dimensions and the consequent expansion of the lungs as they follow the expanding thoracic cavity results in a negative alveolar pressure. The consequence is that the outside air rushes in until the alveolar pressure again equals the atmospheric pressure.

As outside air rushes into the lungs, the muscles of inhalation gradually cease their activity. At this point exhalation begins. The diaphragm starts to relax to its uncontracted state, moving upward. The thoracic muscles also no longer support a state of extension; thus, the thoracic cavity's dimensions decrease. Both of these actions, the upward movement of the diaphragm and the relaxation of the extended wall of the thorax, increase the alveolar pressure to the degree that air is forced out of the lungs, thus, exhalation.

In general, it can be said that during inhalation thoracic muscles support the effect of the descent of the diaphragm by enlarging the thoracic cavity and with it the lungs. During exhalation, abdominal muscles can compress the abdominal cavity, thus aiding in the reduction of the thoracic cavity's size as it returns to a resting position.

The task of the respiratory system during speech production is even more complex. Speech production necessitates a regulated amount of subglottal pressure over a rather wide range of volumes. While the **glottis** is the space between the vocal folds, **subglottal** refers to that area below the vocal folds. For example, if you take a deep breath, i.e., have a high volume of air in the lungs, but only say a word or two, this pressure will have to be regulated if normal loudness is to be maintained. On the other hand, if you utter a longer sentence, a relatively constant amount of subglottal pressure must be maintained from the beginning of the utterance, when there is clearly more air in the lungs (higher lung volume), to its end, when there is far less (lower lung volume). To maintain a constant loudness level during the whole utterance, the outflow of air must somehow be equalized.

This equalization of various lung volumes and pressure levels is done by an interplay, a checks and balances system, between inspiratory and expiratory muscles. For example, action of the expiratory mechanism could result in a loss of air relatively quickly at the beginning of the expiratory phase. This may not be desirable for speech production. In order to counteract this sudden loss of air pressure, action of the inspiratory muscles might slow down the rapid decrease in the dimensions of the thoracic cavity. Therefore, the action of inspiratory muscles would help regulate and maintain the subglottal pressure. On the other hand, if at the end of a long utterance still more air pressure is needed, expiratory muscles might additionally assist in providing a relatively constant flow of air for a longer time period. Based on this interplay of balancing actions, the respiratory system is able to constantly supply the laryngeal system with precisely regulated subglottal pressures.

 FOCUS 2: *How do the inspiratory and expiratory muscles regulate the pressure needed for speech?*

The Phonatory System

The next important system for speech production is the phonatory system. Through controlled expiration, the respiratory system provides a relatively even flow of pressurized air from the lungs, which passes through air passageways into the larynx. The larynx is the principal structure of the phonatory system. The vocal folds, the most important part of the larynx, provide the source of sound for speech. However, this is not the primary function of the larynx. Rather, its primary function is to prevent foreign substances from entering deeper portions of the respiratory airway by forcefully expelling them. This powerful reflex entails the vocal folds coming together so that air is trapped under them, which results in a buildup of air pressure. A sudden release of this closure produces an explosive expulsion of air sufficient enough to expel the foreign substance from the respiratory tract. A cough or a sneeze has similar results.

 Reflect on This: Clinical Application

DYSPHAGIA

Dysphagia is a swallowing disorder characterized by difficulty in preparing for the swallow or in moving material from the mouth to the stomach (ASHA, 1987). In patients with dysphagia, coughing or choking during swallowing might be an indication that food is entering the trachea. However, in some patients with dysphagia, a lack of such a cough does not necessarily mean that food is not entering the trachea. "Silent aspirators" are individuals with food or other foreign substances entering their trachea, although no coughing occurs (Perlman, 2000). One might ask why this important primary function did not occur. Many individuals with swallowing disorders have other medical problems. The most common causes associated with dysphagia in adults are stroke, traumatic brain injury, spinal cord injury, and brain tumor (Cherney, 1994). In these individuals, the neurological problems may decrease their sensitivity to the need to cough or the ability to actually initiate a cough.

When not fulfilling the above-mentioned important primary function, the larynx can function as a sound generator. The larynx is suspended from the hyoid bone in that several of the laryngeal muscles are attached to this bone. The hyoid bone is a horseshoe-shaped bone located at the base of the tongue, above the thyroid cartilage. The larynx itself consists of nine cartilages (one thyroid, one cricoid, one epiglottis, two arytenoid, two corniculate, and two cuneiform) as well as connecting membranes and ligaments (see Figures 2.5 and 2.6).

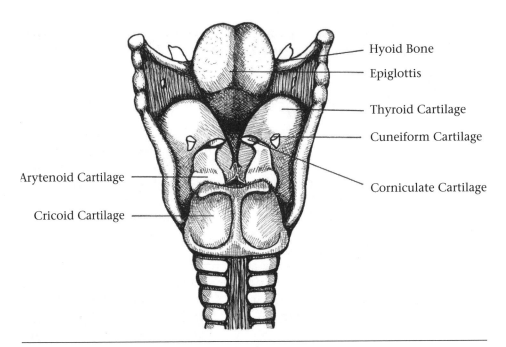

Figure 2.5 Cartilages of the Larynx

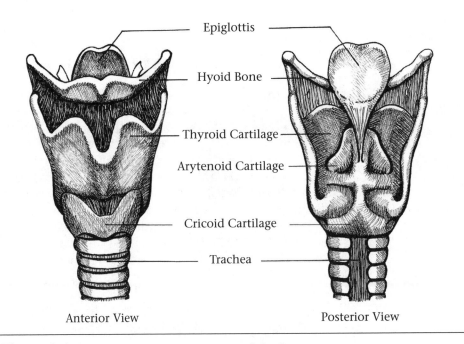

Figure 2.6 Anterior and Posterior View of the Larynx

Primarily **extrinsic muscles** (those having at least one attachment to structures outside the larynx) are responsible for support and fixation of the larynx, while mainly **intrinsic muscles** (those having both attachments within the larynx) are necessary for control during voice production. The extrinsic muscles surround the larynx and anchor it in its position. These external muscles can broadly be divided into the infrahyoids (*infra* = below, beneath), which have their points of attachment at structures below the hyoid bone, and the suprahyoid muscles (*supra* = above, over), which are attached above the hyoid bone. The infrahyoids are the sternohyoid, sternothyroid, thryohyoid, and omohyoid (superior and inferior) muscles. The suprahyoids are the stylohyoid, digastric (posterior and anterior portions), mylohyoid, and geniohyoid muscles. The fascial loop of the digastric muscle is attached to and surrounds the tendon that connects the anterior and posterior portions of this muscle. Figure 2.7 contains the infra- and suprahyoid muscles (with the exception of the sternothyroid and stylohyoid). When contracted, the infrahyoids pull the entire larynx down, while contraction of the suprahyoids elevates the entire larynx. These up-and-down movements occur mainly during swallowing.

The intrinsic muscles are far more interesting during voice production. There are two muscles that help to **adduct,** or close, the vocal folds; thus, they aid in moving the vocal folds toward the midline of the glottis. These are the lateral cricoarytenoid (a paired muscle, the fibers run from the lateral edges of the cricoid cartilage to the arytenoids) and the interarytenoid (a muscle in two portions, the transverse portion runs across the posterior portions of the arytenoid cartilages, while the oblique fibers run from the base of one arytenoid to the apex of the other, crossing each other). The

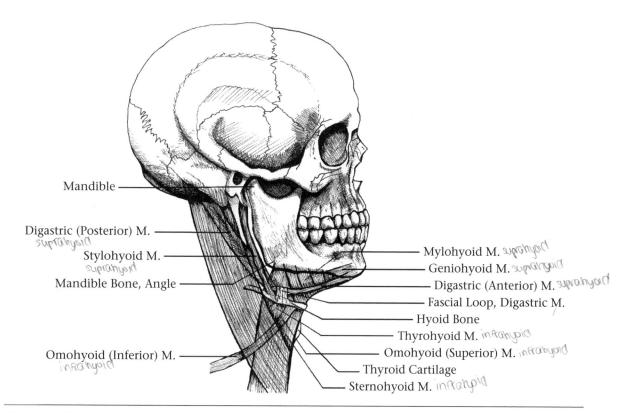

Figure 2.7   Extrinsic Muscles of the Larynx

only muscle that helps to **abduct,** or open, the vocal folds is the posterior cricoarytenoid muscle (in two portions, which run obliquely from the posterior portion of the cricoid cartilage to the arytenoid cartilage). There are also intrinsic muscles that are involved in elongating, thus tensing, the vocal folds. The cricothyroid muscle (in two portions, which both originate on the lateral edges of the cricoid cartilage; one portion, the pars recta, runs at an almost upright angle to insert into the bottom edge of the thyroid cartilage, while the pars oblique runs in a more angled direction up to the top portion of the body of the thyroid cartilage) elongates and tenses the vocal folds. See Figure 2.8 and Table 2.1.

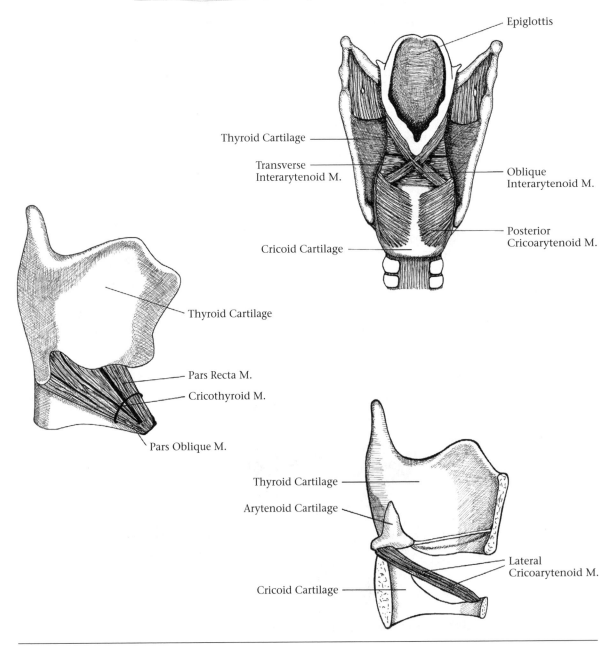

Figure 2.8 Intrinsic Muscles of the Larynx: Transverse and Oblique Interarytenoid Muscles, Posterior Cricoarytenoid Muscle, Cricothyroid Muscle (Pars Recta and Pars Oblique), and the Lateral Cricoarytenoid Muscle

Table 2.1 Intrinsic Muscles of the Larynx

ADDUCTORS—Close the Vocal Folds
　　Lateral Cricoarytenoid
　　Interarytenoid—Transverse and Oblique Portions

ABDUCTORS—Open the Vocal Folds
　　Posterior Cricoarytenoid

ELONGATING, TENSING the Vocal Folds
　　Cricothyroid—Pars Recta and Pars Oblique Portions

The last intrinsic muscle forms the main mass of the vocal folds. It is known as the thyroarytenoid muscle (fibers originate from the inner surface of the thyroid cartilage to two different aspects of the arytenoid cartilages) and functions as a regulator of longitudinal tension. See Figure 2.9.

Although some anatomy books divide this muscle into two distinct portions, as it has been done in Figure 2.9, the vocalis and muscularis, Zemlin (1998) among others has found no anatomical evidence to support this division. This muscle seems able to close or adduct the vocal folds in addition to tensing and relaxing them. It should be kept in mind that rarely do individual muscles act to execute a movement. Rather, they work in pairs or in a group to produce a delicate interplay of various muscle actions producing an appropriate movement.

The primary sound source for speech is derived from the vibration of the vocal folds. Let's examine vocal fold vibration in a simplistic manner: During quiet breathing, the vocal folds are drawn away from the midline. The onset of phonation is marked by the vocal folds moving toward the midline, into an adducted position. In this adducted position, the vocal folds are obstructing expiratory airflow, and subglottal pressure begins to build up. At a critical point of pressure build up, the vocal folds are "blown apart"; the glottis is now open, with the natural consequence of an immediate decrease in subglottal pressure. The folds come together again due to their inherent elasticity, the sudden pressure drop between the folds, and other aerodynamic properties. The vocal folds return once again to their

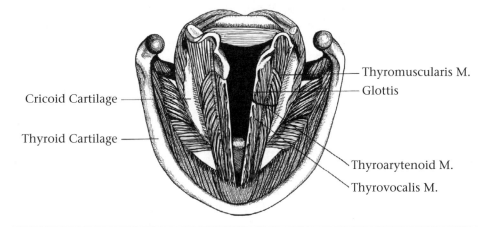

Figure 2.9 Thyroarytenoid Muscle of the Larynx (Thyromuscularis and Thyrovocalis)

adducted position. The subglottal air pressure builds up again and the process is repeated.

FOCUS 3: *What is the mechanism involved in vocal fold vibration?*

The average number of glottal openings per second is known as a person's **fundamental frequency**. The fundamental frequency of an individual is related to his or her perceived vocal pitch. Although every speaker is capable of producing a wide range of fundamental frequencies, females have typically a higher range of fundamental frequencies than males (the fundamental frequency for females is approximately 200 to 260 cycles per second, while for males it is between 120 and 145 cycles per second (Zemlin, 1998). Within this range, changes in the *tension* of the vocal folds are primarily responsible for variations in fundamental frequency. Thus, for any given speaker, increasing the tension of the vocal folds will result in a higher fundamental frequency, a higher perceived pitch, while decreasing the tension will result in a lower fundamental frequency, a lower perceived pitch.

On the other hand, changes in vocal loudness result from *variations in subglottal air pressure,* which varies the *amplitude of the vocal folds' vibratory cycle.* When more subglottal air pressure is present, the vocal folds move farther away from the midline during their vibratory cycles. We perceive this as an increase in loudness. On the other hand, less subglottal air pressure results in less movement of the vocal folds from the midline during vibration. This is perceived as a decrease in loudness.

Vibration of the vocal folds is also important for the voiced-voiceless oppositions of speech sounds as well. This can be exemplified by "s" and "z." During "s" production, the vocal folds are not vibrating, while during "z," there is simultaneous accompanying vibration of the vocal folds. This difference is important for distinguishing between such words as "Sue" versus "zoo" or "sink" versus "zinc," for example.

The consistent cyclic vibration of the vocal folds also plays a role in the quality or timbre of the voice. The term **timbre** refers to the tonal quality that differentiates two sounds of the same pitch, loudness, and duration (Crystal, 1987). If you produce "ah" and your friend says "ah" trying to match your pitch, loudness, and duration, the two utterances will still sound different. This is due to the characteristic vocal quality, or timbre, of each person's voice. If the vocal folds vibrate aperiodically, i.e., not at a reg-

Concept Exercise **FUNDAMENTAL FREQUENCY AND INTENSITY**

Prolong an "ah" vowel at a comfortable pitch. This is probably close to your fundamental frequency. Produce a low tone and then a high tone of about the same loudness level. There is less vocal fold tension at the lower frequencies as compared to the higher ones.

Prolong a soft "ah" and then a loud one. Do you notice the increased pressure that is needed for the louder sound? Feel the independence of pitch and loudness by contrasting "ah" at a low pitch and low volume, a high pitch and low volume, a low pitch and high volume, and a high pitch and high volume.

Reflect on This: Clinical Application

Some abnormal vocal fold conditions can lead to changes in the fundamental frequency. Many of these conditions can be caused by vocal abuse, such as prolonged yelling at a football game. The vocal folds may become thickened, characterized typically by a lowering of the fundamental frequency. Polyps, which are fluid-filled attachments to the vocal folds, and nodules, callous-like formations on the vocal folds, can also cause changes in fundamental frequency. Nodules are often seen in children and have been termed "screamer's nodules" (Boone, McFarlane, & Von Berg, 2004). Also individuals who use and possible abuse their voice a lot, such as singers, public announcers, and teachers who are trying to shout over the classroom noise, may develop these abnormal vocal fold conditions.

ular rate but irregularly, we perceive this as an abnormal voice quality. If, on the other hand, the adduction of the vocal folds is not as complete as it should be and the vocal folds do not approximate the midline, this could be perceived as a breathy voice. Regular cyclic, periodic vocal fold vibration and a functional unity between the respiratory and phonatory systems are necessary for a vocal timbre that is considered to be within normal limits.

Beginning Case Study

JULIE INTERESTED IN HEARING IMPAIRMENTS

In the beginning case study, Julie had noted that the voice quality of the children with more severe hearing impairments was affected. The vocal quality of hearing impaired children has been described as being harsh, breathy, nasal, and/or monotone. Although the phonatory system does not appear to be deviant for these speakers, coordinating the airstream with articulation and voicing does pose a problem. These individuals take in too little air, they begin to speak when the lung volume is low, and they waste air in the often breathy voice quality (Lane, Perkell, Svirsky, & Webster, 1991). It is hypothesized that the lack of auditory feedback plays a role in this lack of coordination.

The Resonatory System

The third important system for voice and speech production, the resonatory system, is comprised of three cavities within the vocal tract. The **vocal tract** consists of all speech-related systems above the vocal folds. The resonatory system includes the pharyngeal, oral, and nasal cavities (see Figure 2.10). The **pharyngeal cavity**, a muscular and membranous tube-like structure, extends from the epiglottis to the soft palate. It is generally divided into three portions: the **nasopharynx (hyperpharynx)**, which

Reflect on This: Clinical Application

DYSARTHRIA AND CONTROL OF PHONATION

The voice quality of many individuals with dysarthria is described as being harsh, strained, or breathy (Darley, Aronson, & Brown, 1975; Dworkin, 1991). This is the direct result of the lack of coordination and/or weakness of the speech musculature that was noted in the original definition of dysarthria. This discoordination also affects the motor control that is necessary for the fine-tuning during phonation. There may be at one time too little muscular action and/or air pressure, in the next instant too much. Strained and harsh voice qualities often result from too much muscular action and tension (**hypertension**), leading to excessive adduction of the vocal folds (**hyperadduction**) (Colton & Casper, 1990; Dworkin, 1991). The breathy voice quality of some dysarthric patients can be due to a lack of muscular tension (**hypotension**), resulting in incomplete closure of the vocal folds and subsequent expiratory air flow, which is perceived as breathiness. However, the breathy voice quality may be the result of a lack of coordination within the respiratory system. In this case, too much subglottal air pressure is suddenly generated, resulting in greater than normal airflow during phonation. This excessive airflow is identified as a breathy voice quality by the listener (Colton & Casper, 1990).

extends from the upper portion of the nasal cavity to the soft palate, the **oropharynx (mediopharynx)**, which extends from the soft palate to the hyoid bone, and the **laryngopharynx (hypopharynx)**, which extends from the oropharynx to the entrance of the esophagus. The **oral cavity**, or mouth area, extends from the lips to the soft palate. The **nasal cavities**, or nose area, consists of two narrow chambers that begin at the soft palate and end at the exterior portion of the nostrils. The floor of the nasal cavities is the hard palate.

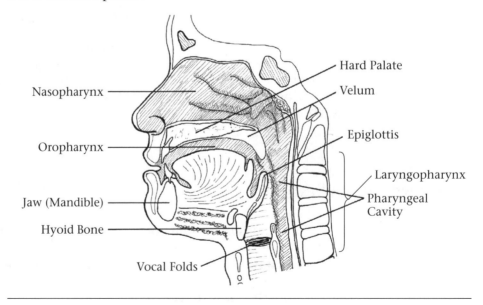

Figure 2.10 The Resonatory System: Nasopharynx, Oropharynx, and Laryngopharynx

Sound energy generated by the larynx is modified as it travels through the pharyngeal, oral, and/or nasal cavities. This portion of the speech mechanism is called the resonatory system because the modification of sound energy is primarily the result of resonance principles. As stated earlier, resonance is the selective radiation and absorption of sound energy at specific frequencies. In other words, certain frequencies are amplified or intensified (radiated) while others are suppressed or damped out (absorbed) according to these principles. Resonance is one major component in determining our characteristic vocal qualities as well as providing the basis for specific speech sounds, especially vowels. If the structures of the resonatory system are examined to find out how resonance works, we find that the pharyngeal, nasal, and oral areas could be described as differently shaped cavities that are variable in size and form. For example, protruding the lips would change the shape of the oral cavity, while muscular action lowering the larynx would change the dimensions of the pharyngeal cavity. Changes in the size and shape of the oral cavity impact the resonance quality and the resulting sound. In addition, variations in the walls of the resonating cavity (i.e., certain structures are softer, more pliable, while others are harder, denser) contribute to the resonating properties. All these types of modifications and differences modify the quality of specific speech sounds.

The resonance properties of the vocal tract are typically studied within acoustic phonetics. Therefore, resonance and its effect on speech sound production will be treated in more detail in the next section of this chapter.

However, there is one structure within this system that does have a direct impact on the resonance quality of specific sounds in American English: the velopharyngeal mechanism. It directly affects speech sound quality by channeling airflow through either the oral or the nasal cavities. The **velopharyngeal mechanism** consists of the structures and muscles of the velum (soft palate) and those of the pharyngeal walls. The **velopharyngeal port,** the passage that connects the oropharynx and the nasopharynx, can be closed by (1) elevation and posterior movements of the velum and (2) some forward and medial movements of the posterior and lateral pharyngeal walls. These combined movements resemble a sphincterlike action. See Figure 2.11.

Closure of the passageway between the oral and nasal cavities is important for three reasons. First, during the primary function of swallowing, the velopharyngeal port closes as the bolus of food or drink passes from the oral into the pharyngeal cavity. This closure prevents the food or drink from entering the nasal cavity. Second, as a secondary function, closure of the velopharyngeal port is important for the production of specific groups of speech sounds, namely nasal versus nonnasal sounds. **Nasal sounds** are those produced with an open velopharyngeal port, allowing airflow through the nasal cavity. In American English, there are only three nasal sounds, "m," "n," and "ng." **Nonnasal sounds** are those produced with the velopharyngeal port closed; airflow passes through the oral cavity only.

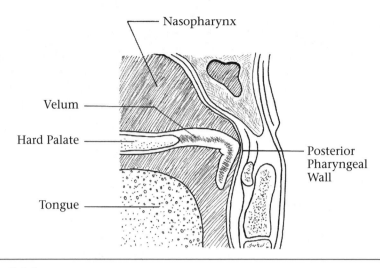

Labels: Nasopharynx, Velum, Hard Palate, Tongue, Posterior Pharyngeal Wall

Figure 2.11   The Velopharyngeal Mechanism

With the exception of "m," "n," and "ng," all other speech sounds in American English are nonnasal sounds. Third, accurately timed and adequate closure of the velopharyngeal port is necessary for normal vocal timbre; without it vocal quality may sound hypernasal. **Hypernasality** refers to an excessive amount of perceived nasal cavity resonance due to lack of necessary velopharyngeal port closure. Hypernasality is predominantly perceived on vowels. Individuals with a cleft palate or dysarthria may demonstrate hypernasality. In both cases, the hypernasality can be traced to inadequacies of velopharyngeal port closure. However, in the two populations distinct differences exist as to why this mechanism fails to function adequately. For the individual with a cleft palate, the roof of the mouth is marked by a cleavage, a split (Shprintzen, 1995). If the clefts are not surgically repaired, these clients demonstrate velopharyngeal port inadequacy primarily due to structural abnormalities: Air escapes through this cleavage from the oral to the nasal cavities. Even after surgery, velopharyngeal insufficiency may still be a problem. Speakers with dysarthria, on the other hand, do not evidence any structural abnormalities; rather, the hypernasality noted is typically due to weakness or incoordination of the velopharyngeal musculature. Certain individuals, for example, may show overall general muscular weakness, which leads to inadequate closure of the velopharyngeal port. Others might lack the coordinated fine tuning necessary to adequately close the velopharyngeal port at the appropriate time. This will also result in the impression of hypernasal speech.

In addition, nasal emission frequently accompanies hypernasality. While nasal emission is not a nasal resonance problem, it is symptomatic of velopharyngeal insufficiency. **Nasal emission** occurs on specific consonants that have a high degree of pressure in the oral cavity during their production. These consonants are produced with a great deal of nasal noise.

FOCUS 4: *Why is the velopharyngeal mechanism important for resonance?*

The Articulatory System

The term *dorsum* has been defined in a variety of ways. For example, the dorsum has been defined as the broad superior surface of the tongue (Ferrand, 2007), the body of the tongue, comprised of the front and back (Small, 2005), or simply as the back of the tongue (Shriberg & Kent, 2003). Although this is somewhat confusing, scholars, as well as many other individuals, often have a hard time agreeing on basic definitions.

Although the mandible is a massive structure, it is exceeded in speed of mobility only by the tip of the tongue. The maximum rate of movement of the mandible is 7.5 per second (pa-pa) while the maximum rate of movement of the tip of the tongue is about 8.2 per second (ta-ta) (Canning & Rose, 1974).

The fourth system within the vocal tract, the articulatory system, is directly involved in forming the individual speech sounds. The structures within this system consist of the lips, tongue, mandible, teeth, hard palate (including the alveolar ridge), velum, and uvula, which are called articulators (see Figure 2.12). Due to their importance for speech realization, a brief review of each of these structures should be helpful for later discussions about specific aspects of speech sound production.

The lips consist primarily of the orbicularis oris muscle. However, there are also many facial muscles that insert into the lips. This allows the lips a wide range of flexibility for facial expression as well as for speech sound production. The lips are the main articulators in sounds such as "b," "p," and "m," for example.

The next articulator, the tongue, is the most important and most active one for speech sound production. Due to the manner of its attachments and the number of intrinsic and extrinsic muscles, the tongue is capable of a wide range of movements. The body of the tongue, which is known as the **dorsum** (Zemlin, 1998) can move horizontally backward and forward, vertically up and down, can assume a concave or a convex shape relative to the palate, can demonstrate central grooving, and can be spread or tapered in its appearance.

Horizontal (forward and backward) and vertical (closer and farther away from the palate) movements are primarily responsible for vowel articulations. In addition, the shape of the tongue plays a major role in both vowel and consonant production. For example, the tip and the sides of the tongue can move independently of the rest of the tongue, curling up and down. There are many sounds in which various portions of the tongue are

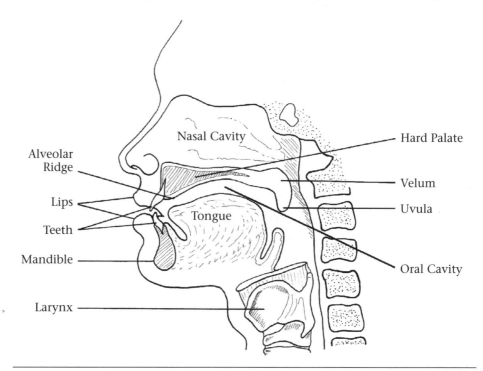

Figure 2.12 The Articulatory System

considered main articulators. The sounds "n" and "t" are produced through the action of the front portion of the tongue, while the typical quality of "k" and "g" is achieved by movement of the back of the tongue.

The mandible or lower jaw houses the lower teeth. Although mandibular movement is very slight during normal speech production, the degree of opening or closing, i.e., various jaw positions, is one dimension used to describe various vowel articulations. Inadequate, inappropriate, or sluggish mandibular movement may contribute to articulatory difficulties (Rosenfeld-Johnson, 2001; Zemlin, 1998).

The primary function of the teeth is the pre-processing of food before it is swallowed and continues on its digestive route. For speech sound production, the secondary function of the teeth is their role as articulators for speech sounds such as "f" and "v" and the th-sounds in "the" or "with." The teeth are also important for other sounds in which they are not considered the primary articulators. For example, the characteristic quality of "s" and "z" is produced by the airstream passing over the edge of the front teeth.

The next group of articulators consists of structures of the roof of the mouth: the hard palate, alveolar ridge, soft palate (velum), and uvula. If you glide your tongue posteriorly from behind the front teeth you will encounter a prominent ridge-like structure known as the **alveolar ridge** or region. This protuberance is formed by the alveolar process, which is a thickened portion of the maxilla (upper jaw) housing the teeth. Moving past the alveolar ridge, the hard bony structure is the hard palate, while farther back you will locate a softer muscular portion, which is referred to as the soft palate or velum. An appendagelike extension of the soft palate is the uvula. All of these structures, alveolar ridge, hard palate, velum, and uvula, play a role in the qualitative end product of speech sounds. For example, "t" and "d" are produced by the tongue tip coming in contact with the alveolar ridge. The first sound in "yes" is considered a palatal sound, while the last sound in "ring," the so-called "ng" sound, has articulatory features that involve the back of the tongue coming in contact with the velum. In American English there are no uvular sounds. However, in French and German there is a uvular trilled-r-type sound. This sound is articulated by raising the back of the tongue close to the uvula, thus creating a narrow opening so that air pressure causes uvular movement.

The preceding section has attempted to describe speech sound production from the viewpoint of physiological phonetics. The structure and function of the respiratory, phonatory, resonatory, and articulatory systems were addressed in respect to their contribution to the generation of speech in general and specific speech sounds. The next section examines speech sound production from the viewpoint of acoustic phonetics. This portion will discuss resonance and its importance in creating the characteristic quality of vowel sounds.

 FOCUS 5: *What are the specific articulations?*

Acoustic Phonetics: An Overview of Principles of Resonance

malocclusions or misaligned teeth.

Since all children go through a period of time when teeth are missing, i.e., primary teeth are replaced by permanent ones, the effect of missing teeth on speech sound production has also been investigated (Bankson & Byrne, 1962; Snow, 1961). Although missing teeth may have an effect on production of certain sounds (for example, simultaneous loss of the two front teeth or what are known as central incisors may affect "s" and "z" sounds), for most children this does not seem to play a decisive role in their speech sound production.

Acoustic phonetics provides information about the physical properties of sounds, specifically speech sounds. One concept within acoustic phonetics that is important in understanding speech production relates to resonance principles. This section will provide a brief review of resonance and then apply these principles to the resonatory system of the vocal tract and specifically to vowel production. This section is seen as only a short review. Other references for acoustic phonetics and acoustics are contained in Further Readings at the end of this chapter.

A good beginning point for understanding resonance starts with a review of different types of vibration and what a resonator actually does. The term **free vibration** is used to describe the natural vibratory response of an object, which is dependent upon the mass, tension, and stiffness of that object (Ferrand, 2007). If you strike a tuning fork of a particular shape and size, it will always vibrate at a certain frequency. The frequency at which the object vibrates is called its **natural** or **resonant frequency**. One object can also set another object into vibration, which is termed **forced vibration**. Forced vibration is effective if the resonant frequencies of the two objects are close to one another. Thus, if you have two tuning forks of the same frequencies and set the first tuning fork into vibration, the second one will be forced to vibrate merely by holding it close to the first. You will also notice that as the first tuning fork forces the second one into vibration the resulting sound is suddenly louder. Because the tuning forks have the same frequency, each vibratory cycle is timed so that they combine and the amplitude of the wave increases, thus creating a louder sound. One principle of resonance is that the closer the resonating frequency of two objects, the greater will be the amplitude response.

There are two types of resonators, mechanical and acoustic. A **mechanical resonator** is when the actual object itself is set into motion. The previous example of the tuning forks is considered a mechanical resonator; tuning fork number 1 sets tuning fork number 2 into vibration. In this instance, the second tuning fork is considered the mechanical resonator. A second type of resonator, an **acoustic resonator**, is a container filled with air that is set into vibration. This type of resonator is very important in the production of speech.

A volume of air within a container can resonate. Everyone has probably had the experience of blowing across the top of a bottle, causing it to emit a tone. You also know that, if you change the size of the air cavity, you change the tone. So by adding water to your empty bottle and blowing, the tone will suddenly be somewhat higher. Different musical instruments are also acoustic resonators. The strings that run across the body of a guitar, when plucked, will cause the air inside the body of the guitar to vibrate. Differently shaped guitars all emit somewhat different types of tones. Based on the same principle, smaller or larger instruments, a violin versus a cello, for example, will each demonstrate characteristic tones created by their resonating cavities. When examining acoustic resonators, we find that frequencies close to the natural, or resonating, frequency of the air-filled cavity will be amplified; others will be damped out or suppressed. The natural or resonating frequency of a particular acoustic resonator depends on several variables: first, the size (larger resonators have lower resonant frequencies, smaller resonators have higher ones), second, the shape of the resonator (more complex or irregularly shaped resonators have a larger range of frequencies to which they respond) and third, the consistency (a hard-walled resonator, such as our bottle, amplifies a smaller range of frequencies, whereas a soft-walled resonator, such as one's vocal tract, responds to a larger range of frequencies) (Ferrand, 2007; Kent, 1997).

These principles of resonance apply to the formation of different vowels. Our vocal tract is, of course, a resonator, with a sound generator at one end (the vibrating vocal folds) and a complex, irregularly shaped soft-walled resonator, the so-called resonating system (which was discussed in the previous section), at the other end. Different degrees of mouth openings and, especially, positioning of the tongue create different cavity sizes within our vocal tract. These different cavity sizes form the basis for creating different vowel qualities. Let's say that a male larynx produces a vowel at a fundamental frequency of 120 cycles per second; i.e., his vocal folds will vibrate 120 times per second. Due to the properties of the vibrating vocal folds, the result will be a so-called **complex wave**, a wave that consists of more than just one frequency, in this case more than just the fundamental frequency. Rather, the fundamental frequency of 120 cycles per second is part of not only this complex wave but also many whole-numbered multiples of that frequency, called **harmonics**. Therefore, harmonics of this fundamental frequency would be 240 Hz, 360 Hz, 480 Hz, etc. Unlike the fundamental frequency, harmonics do not normally create any pitch impression for our ear. Rather, they give the complex wave a special sound quality, a definite timbre. The more harmonics a tone contains, the richer or fuller the tone sounds. Louder harmonics, those with more intensity within the complex wave, will play a more important role in the qualitative end product of the sound in question as opposed to softer, less intense ones. And what causes certain harmonics to be louder than others? These differences are established by the size and the shape of the vocal tract. For example, as the tongue assumes different positions within the oral cavity, the size and shape of the vocal tract will change. Specific sizes and shapes of the vocal tract are mainly (but not exclusively) caused by the many different shapes the tongue can adopt. If the front portion of the tongue is elevated, for example with "ee," the shape of the vocal tract is quite different than if the back portion of the tongue is elevated, which is the case with "oo." As we have seen, depending on their size and form, resonators will reinforce—increase the loudness effect of—certain frequencies and damp out or decrease the loudness effect of others. Vocal tract resonances are called **formants**. The sound source from the vibrating vocal folds with its many harmonics is filtered according to the frequency response of the vocal tract filter. The harmonics that are at or near the resonance frequencies, i.e., near the formants, are reinforced or amplified, while those distant from the resonant frequencies lose energy and are damped. The vocal tract is a variable resonator. As its shape varies because of differences in articulatory placement, the resonances or formants change in frequency, producing a variety of sounds.

One way to actually visually see formants is with sound spectrography.

The number of cycles per second can be abbreviated as cps. *However, the notation* Hz *is commonly used.*

Spectrography is a means of identifying the frequency, intensity, and duration of speech sounds. A **sound spectrogram** is the visual display of this acoustic analysis. On a sound spectrogram, frequency is displayed on the vertical axis, duration on the horizontal axis, and intensity is noted by the darkness of the tracings. A spectrogram allows us to look at formant regions. They will appear as darker, more intense, horizontal bands at certain frequency levels. Formants are customarily numbered: the first formant corresponding to the lowest intense (dark) frequency band, the second to the next highest intense frequency band, etc. Depending on specific sizes and shapes of the vocal tract as a whole, each vowel has a particular pattern of formants. At least two characteristic formant areas are necessary to create the impression of a specific vowel sound. For example, when tongue, lips, and mouth opening are positioned to form "ee," the free space left in the vocal tract establishes several cavity resonators able to reinforce frequencies around 250 and 2400 Hz, the two main formant areas creating the vowel timbre "ee." The formant areas for the vowel "ee" versus "oo" are shown on a sound spectrogram in Figure 2.13.

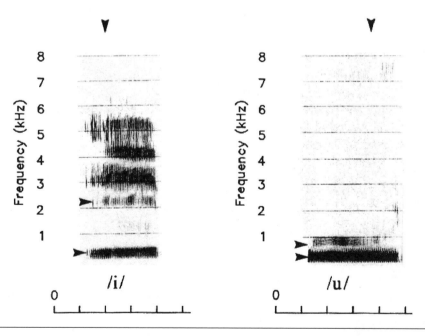

Figure 2.13 Sound Spectrogram of the Vowel [i] (as in "meet") Versus [u] (as in "moon") with the First Two Formants Marked

Source: From *Phonetic Analysis of Normal and Abnormal Speech* (p. 49), by R. N. Ohde and D. J. Sharf, 1992, New York: Merrill. Copyright 1992 by Merrill. Reproduced with permission.

Beginning Case Study

JULIE INTERESTED IN HEARING IMPAIRMENTS

Julie noted that children with more severe hearing impairments had trouble with their vowel qualities, while those with less involvement possibly had difficulty only with sounds such as "s," "sh," and "f." Individuals with hearing impairments have difficulties discriminating between similar acoustic elements. For example, those with milder impairments typically have increased losses in the higher frequencies. It is these high-frequency components that determine the characteristic quality of "s," "sh," and "f." In order to understand and discriminate these sounds from other sounds, an individual must not only be able to hear these high frequencies, he or she must also be able to distinguish various intensity levels of these frequencies. For example, if an individual cannot hear specific intensity differences above 4000 Hz, there is a good chance that "s," "f," and "sh" may be confused. Vowels, on the other hand, contain more intense frequency areas clearly below 4000 Hz. For children with more severe hearing impairments, the perception of these vowels and their production will be affected. Studies have shown that the vowels of individuals with more severe losses are more centralized (moving toward having an "uh" quality), that the vowel formants may overlap considerably so that the acoustic contrasts between vowels are reduced, and that the vowels produced by these individuals are more variable than by speakers with normal hearing (Angelocci, Kopp, & Holbrook, 1964; Osberger, Levitt, & Slosberg, 1979).

Thus, Julie's perception of the speech difficulties of these individuals was based on the acoustic characteristics of what they could perceive and produce. Knowledge of acoustics would aid her in understanding the differences in speech production of these children with varying degrees of hearing loss.

To summarize, the characteristic quality of the vowels is produced by resonance principles functioning within the so-called resonatory system of the vocal tract. Different shapes produced by changes in tongue position, laryngeal movement, mandibular excursions, and lip activity, for example, result in the reinforcement of certain frequency areas, formants, that form the vowel quality. Therefore, the difference between two vowel qualities is a direct result of the shapes of the resonatory system and the resulting reinforced formant areas.

FOCUS 6: *What role does resonance play in the production of vowels?*

Case Study

Peter was 20 years old when he was involved in a serious automobile accident. The head injuries he sustained resulted in a dysarthric condition. When he came to the clinic, he had difficulty sustaining voice for more than 2 or 3 seconds. In addition, his voice sounded strained, and it was difficult to understand what he was saying. One of Peter's major difficulties was coordinating the various components of the speech mechanism. His respiratory efforts were not synchronized with his attempts at phonation, while resonatory and articulatory efforts demonstrated a musculature that was weak and not functionally working together. We focused on normalizing and coordinating his breathing with voice production so that phonation could be maintained for a longer period of time. The resonatory system was also affected. The weakened musculature caused hypernasality, because the muscles of the velopharyngeal mechanism were often not functionally able to close off the oral from the nasal cavities. This weakened musculature also affected the articulatory system; certain consonants were imprecise. In this case, it was clear that all four systems, the respiratory, phonatory, resonatory, and articulatory, were impacted by the dysarthric condition.

Summary

 FOCUS 1: *What are the structures and general functions of each of the four subsystems of the speech mechanism?*

The speech mechanism comprises all structures that are involved in producing speech. These structures are commonly divided into the (1) respiratory, (2) phonatory, (3) resonatory, and (4) articulatory systems. The respiratory system consists primarily of the lungs and airways, including the trachea, rib cage, abdomen, and diaphragm. The phonatory system consists of the larynx, while the resonatory system is composed of a series of cavities, the oral, nasal, and pharyngeal cavities. The articulatory system contains the mandible, tongue, lips, teeth, alveolar ridge, hard palate, and velum.

When studying the respiratory system, one must include information about breathing and its adequacy for speech as well as how these structures function to generate the airflow that makes voice and speech possible. The function of the vocal folds, which are the sound source for speech, would be a portion of the study of the phonatory system, while the way the various cavities of the head and neck modify this sound source would be considered when studying the resonatory system. Study of the articulatory system would include examining the structure and function of the articulators as they form the various speech sounds.

 FOCUS 2: *How do the inspiratory and expiratory muscles regulate the pressure needed for speech?*

Speech production necessitates a regulated amount of subglottal pressure over a rather wide range of volumes. For example, if you take a deep breath but only say a word or two, this pressure will have to be regulated if normal loudness is to be maintained. On the other hand, if you utter a longer sentence, a relatively constant amount of subglottal pressure must be maintained from the beginning of the utterance, when there is clearly more air in the lungs, to its end, when there is far less. To maintain a constant loudness level during the whole utterance, the outflow of air must somehow be equalized.

This equalization of various lung volumes and pressure levels is done by an interplay, a checks and balances system, between inspiratory and expiratory muscles. For example, action of the expiratory mechanism could result in a loss of air relatively quickly at the beginning of the expiratory phase. This may not be desirable for speech production. In order to counteract this sudden loss of air pressure, action of the inspiratory muscles might slow down the rapid decrease in the dimensions of the thoracic cavity. Therefore, the action of inspiratory muscles would help regulate and maintain the subglottal pressure. On the other hand, if at the end of a long utterance still more air pressure is needed, expiratory muscles might assist in providing a relatively constant flow of air for a longer time period. Based on this interplay of balancing actions, the respiratory system is able to constantly supply the laryngeal system with precisely regulated subglottal pressures.

FOCUS 3: *What is the mechanism involved in vocal fold vibration?*

At the onset of phonation, the vocal folds move toward the midline into an adducted position. In this adducted position, the vocal folds are obstructing expiratory airflow, and subglottal pressure begins to build up. As subglottal pressure increases, the vocal folds are forced apart by the air pressure. The open glottis decreases the subglottal pressure. The folds come together again due to their inherent elasticity, the sudden pressure drop between the folds, and other aerodynamic properties. The vocal folds return once again to their adducted position. The subglottal air pressure builds up again and the process is repeated.

FOCUS 4: *Why is the velopharyngeal mechanism important for resonance?*

Closure of the velopharyngeal port is important for the differentiation between specific groups of speech sounds, namely nasal versus nonnasal sounds. Nasal sounds are those produced with an open velopharyngeal port, allowing airflow through the nasal cavity. Nonnasal sounds are those produced with the velopharyngeal port closed; airflow passes through the oral cavity only. With the exception of "m," "n," and "ng," which are nasal sounds, all other speech sounds in American English are nonnasal sounds. In addition, accurately timed and adequate closure of the velopharyngeal port is necessary for normal vocal quality. Without this accurate timing of the velopharyngeal mechanism, the voice may sound as if there is too much or too little nasality.

FOCUS 5: *What are the specific articulators?*

The articulators consist of the lips, tongue, mandible, teeth, hard palate (including the alveolar ridge), velum, and uvula. These structures are directly involved in the production of speech sounds, both vowels and consonants.

FOCUS 6: *What role does resonance play in the production of vowels?*

The vocal tract is an acoustic resonator with a sound generator at one end (the vibrating vocal folds) and a complex, irregularly shaped soft-walled resonator (which consists of the area above the vocal folds, including the pharyngeal, oral, and nasal cavities) at the other end. Different degrees of mouth openings and, especially, positioning of the tongue create different cavity sizes within our vocal tract. These different cavity sizes form the basis for creating different vowel qualities. For example, as the tongue assumes different positions within the oral cavity, the size and shape of the vocal tract will change. Depending on their size and form, resonators will reinforce—increase the loudness effect of—certain frequencies and damp out or decrease the loudness effect of others. Vocal tract resonances are called *formants*. The sound source from the vibrating vocal folds with its many harmonics is filtered according to the frequency response of the vocal tract filter. The harmonics that are at or near the resonance frequencies i.e., near the formants, are reinforced or amplified, while those distant from the resonant frequencies lose energy and are damped. As the vocal tract's shape varies, because of differences in articulatory placement, the resonances or formants change in frequency, producing a variety of sounds.

Further Readings

Borden, G., Harris, K., & Raphael, L. (2003). *Speech science primer: Physiology, acoustics, and perception of speech* (4th ed.). Baltimore: Lippencott Williams & Wilkins.

Ferrand, C. T. (2007). *Speech science: An integrated approach to theory and clinical practice* (2nd ed.). Boston: Pearson/Allyn and Bacon.

Kent, R. (1997). *The speech sciences*. San Diego: Singular.

Seikel, J., Drumright, D., & Seikel, P. (2004). *Essentials of anatomy and physiology for communication disorders*. Clifton Park, NY: Thomson Delmar Learning.

Zemlin, W. (1998). *Speech and hearing science: Anatomy and physiology* (4th ed.) Boston: Allyn and Bacon.

Key Terms

abduct p. 32
acoustic resonator p. 41
adduct p. 31
alveolar pressure p. 27
alveolar ridge p. 40
articulatory system p. 22
atmospheric pressure p. 27
complex wave p. 42
dorsum p. 39
dysarthrias p. 25
dysphagia p. 29
extrinsic muscles p. 31
forced vibration p. 41
formants p. 42
free vibration p. 41
fundamental frequency p. 34
glottis p. 28
harmonics p. 42
hyperadduction p. 36

hypernasality p. 38
hypertension p. 36
hypotension p. 36
intrinsic muscles p. 31
laryngopharynx (hypopharynx) p. 36
malocclusion p. 40
mechanical resonator p. 41
nasal cavities p. 36
nasal emission p. 38
nasal sounds p. 37
nasopharynx (hyperpharynx) p. 35
natural frequency p. 41
nonnasal sounds p. 37
occlusion p. 40
oral cavity p. 36
oropharynx (mediopharynx) p. 36
overbite p. 40
overlaid function p. 24
pharyngeal cavity p. 35

Think Critically

1. Follow your breathing as you are sitting and reading this sentence. Next, follow your breathing as you inhale and read these sentences out loud. What differences in respiration do you note between quiet breathing without speech and when speaking?

2. Lack of respiratory control is often noted in dysarthric speakers. How would this translate into problems controlling pitch and loudness during phonation?

3. Which sounds are considered nonnasal? Devise a sentence that you could use to test only nonnasal sounds.

4. Which articulators are used for the following sounds: "m," "l," "s," "g," and "v"? Which of those sounds has simultaneous vocal fold vibration; i.e., which of those sounds are voiced?

5. Formants are vocal tract resonances. Explain what this means.

Test Yourself

1. Which one of the systems of the speech mechanism contains the diaphragm?
   a. respiratory system
   b. phonatory system
   c. resonatory system
   d. articulatory system

2. Which one of the systems of the speech mechanism examines the specific structures used when producing [s]?
   a. respiratory system
   b. phonatory system
   c. resonatory system
   d. articulatory system

3. Which one of the systems of the speech mechanism examines vocal fold function?
   a. respiratory system
   b. phonatory system
   c. resonatory system

d. articulatory system

4. The velopharyngeal mechanism is contained in which system of the speech mechanism?

    a. respiratory system

    b. phonatory system

    c. resonatory system

    d. articulatory system

5. The average number of glottal openings per second is the

    a. timbre.

    b. harmonic.

    c. fundamental frequency.

    d. natural frequency.

6. The selective absorption and reinforcement of sound energies that create the characteristic quality of certain speech sounds is

    a. forced vibration.

    b. free vibration.

    c. timbre.

    d. resonance.

7. The velopharyngeal port is a passage between the nasopharynx and the

    a. oropharynx.

    b. laryngopharynx.

    c. vocal tract.

    d. dorsum.

8. During inhalation, the alveolar pressure is

    a. equal to the atmospheric pressure.

    b. more than the atmospheric pressure.

    c. less than the atmospheric pressure.

    d. always positive.

9. Harmonics are related to the

    a. subglottal air pressure.

    b. fundamental frequency.

    c. nasal cavity.

    d. velopharyngeal mechanism.

10. During production of the nasal sounds, the velopharyngeal port is

    a. closed.

    b. open.

    c. vibrating.

    d. abducted.

Answers: 1. a 2. d 3. b 4. c 5. c 6. d 7. a 8. c 9. b 10. b

For additional information, go to www.phonologicaldisorders.com

CHAPTER 3

An Introduction to Phonetic Transcription

Chapter Highlights

- What three necessities must a phonetic notation system fulfill?
- What is the difference between phonetic and phonemic transcription?
- Which theoretical concepts form the basic premise for the IPA notation?
- Why is the orthographic letter system not a good possibility for phonetic transcription?
- Which three guidelines are important to remember when learning phonetic transcription?

Chapter Application: Case Study

Lilly was a darling child who had just moved to the United States with her mother from the Canton Province of Southern China. She came wide-eyed into Peter's first-grade classroom without one word of English. Peter was trained as a teacher of English as a second language and was a new arrival from Texas to the San Francisco Bay area. He felt very comfortable speaking Spanish but had to admit that he really didn't know much about the Chinese language. Although his school had a high percentage of Chinese children, this was the first time that he had a child in his class that could not speak any English. However, Lilly seemed to be a bright child and tried within the first week to say some words in English. Within a short time Lilly had a small core vocabulary, but he noticed that her pronunciation was definitely different. For example, for "the" she said something like "fa" and "shoe" sounded more like "Sue." Peter decided to do some research into Chinese to see how the vowels and consonants of Lilly's language might differ from American English. First, Peter learned that there are several dialects of Chinese. He finally found out that Lilly's native dialect was Cantonese: She and her mother were from Hong Kong. Looking further, Peter found a list of consonants and vowels that represented those that are present in the Cantonese dialect. He found a reference to the International Phonetic Alphabet and saw that many of the symbols were represented on a chart that he found. While he was somehow able to figure out some of the sounds, many of the symbols that he saw were so different that they might have been written in Chinese. He wondered how he would be able to figure out the sounds according to this chart.

The purpose of this chapter is to introduce the reader to phonetic transcription and to the International Phonetic Alphabet. *Phonetic transcription* is the term generally used to refer to the written notation of speech sounds. For many individuals and professions, knowledge of certain aspects of phonetic transcription is an important aspect of what they do. Linguists may use phonetic transcription to document specific sounds within a foreign language; while experts in English as a second language will use their knowledge of transcription to determine which speech sound differences might exist between American English and the child's native language. Foreign language teachers might use examples from phonetic transcription in an attempt to teach their students better pronunciation of the different sounds of that foreign language, i.e., those sounds that do not exist in American English but do in Spanish, for example. Transcription is also very useful when transcribing dialects for the stage and for trained singers who are learning songs in other languages. And speech-language clinicians will use transcription to write down the differences that they hear when assessing an adult or a child with a possible speech disorder. All in all, phonetic transcription is a very useful tool for many individuals and professions.

This chapter will introduce the International Phonetic Alphabet, which is the most widely used system to document individual speech sounds and their variations. This chapter is seen solely as an introductory chapter; many of the concepts will be re-examined and further developed in later chapters. Learning phonetic transcription is a challenge. It necessitates that certain "writing rules" are unlearned and that unknown symbols representing specific speech sounds are learned. It is not only a skill that requires that symbols be written but also one that requires careful tuning of our auditory perceptual skills. However, with the acquisition of this skill, students and professionals will have a useful tool that can be used in a variety of circumstances and professions.

Phonetic Transcription as a Notation System

Speech is a fleeting event; it exists only in the briefest moment of its realization. After this very short time it is gone. If our goal is to document a speech event, then we must grapple with the concept of how to preserve speech. Keeping in mind that we have a special purpose, be it the documentation of a foreign language or the assessment of individuals with deviant speech patterns, certain system requirements need to be fulfilled to preserve the speech event.

First, the system that we use must *accurately* preserve speech. If our system is not accurate, then our record of the speech event is faulty from the beginning. Accuracy implies that the notation system that we use must be broad enough to be practical yet detailed enough to allow fine distinctions between sound productions. The balance between these two positions, user friendly, on the one hand, and having adequate detail, on the other hand, is not always an easy one. The system that we choose should attempt to deal with this balance.

The second necessity our notation system must satisfy is one of *documentation*. In speech-language pathology, documentation refers to records that give evidence of outcomes of performance-based assessment and/or treatment effectiveness (Blosser & Neidecker, 2002). Thus, our notation system must be able to provide records that allow us to note the present speech status as well as outcome measures. For example, as speech-language clinicians, we will need to document not only why we arrived at a clinical decision, norm versus disordered speech, but treatment results as well. Or the teacher of English as a second language may need to document the progress the child has made in acquiring American English speech sounds. The notation system that we choose must allow us to document and provide records of the speech event.

The third necessity for our notation system is *communication*; the system must allow communication with other professionals. Other professionals must be able to readily identify and understand our record keeping. The system that we use must be one that is immediately recognized and can be interpreted by any other professional in the United States or around the globe. The notation system that will be introduced in this chapter is the International Phonetic Alphabet. It is recognized worldwide as such a system. It is well documented in many books and scholarly works; therefore, it is a system that facilitates communication among professionals.

 FOCUS 1: *What three necessities must a phonetic notation system fulfill?*

What Is Phonetic Transcription?

Broadly defined, **phonetic transcription** is the use of phonetic notation to record utterances or parts of utterances (Abercrombie, 1967). **Phonetic notation** refers to a set of symbols that stand for sound segments. In other words, phonetic notation uses a specific type of symbol system to describe each speech sound within a given language. Over the years, a variety of phonetic notation systems have been invented. The notation system that will be presented in this chapter, the **International Phonetic Alphabet** (IPA), is the most widely used system. In general, one speaks about "transcribing" a speech sample or using "phonetic transcription" to verify a speech disorder.

However, there is a more specific way in which the term *phonetic transcription* is often denoted. Transcription can be of two types: phonetic or phonemic. In this case, phonetic transcription entails the use of a phonetic categorization that includes as much production detail as possible. This detail encompasses the use of the broad classification system noted in the IPA as well as extra symbols that can be added to give a particular phonetic value, in other words, to characterize specific production features. These additional symbols are termed *diacritics* and will be introduced in a later chapter. Phonetic transcription, thus defined, is called **narrow transcription** (Abercrombie, 1967; Grunwell, 1987). For phonetic transcription, the symbols are placed within brackets [ ]. For example, [p] would be a phonetic transcription. On the other hand, **phonemic transcription** is based on the phoneme system of that particular language; each symbol represents a phoneme (MacKay, 1987). It is a more general type of transcription and is,

Reflect on This: Clinical Application

BROAD VERSUS NARROW TRANSCRIPTION

Both broad and narrow transcriptions are used by clinicians when summarizing the results of a speech evaluation. When do we need more detail (narrow transcription), and when is less detail (broad transcription) sufficient? The following clinical examples are given to exemplify when each could be used.

Tonya is 4 years old and uses a "w" sound in all of the words that are typically produced with an "l": For example, "lamp" becomes "wamp," "light" becomes "wight," and "leg" becomes "weg." In this case, a summary using broad transcription would probably be adequate. Tonya is replacing one phoneme with another. We would note this by saying Tonya uses /w/ instead of /l/.

Sherri is 6 years old and has an "s" that is clearly perceptually off. It sounds somehow between an "s" and a "th"; in other words, it is not a clear "s" or a regular "th." Here a more specific phonetic transcription would be required. It would be inaccurate to transcribe Sherri's production as an "s" or a "th." In this case, narrow transcription would be necessary.

thus, referred to as **broad transcription.** For phonemic transcription, the symbols are placed within slashes / /, which are termed *virgules*. Thus, /p/ would indicate phonemic transcription.

This dichotomy between phonetic and phonemic transcription often leads to transcribers using brackets [ ] and slashes / / interchangeably. However, as noted in the previous chapter, brackets [ ] should be used when listening to and transcribing actual productions. This notation indicates actual realizations, the concrete productions of a speech sound. Therefore, if we are transcribing a child's speech, the brackets [ ] should be used. However, if we are summarizing our results, it may not be necessary to use phonetic transcription, i.e., to use as much detail as possible. If we are summarizing a phonemic inventory, especially of normal speech, then phonemic, or broad, transcription might be sufficient. As speech-language clinicians, however, we will often be assessing disordered speech. In this case, phonetic transcription will probably be used to note as much detail as possible. Phonetic transcription is a necessity when the individual's speech patterns demonstrate errors that cannot be perceptually classified as phonemes of that given language.

Throughout the years, a variety of notation systems have been developed to transcribe the speech event. The International Phonetic Alphabet is one of the more contemporary systems. The following brief overview demonstrates the various types of notation systems.

 FOCUS 2: *What is the difference between phonetic and phonemic transcription?*

Types of Transcription Systems

Experiments attempting to develop various types of phonetic notation systems date back centuries. These notations fall broadly into two types of systems: alphabetic and analphabetic. **Alphabetic systems** are based on the same principles that govern ordinary alphabetic writing consisting of the use of a single symbol to represent a speech sound. There exists a one-to-one relationship between the symbol and the sound. In **analphabetic systems** (those that are not alphabetic), each sound segment is represented by a composite notation made up of a number of symbols. These symbols are abbreviated descriptive labels for the sound segment. Analphabetic systems of phonetic notation used certain symbols to represent the presence or absence of voicing, velar activity, the nature of the constriction, which articulators are used, and any additional production features the author thought were important. The more symbols used typically indicated a more detailed explanation of the production properties.

The Alphabet of the International Phonetic Association: IPA

The International Phonetic Association (first known as the Phonetic Teachers' Association) was founded in 1886 in France by a group of language teachers under the leadership of Paul Passy. These professionals found phonetic transcription to be especially helpful in teaching foreign languages and wanted to popularize this particular method. One of the first things that the association did was publish a journal in which the contents were entirely written in phonetic transcription. Both the International Phonetic Alphabet and the International Phonetic Association are abbreviated with the same letters: IPA. Typically, the alphabet is referred to as "the IPA."

The concept of establishing an international phonetic alphabet is attributed to Otto Jespersen, and the first version of the International Phonetic Alphabet was published in 1888 (Crystal, 1987). The aim of the International Phonetic Alphabet was to allow anyone who was familiar with the system the possibility of having a fairly accurate idea of how to pronounce any language in the world. The symbols should be convenient to use but comprehensive enough to deal with the wide variety of sounds that occur across all the languages. The symbols are based on the Roman alphabet, but, since there are more sounds than letters within that alphabet, letters and symbols from additional sources have been incorporated.

In actuality, the IPA system is a compromise between alphabetic and analphabetic systems. There is a one-to-one correspondence between phoneme realizations and sound symbols; however, at the same time, many additional signs can be used to identify modifications in the original production. These additional signs, called diacritics, are placed above, below, to the right, or as superscripts to the right of the symbols.

The IPA has not been without controversy, and as the goals and scope of the International Phonetic Association changed, so did the alphabet. Although the notation system as a whole has stayed fairly intact, the most recent changes were made in 2005. The IPA is presented in Figure 3.1. Although many of the symbols are as yet unfamiliar, the reader will probably recognize some of the consonants in the upper box. The vowels are

CONSONANTS (PULMONIC)

	Bilabial	Labiodental	Dental	Alveolar	Postalveolar	Retroflex	Palatal	Velar	Uvular	Pharyngeal	Glottal
Plosive	p b			t d		ʈ ɖ	c ɟ	k g	q ɢ		ʔ
Nasal	m	ɱ		n		ɳ	ɲ	ŋ	N		
Trill	ʙ			r					R		
Tap or Flap				ɾ		ɽ					
Fricative	ɸ β	f v	θ ð	s z	ʃ ʒ	ʂ ʐ	ç ʝ	x ɣ	χ ʁ	ħ ʕ	h ɦ
Lateral fricative				ɬ ɮ							
Approximant		ʋ		ɹ		ɻ	j	ɰ			
Lateral approximant				l		ɭ	ʎ	ʟ			

Where symbols appear in pairs, the one to the right represents a voiced consonant. Shaded areas denote articulations judged impossible.

CONSONANTS (NON-PULMONIC)

Clicks		Voiced implosives		Ejectives	
ʘ	Bilabial	ɓ	Bilabial	’	Examples:
ǀ	Dental	ɗ	Dental/alveolar	p’	Bilabial
ǃ	(Post)alveolar	ʄ	Palatal	t’	Dental/alveolar
ǂ	Palatoalveolar	ɠ	Velar	k’	Velar
ǁ	Alveolar lateral	ʛ	Uvular	s’	Alveolar fricative

OTHER SYMBOLS

ʍ	Voiceless labial-velar fricative	ɕ ʑ	Alveolo-palatal fricatives
w	Voiced labial-velar approximant	ɺ	Voiced alveolar lateral flap
ɥ	Voiced labial-palatal approximant	ɧ	Simultaneous ʃ and x
ʜ	Voiceless epiglottal fricative		
ʢ	Voiced epiglottal fricative		Affricates and double articulations can be represented by two symbols joined by a tie bar if necessary. k͡p t͡s
ʡ	Epiglottal plosive		

VOWELS

Where symbols appear in pairs, the one to the right represents a rounded vowel.

SUPRASEGMENTALS

ˈ	Primary stress	ˌfoʊnəˈtɪʃən
ˌ	Secondary stress	
ː	Long	eː
ˑ	Half-long	eˑ
˘	Extra-short	ĕ
ǀ	Minor (foot) group	
ǁ	Major (intonation) group	
.	Syllable break	ɹi.ækt
‿	Linking (absence of a break)	

DIACRITICS

Diacritics may be placed above a symbol with a descender, e.g. ŋ̊

̥	Voiceless	n̥ d̥	̤	Breathy voiced	b̤ a̤	̪	Dental	t̪ d̪
̬	Voiced	s̬ t̬	̰	Creaky voiced	b̰ a̰	̺	Apical	t̺ d̺
ʰ	Aspirated	tʰ dʰ	̼	Linguolabial	t̼ d̼	̻	Laminal	t̻ d̻
̹	More rounded	ɔ̹	ʷ	Labialized	tʷ dʷ	̃	Nasalized	ẽ
̜	Less rounded	ɔ̜	ʲ	Palatalized	tʲ dʲ	ⁿ	Nasal release	dⁿ
̟	Advanced	u̟	ˠ	Velarized	tˠ dˠ	ˡ	Lateral release	dˡ
̠	Retracted	e̠	ˤ	Pharyngealized	tˤ dˤ	̚	No audible release	d̚
̈	Centralized	ë	̴	Velarized or pharyngealized	ɫ			
̽	Mid-centralized	e̽	̝	Raised	e̝ (ɹ̝ = voiced alveolar fricative)			
̩	Syllabic	n̩	̞	Lowered	e̞ (β̞ = voiced bilabial approximant)			
̯	Non-syllabic	e̯	̘	Advanced Tongue Root	e̘			
˞	Rhoticity	ɚ a˞	̙	Retracted Tongue Root	e̙			

TONES AND WORD ACCENTS

LEVEL			CONTOUR		
e̋ or ˥	Extra high		ě or ˇ	Rising	
é or ˦	High		ê or ˆ	Falling	
ē or ˧	Mid		e᷄ or ˏ	High rising	
è or ˨	Low		e᷅ or ˎ	Low rising	
ȅ or ˩	Extra low		e᷈ or ˜	Rising-falling	
↓	Downstep		↗	Global rise	
↑	Upstep		↘	Global fall	

Figure 3.1 The International Phonetic Alphabet (1993, revised 2005). Copyright © 2005 by the International Phonetic Association.

located below and to the right of the consonants. Keep in mind that these symbols were developed in an attempt to document all the speech sounds of all the languages of the world, a rather daunting task.

Several theoretical concepts underlie the notation known as the IPA. These include:

- Some aspects of speech have linguistic relevance, i.e., have phonemic value, while others, such as one's personal voice quality, do not.
- Speech can be represented as a sequence of discrete sounds.
- Sound segments can be divided into two major categories, consonants and vowels.
- The phonetic description of sound segments can be referenced according to their production and auditory characteristics.
- In addition to the sound segments, a number of "suprasegmental" aspects of speech need to be independently represented (International Phonetic Association, 1999).

 FOCUS 3: *Which theoretical concepts form the basic premise for the IPA notation?*

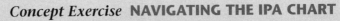

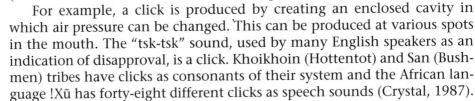 *Concept Exercise* **NAVIGATING THE IPA CHART**
To aid in navigating this chart, some definitions and explanations might be helpful. The top box (see Figure 3.2) contains pulmonic consonants.

Pulmonic sounds are those that use air from the lungs for sound production. Both vowels and consonants in American English are pulmonic. The grids of the large box provide production details about the specific consonants: Along the left-hand column is the type of consonant, while across the top are the specific articulators that are used for the sound production. If two symbols appear in one box, the first one is the voiceless sound, and the second its voiced counterpart. The small box labeled "Consonants (**Non-pulmonic**)" refers to those sounds that are produced using "other airstream mechanisms" (International Phonetic Association, 1999, p. 9). See Figure 3.3.

For example, a click is produced by creating an enclosed cavity in which air pressure can be changed. This can be produced at various spots in the mouth. The "tsk-tsk" sound, used by many English speakers as an indication of disapproval, is a click. Khoikhoin (Hottentot) and San (Bushmen) tribes have clicks as consonants of their system and the African language !Xũ has forty-eight different clicks as speech sounds (Crystal, 1987).

To the right of the non-pulmonic consonants are the vowels. The vowels are noted according to the relative position of the tongue during their production. If two vowels appear on the same level, one to the right and one to the left of the dot, then this indicates that the vowel to the right of the dot has the same tongue placement as the vowel to the left but with lip rounding. Thus, the vowel to the left is produced with lip spreading. Vowels and their phonetic transcription symbols will be discussed in more detail in the next chapter. See Figure 3.4.

CONSONANTS (PULMONIC)

	Bilabial	Labiodental	Dental	Alveolar	Postalveolar	Retroflex	Palatal	Velar	Uvular	Pharyngeal	Glottal
Plosive	p b			t d		ʈ ɖ	c ɟ	k g	q ɢ		ʔ
Nasal	m	ɱ		n		ɳ	ɲ	ŋ	ɴ		
Trill	ʙ			r					ʀ		
Tap or Flap				ɾ		ɽ					
Fricative	ɸ β	f v	θ ð	s z	ʃ ʒ	ʂ ʐ	ç ʝ	x ɣ	χ ʁ	ħ ʕ	h ɦ
Lateral fricative				ɬ ɮ							
Approximant		ʋ		ɹ		ɻ	j	ɰ			
Lateral approximant				l		ɭ	ʎ	ʟ			

Where symbols appear in pairs, the one to the right represents a voiced consonant. Shaded areas denote articulations judged impossible.

Figure 3.2 Pulmonic Consonants

Source: From *The International Phonetic Alphabet* (revised to 1993, updated 2005). Copyright © 2005 by the International Phonetic Association.

CONSONANTS (NON-PULMONIC)

Clicks		Voiced implosives		Ejectives	
ʘ	Bilabial	ɓ	Bilabial	ʼ	Examples:
ǀ	Dental	ɗ	Dental/alveolar	pʼ	Bilabial
ǃ	(Post)alveolar	ʄ	Palatal	tʼ	Dental/alveolar
ǂ	Palatoalveolar	ɠ	Velar	kʼ	Velar
ǁ	Alveolar lateral	ʛ	Uvular	sʼ	Alveolar fricative

Figure 3.3 Non-Pulmonic Consonants

Source: From *The International Phonetic Alphabet* (revised to 1993, updated 2005). Copyright © 2005 by the International Phonetic Association.

VOWELS

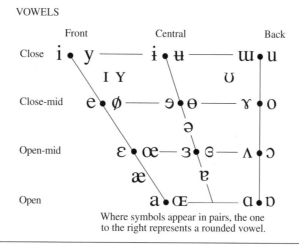

Where symbols appear in pairs, the one to the right represents a rounded vowel.

Figure 3.4 Vowels

Source: From *The International Phonetic Alphabet* (revised to 1993, updated 2005). Copyright © 2005 by the International Phonetic Association.

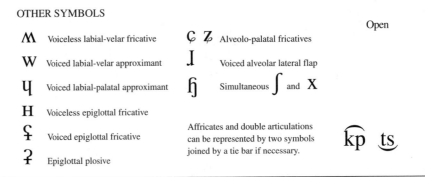

ʍ	Voiceless labial-velar fricative	ɕ ʑ	Alveolo-palatal fricatives		Open
w	Voiced labial-velar approximant	ɺ	Voiced alveolar lateral flap		
ɥ	Voiced labial-palatal approximant	ɧ	Simultaneous ∫ and X		
ʜ	Voiceless epiglottal fricative				
ʢ	Voiced epiglottal fricative	Affricates and double articulations can be represented by two symbols joined by a tie bar if necessary.		k͡p t͡s	
ʡ	Epiglottal plosive				

Figure 3.5 Other Symbols

Source: From *The International Phonetic Alphabet* (revised to 1993, updated 2005). Copyright © 2005 by the International Phonetic Association.

Underneath the non-pulmonic consonants are "other symbols." These are consonants that could not fit easily into the large upper grid due to their production features. For example, the /w/ (typically heard in "win" or "wing") involves two types of articulation that are produced simultaneously. See Figure 3.5.

Underneath the "other symbols" are the diacritics: those symbols that are added to the original one to modify or refine its meaning in various ways. Several of these diacritics will be introduced in Chapter 7. See Figure 3.6.

To the right of the "other symbols" are the suprasegmentals. These are the symbols that are used to note pitch, loudness, and timing of speech. Symbols that can be used for words and for longer units are represented.

DIACRITICS   Diacritics may be placed above a symbol with a descender, e.g. ŋ̊

̥	Voiceless	n̥ d̥	̤	Breathy voiced	b̤ a̤	̪	Dental	t̪ d̪
̬	Voiced	s̬ t̬	̰	Creaky voiced	b̰ a̰	̺	Apical	t̺ d̺
ʰ	Aspirated	tʰ dʰ	̼	Linguolabial	t̼ d̼	̻	Laminal	t̻ d̻
̹	More rounded	ɔ̹	ʷ	Labialized	tʷ dʷ	̃	Nasalized	ẽ
̜	Less rounded	ɔ̜	ʲ	Palatalized	tʲ dʲ	ⁿ	Nasal release	dⁿ
̟	Advanced	u̟	ˠ	Velarized	tˠ dˠ	ˡ	Lateral release	dˡ
̠	Retracted	e̠	ˤ	Pharyngealized	tˤ dˤ	̚	No audible release	d̚
̈	Centralized	ë	̃	Velarized or pharyngealized	ɫ			
̽	Mid-centralized	e̽	̝	Raised	e̝ (ɹ̝ = voiced alveolar fricative)			
̩	Syllabic	n̩	̞	Lowered	e̞ (β̞ = voiced bilabial approximant)			
̯	Non-syllabic	e̯	̘	Advanced Tongue Root	e̘			
˞	Rhoticity	ɚ a˞	̙	Retracted Tongue Root	e̙			

Figure 3.6 Diacritics

Source: From *The International Phonetic Alphabet* (revised to 1993, updated 2005). Copyright © 2005 by the International Phonetic Association.

SUPRASEGMENTALS

ˈ	Primary stress	
ˌ	Secondary stress	
		ˌfoʊnəˈtɪʃən
ː	Long	eː
ˑ	Half-long	eˑ
˘	Extra-short	ĕ
ǀ	Minor (foot) group	
‖	Major (intonation) group	
.	Syllable break	ɹi.ækt
‿	Linking (absence of a break)	

Figure 3.7 Suprasegmentals

Source: From *The International Phonetic Alphabet* (revised to 1993, updated 2005). Copyright © 2005 by the International Phonetic Association.

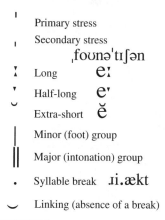

TONES AND WORD ACCENTS

LEVEL			CONTOUR		
e̋ or ˥	Extra high		ě or ꜛ/	Rising	
é ˦	High		ê ꜜ\	Falling	
ē ˧	Mid		e᷄ ꜛ/	High rising	
è ˨	Low		e᷅ ꜜ/	Low rising	
ȅ ˩	Extra low		e᷈ ꜛ/	Rising-falling	
↓	Downstep		↗	Global rise	
↑	Upstep		↘	Global fall	

Figure 3.8 Tones and Word Accents

Source: From *The International Phonetic Alphabet* (revised to 1993, updated 2005). Copyright © 2005 by the International Phonetic Association.

Suprasegmentals and the diacritics used to signify them will be discussed in Chapter 7. See Figure 3.7.

Finally, the small group in the lower right-hand corner of this chart contains symbols to note tones and word accents. There are languages in which pitch variation, at the morpheme level, distinguishes meaning; thus, a pitch change has phonemic value. Although American English is not a tone language, many of the languages around the world, such as Thai and forms of Chinese, are tone languages. These symbols are used to indicate these pitch variations. See Figure 3.8.

Beginning Case Study

PETER, THE ENGLISH AS A SECOND LANGUAGE TEACHER

Peter is still working on the IPA chart. He finds the consonants of Cantonese and compares them to another chart with the consonants of American English. First, he sees that there are similar consonants. For example, "p," "t," and "k" exist in both Cantonese and American English. However, "b," "d," and "g" are not part of the Cantonese consonant inventory. So, he is making progress. He is also able to note that "f" is present in Cantonese but not "v," "s" but not "z," and that the "sh" and "th" sounds are not a part of the Cantonese consonant system. And there is not an "r" in Cantonese; he had anticipated that after listening to Lilly struggle with r-words. This would explain some of her other problems as well, such as using "s" for the word "shoe" or "f" for "th." There were still some things he didn't quite understand: For example, what did the little raised "h" and "w" letters mean following "p," "t," and "k"? He would find them somewhere on the chart.

Why Use Phonetic Transcription?

Accurate phonetic transcription is an indispensable tool for many professionals. Its importance is underlined by the fact that students' skill preparation in several different fields such as linguistics, communication, foreign language studies, and communicative disorders often involves coursework directed toward learning and becoming proficient in phonetic transcription. In the field of communication disorders, these skills form the basis of assessment and remediation of impaired speech. Without a reliable record of how a child or adult realized a particular speech sound, we simply do not have enough information for goal-directed intervention. Phonetic transcription provides a reasonably accurate written record of what was said and what it sounded like.

Why not make a high-quality audio or video recording? With present-day technology, it should create an acceptable likeness of not only what was said but also how it sounded. Such a recording could be easily done; the procedure is repeatable and relatively durable. Audio and video recordings are important aids in our field. However, they can never take the place of reliable phonetic transcription, which is done as we listen to the speaker.

There is typically a direct relationship between how a sound was produced and its audible result. An [s] with the tongue tip either too far forward in the mouth or too far back will have a characteristic quality. If the tongue tip is too far forward, the [s] loses its characteristic sharp tone and sounds "dull." This is a direct result of the tongue position. However, specific conditions can also create an [s] that sounds "dull," similar to our [s] with the tongue tip too far forward. For example, this impression may be the result of air pressure that is too low, a so-called weak articulation.

Poor-quality recording equipment, a microphone that is positioned too close, or improper adjustment of input levels may also lead to a recording that sounds as if [s] is produced with the tongue tip too far forward. Therefore, taped transcriptions should only complement those obtained from live transcriptions. Phonetic transcription done in this manner will secure a reliable record of the status quo, which is a prerequisite for accurate documentation of normal and disordered speech.

Why not use the letters of American English orthography to represent the sounds? First, there are far more sounds than letters. Although our English orthography system is considered to be an alphabetic system, it does not use a true one-to-one correspondence between distinctive speech sounds and letters of the alphabet. Examples of these problems include the following (MacKay, 1987):

1. One sound is often represented by several different spellings. For example, the vowel sound in "m<u>ay</u>," which in this example is spelled "ay," can be spelled as "a" in "able," "a–e" in "cake," "ai" in "chain," "ea" in "steak," "au" in "gauge," "et" in "ballet," and "ee" in "matinee."
2. The same letter can represent several different sounds. For example, listen to the different vowel qualities that are all spelled with the letter "o": "toe," "today," "women," "clock," and "glove."
3. Alphabetic notations are noted as having a one-symbol-to-one-sound correspondence. The use of digraphs in spelling violates this principle. A **digraph** is a combination of two letters representing one sound. For example, the spelling "ph" is the "f" sound in "elephant" or "telephone." The letters "th" in "the," "this," and "then" are actually one sound, in this case the voiced "th" sound. There are also vowel digraphs such as "ee" in "beet" or "oo" in "moon." In these examples, two letters represent one vowel sound.
4. English spelling is not alphabetic, as we often use letters to represent no sound at all. These "silent" letters appear in words such as "thought," "knee," "fight," "psychology" (which also contains a digraph "ch"), "doubt," "whistle," and "pneumonia."
5. Finally, there are sounds that are not represented by the spelling of English words. For example, the first sound in "use" is the same sound as in "yes." If "fool" and "fuel" are compared, it is clear that this sound appears to be missing in the spelling of "fuel" as well.

And what about pronunciation guides in dictionaries? These guides typically report most but not all of the vowel and consonant sounds. In addition, the symbols used in dictionaries are not universal. For example, the *New Webster's Dictionary* (1986) uses the symbol u̜ to denote the vowel in "book," while the *Random House Dictionary* (Flexner, 1987) uses the symbol oo for the same sound. Even if a dictionary notation system would be adopted, confusion would immediately arise as to which sound a particular notation signified. Using phonetic transcription and the International Phonetic Alphabet guarantees a symbol system that is universally agreed upon.

Beginning transcribers sometimes forget which symbols go with which sounds. Like any competency, phonetic transcription needs to be maintained; it is a "use it" or "lose it" skill. As you master this system, remember to use it, teach it to your friends, and write notes in phonetic transcription. You will find that the more you practice transcription, the more you will feel comfortable with it. As your comfort level increases, it will become easier to remember and use. Possibly based on forgetting which symbol to use, clinicians often "create" their own symbols. This can be a serious problem for communication among professionals. In speech-language pathology, your documentation for a client, including the transcription of an articulation test, initial assessment results, and therapeutic changes, will partially or totally rely upon phonetic transcription. In other professions such as linguistics or teaching of English as a second language, these results will provide the foundation for analysis and further documentation. They may be sent to other professionals just as you will obtain

Reflect on This: Clinical Application

The written letters of the alphabet, singly or in combination, make up graphemes. A **grapheme** is a letter or combination of letters that supposedly represents a speech sound. However, clinically it is important that we separate graphemes from sounds. Here are some guidelines to remember when beginning to learn to transcribe (MacKay, 1987).

1. Keep the concepts *sounds* and *letters* separate. There are two sounds in "though" and six letters. When we are talking about the pronunciation of children's or adult's speech, use *sounds* not *letters*.

2. There is no "correct" pronunciation, but transcription should be based on what you hear, not how you think it should be pronounced. Within American English, the norm or typical pronunciation is referred to as **General American English** or **Standard American English**. However, often a pronunciation may reflect regional dialects, cultural dialects, or just pronunciation differences. For example, the author says the first vowel in "Denver," where she was born, similar to the vowel in "hit." Although preserved in certain areas of the country, many individuals do not differentiate between the vowel quality in "caught" and "cot."

3. Your knowledge of spelling should not distort your perception of speech sounds. Words with double letters such as "hammer" or "sitting" are not pronounced with two sounds, and there is not a [p] in the word "diphthong." The letters "ch" in "church" do not represent two sounds, and "sandwich" is typically not pronounced with a [d] before "wich."

4. What vowels and consonants a word contains are tallied according to the pronunciation and not the spelling. Be aware that different pronunciations, especially different from your own pronunciation, will need to be transcribed accordingly.

records from other sources. The ability to communicate with other professionals is the advantage of using the IPA and not another type of invented or devised system. Using the IPA, we can easily document how a client produces a particular sound. With one symbol (and maybe a diacritic), we can relay the production features that we observed and heard. In the following section, we will look a bit closer at how phonetic transcription is actually used in the assessment and treatment of speech disorders.

FOCUS 4: *Why is the orthographic letter system not a good possibility for phonetic transcription?*

How to Use Phonetic Transcription

This section will introduce the reader to some general guidelines that are important when transcribing the International Phonetic Alphabet. Examples will also be given as to how speech-language pathologists can use phonetic transcription in their assessment and intervention procedures. This is only an introduction to the basic concepts surrounding transcription; more in-depth explanations will be provided in the following chapters and in the transcription workbook. For example, each of the vowels and consonants of American English will be presented in detail within the next two chapters.

The first requirement for learning phonetic transcription is that we begin to think in terms of sounds and not letters. Each sound within a word is represented by a symbol of the IPA. That seems relatively easy but can get confusing quite quickly. In some words, there is a correspondence between the number of letters and sounds. For example, "it" has two letters and contains two sounds. However, there are words in which two letters represent only one sound. A word such as "seat" demonstrates this: Two letters, "ea," represent only one sound. Other words, such as "high" or "knee," have silent letters, while others are written with only one letter but contain two sounds. In the word "box," the letter "x" actually represents two sounds, "k" + "s." This will be explained in more detail, but it is important to begin thinking in terms of speech sounds and not alphabetic letters. First, phonetic transcription is the process of translating speech sounds into symbols contained within the IPA.

The second requirement necessitates learning which symbol represents which sound. For many of the sounds, the alphabetic letter and the IPA symbol will be the same. The first sound in "pipe" is /p/, and the last sound in "coat" is /t/, for example. However, there will be some sounds that are symbolized by new notations: The symbol /ʃ/ is the first sound in "ship" and "shop," in both cases represented by the letters "sh." The vowels become a bit more complicated and can be at first confusing. The first sound in "it" is represented by /ɪ/, while the first sound in "eat" is /i/. Second, phonetic transcription is translating specific sounds into the IPA symbols that represent these sounds. The transcription of the various vowels and consonants together with examples of words in which these sounds can be heard are contained in Table 3.1. This table shows the vowels and consonants that are commonly used in American English. Possible dialectal or general pronunciation variations are marked with an asterisk.

The third requirement is to listen carefully and try to avoid our auditory biases. In addition to receiving the incoming speech signal, we interpret the signal as well; this is perception. Our perceptions are based on our experience. That means that we sometimes unwillingly "distort" the perception of the incoming acoustic signal in the direction of our former experiences: in this case, how the listener would have produced the word or thinks the word should have been produced. This "built-in" tendency is one of the greatest dangers to any serious transcription effort. A high degree of transcription accuracy is difficult to attain if perceptual biases rule transcription efforts. It is important to listen to how the speech sound is actually produced, and try not to rely on preconceived expectations.

How do we use phonetic transcription as clinicians? Using phonetic transcription as a portion of our speech assessment procedures usually begins with an articulation test. Typically, a child is shown pictures that she or he can identify, whereas an adult may be given sentences or a short passage to read. Words are transcribed that contain sounds differing from those normally noted in General American English. These changes may be reflected in consonant or vowel productions; their differences are noted using symbols within the IPA. This requires that the clinician complete several tasks at the same time: first, administering the articulation test; second, listening to the production of the client; third, judging its production

According to the symbols of the International Phonetic Alphabet, "r" is officially transcribed as /ɹ/ or /ɻ/ (an upside-down "r" or an "r" with a tiny hook indicating the diacritic for retroflexed). The /r/ symbol is officially reserved for the alveolar trilled "r" sound, which occurs in Spanish, for example. Because trilled "r" sounds do not exist in General American English, and in order not to complicate matters unnecessarily, it is customary to use the /r/ symbol for both the bunched and retroflexed "r" sounds. This is further discussed in Chapter 5. However, students using this text should consult with their instructor as to how the "r" should be transcribed.

Table 3.1 IPA Symbols

Consonants		Vowels	
Symbol	Commonly realized in:	Symbol	Commonly realized in:
/p/	pay	/i/	eat
/b/	boy	/ɪ/	in
/t/	toy	/eɪ/	ape
/d/	doll	/ɛ/	egg
/k/	coat	/æ/	at
/g/	goat	/a/	father*
/m/	moon	/u/	moon
/n/	not	/ʊ/	wood
/ŋ/	sing	/oʊ/	boat
/θ/	think	/ɔ/	father*
/ð/	those	/ɑ/	hop
/f/	far	/aɪ/	tie
/v/	vase	/aʊ/	mouse
/s/	sun	/ɔɪ/	boy
/z/	zoo	/ɜ/	girl*
/ʃ/	shop	/ɝ/	bird
/ʒ/	beige	/ɚ/	winner
/h/	hop	/ʌ/	cut
/tʃ/	chop	/ə/	above
/dʒ/	job		
/j/	yes		
/w/	win		
/ʍ/	what*		
/l/	leap		
/r/	red		

Source: From Wise (1958).

*May be regional or individual pronunciations

Reflect on This: Clinical Application

PERCEPTUAL BIASES

In one beginning transcription class, the author was having the students transcribe the vowels of single-syllable words. The word given was "tan." After showing the transcription on the board, one of the students was very confused. Being a native from Pittsburgh, her pronunciation of "tan" rhymed with "men." Not being a native of Pittsburgh, the author's version of "tan" rhymed with "man." The student's perception of "tan" (based on her production) was clearly different than the author's.

Reflect on This: Clinical Application

Ann, a speech and drama major, is going to be in a production of a play that is staged in southeast England. The stage accent for this play will be British **received pronunciation**, which until fairly recently was considered to be the most "official" version of English spoken in the British Isles, commonly used by most announcers on radio and television (Roach, 2004; Wells, 1997). (A note: In the meantime received pronunciation "the cut-glass accent . . . is to be banished from the air waves by the BBC in favour of more energetic and vigorous voices from the regions" (*Guardian*, London, 27 January 1994).) To prepare for this part, Ann must examine the differences in pronunciation between her Midwest American and this English pronunciation. Ann does get a copy in phonetic transcription of some of the vowel and consonant differences. Here are several examples:

Vowels:

Instead of [ɑ] as in "shop" or "not," this is to be produced as [ɒ].

Instead of [aɪ] as in "science," this is to be replaced by [aə], thus [saəns].

Vowels such as "ire" in "fire," and "au" as in "power" should be replaced by [a], thus "fire" becomes [faə] and "power" [paə] (Wells, 1997).

Ann had a course in phonetic transcription but had to go back and look through her notes. She found that [ɒ] is similar to the American English vowel in "hot" but with lip rounding; the [a] vowel is similar to those "ah" vowels heard in New England dialects (technically a vowel that is produced with the tongue in a lower position than "a" as in "cat"); and the [ə] symbol represents the "uh" vowel, which is heard as the first vowel in "away." So words such as "power" and "fire" did not have the r-quality that is typically found in the Midwest. Ann's knowledge of phonetic transcription was very helpful. Ann's accuracy in depicting this accent would depend on her understanding of specific phonetic variations that occur in this British pronunciation.

accuracy; and fourth, if the production is in error, transcribing what was heard. This necessitates that clinicians be both competent and time-efficient transcribers.

FOCUS 5: *Which three guidelines are important to remember when learning phonetic transcription?*

Phonetic transcription is also used by speech-language pathologists when assessing individual words and spontaneous speech. Evaluating spontaneous speech is important, as clients may demonstrate a disparity between the results obtained from an articulation test, referred to as citation-form testing, and spontaneous speech. **Citation form** refers to the spoken form of a word produced in isolation, as distinguished from the form it would have when produced in conversational speech. Since single words are relatively easier to produce than connected speech, an individual's speech sound performance on a citation-form articulation test may be better than that noted in spontaneous conversation. Phonetic transcription will be used to document these differences.

Skills developed in phonetic transcription will also be an important aspect of the documentation of speech sound production throughout the intervention process. In each therapy session, we will be listening to and making judgments about the accuracy of these features. Accuracy of production is typically reported as a percentage: the number of times the client attempted the speech sound(s) versus the number of correct productions. There are several ways to report these measures. It may be as simple as making a plus for a correct response and a minus for a mismatch or more detailed, in which a portion of the therapy session is transcribed. These percentages will often be a determining factor when deciding to increase the difficulty of the task in therapy, for example, when moving from single-syllable words to more complex words or structured spontaneous speech. The increased accuracy of speech sound production will also be one way of documenting therapeutic effectiveness. Figure 3.9 is an example of a recording sheet that could be used to record production accuracy.

Case Study

CITATION-FORM ARTICULATION TEST VERSUS SPONTANEOUS SPEECH

Ben, age 6, had just completed the articulation test. He had been very shy at first, so we were happy that he had at least named the pictures of the test and we had a good sample of his citation-form abilities. Looking at his results, we noted that there were several consonant sounds in error; however, most of the sounds were later-developing sounds, and our prognosis was a fairly optimistic one. We were a bit surprised that his teacher had said that she was very concerned about his articulation skills. We decided to try to elicit some conversation. Knowing that he liked baseball, we had brought in some pictures of the Chicago Cubs, his favorite team. Ben immediately opened up and began to point to the various pictures and try to tell us about them. In spontaneous speech, his articulation skills were drastically reduced; we had a very hard time understanding any of what he was saying. This was a child that demonstrated an obvious difference between citation-form abilities and spontaneous speech.

Summary

FOCUS 1: *What three necessities must a phonetic notation system fulfill?*

The three necessities are accuracy, documentation, and communication. First, the system that we use must *accurately* preserve speech. If our system is not accurate, then our transcription is faulty from the beginning. Accu-

Client's Name_____ Therapist_____

Target Sound_____ Target Behavior_____

RESPONSE	1	2	3	4	5	6	7	8	9	10

EXAMPLE

DATE _1/10/08_

Client's Name _George M._   Therapist _Amy S._

Target Sound _r_   Target Behavior _w_

RESPONSE	1	2	3	4	5	6	7	8	9	10
run	r	r	r	r	r	r				
rug	r	r	r	r	r	r				
rough	r	r	r	r	r	r				
reach	w	w	w	w	w					
race	w	w	r	w	w					
red	w	w	w	r	r	r	r			
rub	r	r	r	r	r	r				
room	w	w	w	w	w					
row	w	w	r	r	w	w	w			
rock	r	r	r	r	r	r				

Figure 3.9 Recording Sheet for Charting Production Accuracy

racy implies that the notation system that we use must be broad enough to be practical yet detailed enough to allow fine distinctions between sound productions.

The second necessity our notation system must satisfy is one of *documentation*. Our notation system must be able to provide records that allow us to note the present speech status as well as changes that might occur if necessary. For example, as speech-language clinicians, we will need to document not only why we arrived at a clinical decision but treatment results as well. As teachers of English as a second language, we might need to document the progress the child has made in American English pronunciation. The notation system that we choose must allow us to document and provide records of the speech event.

The third necessity for our notation system is *communication*; the system must allow communication with other professionals. Other professionals must be able to readily identify and understand our record keeping. The system that we use must be one that is immediately recognized and can be interpreted by any other professionals within the United States or around the globe.

FOCUS 2: *What is the difference between phonetic and phonemic transcription?*

Phonetic transcription, or narrow transcription, entails the use of a phonetic categorization that includes as much production detail as possible. This detail encompasses the use of the broad classification system noted in the International Phonetic Alphabet as well as extra symbols that can be added to give a particular phonetic value. Phonemic transcription (or what can be called broad transcription) is a more general type of transcription. It is based on the phoneme system of a language and, therefore, is a notation system that notes vowel and consonant phonemes within a language.

FOCUS 3: *Which theoretical concepts form the basic premise for IPA notation?*

1. Some aspects of speech have linguistic relevance, i.e., phonemic value, while others, such as one's personal voice quality, do not.
2. Speech can be represented as a sequence of discrete sounds.
3. Sound segments can be divided into two major categories, consonants and vowels.
4. The phonetic description of sound segments can be referenced according to their production and auditory characteristics.
5. In addition to the sound segments, a number of "suprasegmental" aspects of speech need to be independently represented (International Phonetic Association, 1999).

FOCUS 4: *Why is the orthographic letter system not a good possibility for phonetic transcription?*

Although the English orthography system is considered to be an alphabetic system, it does not use a true one-to-one correspondence between distinctive speech sounds and letters of the alphabet. Examples of these problems include the following:

1. One sound is often represented by several different spellings.
2. The same letter can represent several different sounds.
3. Alphabetic notations are noted as having a one-symbol-to-one-sound correspondence. The use of digraphs in spelling violates this principle.

4. English spelling is not alphabetic, as we often use letters to represent no sound at all. These "silent" letters appear in many words.
5. Finally, there are sounds that are not represented by the spelling of English words. For example, the first sound in "use" is the same sound as in "yes"; there is no letter to represent this sound in these words.

FOCUS 5: *Which three guidelines are important to remember when learning phonetic transcription?*

The first requirement for learning phonetic transcription is that we begin to think in terms of sounds and not letters. Each sound within a word is represented by a symbol of the IPA.

The second requirement is learning which symbol represents which sound. For many of the sounds, the alphabetic letter and the IPA symbol will be the same. However, there will be some sounds that are symbolized by new notations: For example, the symbol /ʃ/ is the first sound in "ship" and "shop," in both cases represented by the letters "sh."

The third requirement is to listen carefully and try to avoid our auditory biases. In addition to receiving the incoming speech signal, we interpret the signal as well; this is perception. Our perceptions are based on our experience. That means that we sometimes unwillingly "distort" the perception of the incoming acoustic signal in the direction of our former experiences: in this case, how the listener would have produced the word or thinks the word should have been produced. This "built-in" tendency is one of the greatest dangers to any serious transcription effort.

Further Readings

Edwards, H. T. (2003). *Applied phonetics: The sounds of American English* (3rd ed.). Clifton Park, NY: Thomson Delmar Learning.
International Phonetic Association (1999). *Handbook of the International Phonetic Association: A guide to the use of the International Phonetic Alphabet.* Cambridge: Cambridge University Press.
Pagel-Paden, E. (1989). *Exercises in phonetic transcription: A programmed workbook.* New York: Elsevier Science and Technology Books.
Shriberg, L., & Kent, R. (2003). *Clinical phonetics* (3rd ed.). Boston: Allyn and Bacon.
Small, L. (2005). *Fundamentals of phonetics: A practical guide for students* (2nd ed.). Boston: Allyn and Bacon.

Key Terms

alphabetic systems p. 54
analphabetic systems p. 54
broad transcription p. 53
citation form p. 65
digraph p. 61
General American English p. 62
grapheme p. 62
International Phonetic Alphabet p. 52

narrow transcription p. 52
non-pulmonic sounds p. 56
phonemic transcription p. 52
phonetic notation p. 52
phonetic transcription p. 52
pulmonic sounds p. 56
received pronunciation p. 65
Standard American English p. 62

Think Critically

1. Write down how many sounds, not letters, are in the following words:

   though _____   clock _____

   judge _____   knowledge _____

   psychology _____   mislead _____

2. Write down a word that has 4 letters but only 3 sounds.

   _____

   Write down a word that has 5 letters but only 3 sounds.

   _____

   Write down a word that has 5 letters and 4 sounds.

   _____

3. In "keep," the vowel sound is spelled "ee." Find four other spellings that have the same vowel sound.

4. There are over ten different vowel sounds in American English. Can you find words that represent seven different vowel sounds of American English?

5. Why would you need a notation system to document disordered speech?

Test Yourself

1. Which one of the following is not a necessity when choosing a phonetic notation system?

   a. that it is an accurate system

   b. that it can be used with no previous training

   c. that it can be used for documentation

   d. that it can be used to communicate between professionals

2. If we wanted to transcribe as much detail as possible, we would use which type of notation system?

   a. analphabetic

   b. phonemic transcription

   c. phonetic transcription

   d. broad transcription

3. Broad transcription can also be called

   a. analphabetic transcription.

   b. phonemic transcription.

   c. phonetic transcription.

   d. citation-form transcription.

4. Orthographically, in the word "think," the "th" is considered a

   a. digraph.

   b. phoneme.

c. non-pulmonic letter.

d. one letter–one sound correspondence.

5. IPA is the label given to the

a. International Phonetic Association.

b. International Phonetic Alphabet.

c. all of the above.

d. none of the above.

6. Which one of the following exemplifies the fact that the English orthography system is not a good alphabetic system?

a. there are 3 sounds in "hat"

b. "sight" has 3 sounds

c. "tops" has 4 sounds

d. "so" has 2 sounds

7. Which one of the following is not important when learning how to transcribe?

a. one needs to think in terms of sounds, not letters

b. one needs to learn new symbols for some of the sounds

c. one needs to be careful about perceptual biases

d. one needs to know the correct pronunciation as noted in the dictionary

8. General American English is

a. the norm or typical pronunciation.

b. also called Standard American English.

c. not a description of "correct" pronunciation.

d. all of the above.

9. The International Phonetic Alphabet

a. attempts to describe all the speech sounds of all the languages of the world.

b. attempts to describe speech sounds according to their specific production features.

c. has diacritics that can be used to add special production characteristics to a specific sound.

d. all of the above.

10. The International Phonetic Alphabet is

a. a compromise between alphabetic and analphabetic systems.

b. a completely analphabetic system.

c. a citation-form system.

d. a grapheme system.

Answers: 1. b 2. c 3. b 4. a 5. c 6. b 7. d 8. d 9. d 10. a

For additional information, go to www.phonologicaldisorders.com

Articulatory Phonetics

PRODUCTION FEATURES OF VOWELS

Chapter Highlights

- What are the productional and functional differences between vowels and consonants?
- What are the three dimensions used to describe vowel articulation?
- What is meant by tense–lax, close–open, and long–short in relationship to vowels?
- What are the divisions for categorizing vowels according to the IPA?
- What are diphthongs, and how are they categorized?
- How are each of the vowels of American English described according to the horizontal and vertical planes of the tongue as well as lip rounding?

Chapter Application: Case Study

Lori is a bilingual teacher who was asked to teach an English class to adult speakers of Spanish. She had worked with children for two years in a transitional classroom and felt fairly comfortable with the job, but she had never worked with adult speakers of Spanish. The first night arrived, and she was greeted by fifteen adults, who were all eager to learn better English. With just a few exceptions, these were all adults who had good vocabularies, and their sentence structure appeared to be adequate. Their main complaint was their accent. They said that they often could not get better jobs because their Spanish accent was too pronounced. Lori was a little surprised. She had always worked with children on vocabulary and grammar, and it seemed as if they had learned English with hardly any accent. One thing that Lori noticed was the vowel quality of the speakers. She knew that Spanish had five basic vowels, but she was not sure about all the vowel variations in American English. She thought that she should go back and learn a bit more about the vowels of American English.

Speech sounds are typically divided into two major categories, vowels and consonants. This chapter discusses the first of these categories, the vowels of General American English. It is often a surprise to realize that there are far more vowels than just *a, e, i, o,* and *u* in American English. If we count the vowels that are commonly used and throw in two or three variations that might be heard in some parts of the United States, we arrive at anywhere between fifteen and nineteen different vowel sounds. That means that there are almost as many vowels as consonants in American English. Vowels are very important as speech sounds. Although consonants are often the main target in speech-language therapy, their role in learning English as a second language or linguistically analyzing vowels of other languages is essential. And with some children with phonological disorders, vowels may be distorted or their inventory of vowels might be greatly reduced.

We will find that, in most cases, vowels occupy the most prominent portion of the syllable. Thus, they are labeled the **nucleus** of the syllable. As syllable nuclei, vowels are louder than the other components of the syllable; they are more *intense* than the surrounding consonants. Their physical production features and their function within the language give vowels a central role in our study of phonetics and phonology.

The goal of this chapter is twofold. First, the factors that distinguish vowels from consonants will be addressed. Vowels and consonants not only differ in their speech sound *form,* they also *function* differently within a language. These characteristics will be discussed in the first part of the chapter. Second, the production features of American English vowels will be examined in detail. Vowel productions are typically categorized according to very specific parameters. These parameters will be introduced and applied to the vowels of American English. Clinical applications will be provided throughout the chapter.

Vowels Versus Consonants

In quick review, vowels are produced with a relatively open vocal tract; *no significant constriction* of the oral (and pharyngeal) cavities exists. The airstream from the vocal folds to the lips is relatively unimpeded. Therefore, vowels are considered to be *open sounds*. In contrast, consonants are produced with a *significant constriction* in the oral and/or pharyngeal cavities during their production. For consonants, the airstream from the vocal folds to the lips and nostrils encounters some type of obstacle along the way. Therefore, consonants are considered to be *constricted sounds*. For most consonants, this constriction occurs along the so-called sagittal midline of the vocal tract. The **sagittal midline** refers to the median plane that divides the body, or in this case the vocal tract, into right and left halves. This constriction for consonants can be exemplified by the first sound in "top," /t/, or "soap," /s/. For /t/, the contact of the front of the tongue with the alveolar ridge occurs along the sagittal midline, while the characteristic s-quality is made by air flowing along this median plane as the tongue approximates the alveolar ridge. In contrast, during all vowel productions, the sagittal midline remains free. In addition, under normal speech conditions, American English vowels are always produced with vocal fold vibration; they are voiced speech sounds. Only during whispered speech are vowels unvoiced. Consonants, on the other hand, may be generated with or without simultaneous vocal fold vibration; they can be voiced or voiceless. Pairs of sounds such as /t/ and /d/ exemplify this relevant feature. Pairs of similar sounds, in this case differing only in their voicing feature, are referred to as **cognates**; however, the term *cognate* can also be applied to similar vowels.

Vowels can also be distinguished from consonants according to the patterns of acoustic energy they display. Vowels are highly resonant, demonstrating at least two formant areas. Thus, vowels are more intense than most consonants; in other words, they are typically louder than consonants. In this respect, we can say that vowels have greater sonority than consonants. **Sonority** of a sound is its loudness relative to that of other sounds with the same length, stress, and pitch (Ladefoged, 2006).

The production features differentiating vowel and consonant form are summarized in Table 4.1.

There are also functional differences between vowels and consonants. In other words, vowels and consonants play different linguistic roles. The term *consonant* actually indicates this: *con* meaning "together with," and *-sonant* reflecting the tonal qualities that characterize vowels. Thus, consonants are those speech sounds that function linguistically *together with* vowels. As such, vowels serve as the center of syllables, as syllable nuclei. Vowels can constitute syllables all by themselves, for example, in the first syllable of the words "a-go" or "e-lope." Vowels can also appear together with one or more consonants, exemplified by "blue," "bloom," and "blooms." Although there are many different types of syllables, vowels are typically the center of the syllable, its nucleus. A notational system is often used to signify the sound syllable structure. V is used for a vowel sound, C for a consonant sound. The word "shop" has a CVC structure, while "off" has a VC structure. In both cases, the vowel is considered to be the nucleus of the syllable.

However, in certain circumstances, consonants can function as syllable nuclei. These consonants are labeled syllabics to indicate their role as the nucleus of the syllable. Syllabics are discussed in more detail in Chapter 7 (pages 220–221), and audio examples are provided in Module 11 of the accompanying phonetic workbook (pages 388–389).

FOCUS 1: *What are the productional and functional differences between vowels and consonants?*

Table 4.1 Production Features Differentiating Vowel and Consonant Form

Vowels	Consonants
No significant constriction of vocal tract	Significant constriction of the vocal tract
Open sounds	Constricted sounds
Sagittal midline of the vocal tract remains open	Constriction occurs along sagittal midline of vocal tract
Voiced	Voiced or unvoiced
Acoustically more intense	Acoustically less intense
Demonstrate more sonority	Demonstrate less sonority

American English Vowels

Vowel quality is determined by the shape and configuration of the vocal tract. Using the vowel in "<u>ea</u>t" as an example, if the vocal tract is adjusted so that the specific formant frequencies for this vowel are reinforced, then we will perceive an e-type sound. Obviously, the tongue plays a role in forming this quality. Compare where your tongue is for the vowel in "eat" versus the one in "at" and you will notice how it changes position. This change in tongue position affects the shape of the vocal tract and, thus, will impact the quality of the tone that is heard.

How does one describe these changes in tongue position for vowel productions? The articulation of vowels is more difficult to describe than the articulation of consonants. Due to their relative lack of constriction of the vocal tract, there is no contact or near contact between the articulators. Therefore, vowels and consonants have completely different systems for describing the production detail. With the wide articulatory channel, there is a comparatively large area within the oral cavity that allows for the tongue positioning when producing vowels. This vowel area (Ball & Rahilly, 1999) is shown in Figure 4.1. As one can see from this diagram, the vowel area is fairly large. Within this area, the tongue can move from a fairly high to a low position and from a front to a back position. If the tongue is raised above the upper front or back boundaries of the vowel area, the resulting sound will be a consonant (i.e., those consonants known as approximants or fricatives, which will be discussed in the next chapter).

Traditionally, phoneticians have described vowels in part by stating where the tongue is placed within the vowel area. Since the tongue is a rather large articulator, the highest point of the tongue is used first as a reference during the vowel production. Second, the position of the tongue is contrasted to other vowels, especially those vowel sounds that have similar articulations. The following vowel categorization is based on the work of Bauman-Waengler (2008), Garn-Nunn and Lynn (2004), Shriberg Kent (2003), and Small (2005). The system used by the International Phonetic Alphabet varies slightly from the one presented in this text and will be discussed in a later section.

During the vowel articulation, the highest point of the tongue is referenced according to the following dimensions:

1. *The tongue's position relative to the palate*, i.e., closer or further away from the palate, which provides the references of *high, mid*, and *low*. According to this dimension, vowels are high, indicating the tongue is fairly close to the palate, mid, further away from the palate, or low. The **high vowels** have the greatest degree of tongue elevation, while the **low vowels** have the least. Although no distinct boundary exists to distinguish the **mid vowels** relative to the other vowels, the tongue is located approximately midway between the highest and the lowest vowel articulation. The position of the mandible or lower jaw is also sometixmes described relative to specific vowel productions. However, whether the angle of the jaw is relatively open or closed follows from the tongue height relative to the palate. High vowels demonstrate a relatively closed jaw position, while low vowels have a relatively low or open jaw position.

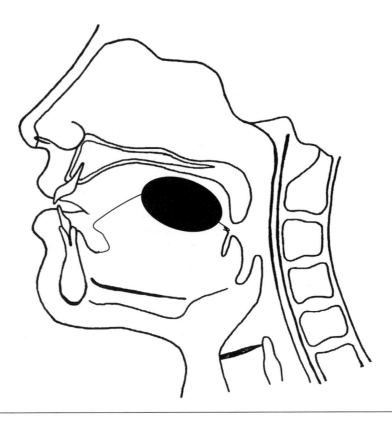

Figure 4.1   The Vowel Area

2. *The anterior/posterior dimensions of the tongue* provide the references of *front*, *central*, and *back*. Vowels are labeled front, central, and back representing the location of the hump or bulge of the tongue in a front-to-back dimension. For the **front vowels**, the most observable characteristic is the more forward location of this bulge in the tongue, while for the **back vowels**, the hump of the tongue is farther back, creating a narrowing in the upper pharynx. The **central vowels** are characterized by a centralized positioning of the hump of the tongue. When contrasted to the front or the back vowels, the central vowels have a more neutral tongue position.

A four-sided form called a vowel quadrilateral is often used to schematically demonstrate the front-back and high-low positions. The form roughly represents the tongue position in the oral cavity. See Figure 4.2 for a schematic drawing of the vowel quadrilateral.

Note in Figure 4.2 the labels along the horizontal axis: *front*, *central*, and *back*. These labels refer to where the bulge of the tongue is located, whether the hump of the tongue is more toward the front of the mouth, the central portion, or the back of the mouth. The vertical labels *high*, *mid*, and *low* refer to the *extent* to which the tongue is raised. The highest tongue position is relatively close to the palate, somewhat lowered is considered *mid*, and farther away from the palate would be a *low* tongue position. You can also see from Figure 4.2 that as you move from high to mid to low, the front axis of the quadrilateral is more slanted than the back. This again relates to articulatory properties. The front portion of the tongue is capable of a wider range of movement when compared to the relatively limited possibilities for the back of the tongue. The more slanted line at the front of the quadrilateral is a schematic attempt to indicate this.

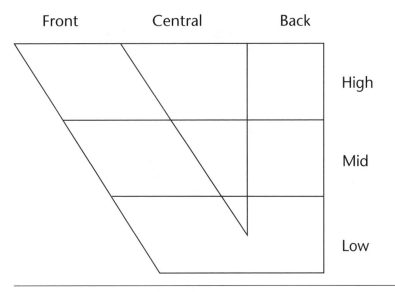

Figure 4.2 The Vowel Quadrilateral

Although these two dimensions will give you a fairly accurate description, one more categorization is necessary. This third dimension can be exemplified by noting the position of your lips when saying the vowels in "b<u>ea</u>t" versus "b<u>oo</u>t." You will find that the lips are not rounded for the first vowel sound but are rounded for the vowel in "boot." The lip shape also provides an adjustment to the vocal tract that will again impact the final vowel quality. Therefore, another dimension is used to describe the articulation of vowels:

3. The *degree of lip rounding or unrounding*: **Unrounded vowels** (which can also be labeled vowels with **lip spreading** or **lip retraction**) are produced either with the muscles of the lips quite inactive or neutral or with the contraction of specific muscles that draw back the corners of the lips. **Rounded vowels** are produced when the mouth opening is reduced by contraction of the muscles of the lips.

A fourth dimension, the position of the soft palate—raised for oral vowels and lowered for nasalized ones—is also used in vowel dsescriptions. However, since there are no nasalized vowels in American English that have phonemic value, this dimension is commonly omitted when describing these vowels.

 FOCUS 2: *What are the three dimensions used to describe vowel articulation?*

As we proceed to describe the vowels according to these parameters, it must be kept in mind that there are several inherent problems when using this system. Although vowel quality is affected by the configuration of the vocal tract, our identification of a particular vowel is ultimately tied to our perceptual judgment of its quality. That might sound relatively straightforward; we perceptually identify one vowel as being "ee," for example, and one as being "oo." However, there are no clear-cut divisions between vowel qualities. This can be easily demonstrated by prolonging the vowel "ee" then slowly moving your tongue to the first vowel sound in "is." Can you hear at which point the vowel is no longer "ee"? Is there a point at which the vowel you are producing sounds a little like both vowel qualities? Since perception is individually based, if you were to ask someone else at which point the vowel no longer sounded like "ee," a slightly different judgment might be made than yours. One problem in describing vowel articulation has to do with its perceptual basis and the fact that clear divisions do not exist between vowel qualities.

A second problem when trying to describe vowel articulation is the difficulty of trying to judge and describe tongue positions. Unlike with consonants, the characteristic vowel articulation does not demonstrate a point of contact or even a constriction within the vocal tract that could be used as a reference point. We must rely on rather imprecise descriptions that are fairly inadequate given the constant changes that occur in individual speakers and in varying speech contexts. The terms that are used should be seen simply as labels that describe how vowels are produced *relative to one another*. They are not, and cannot be, absolute descriptions of the tongue during vowel productions.

Figure 4.3 is a vowel quadrilateral with the individual vowel symbols listed according to the tongue's position relative to the palate (high–low dimensions) and where the bulge of the tongue is located (anterior–posterior dimensions).

There are several other ways to describe vowels. Vowels have been categorized according to the amount of muscular tension necessary to produce the vowel, the position of the body of the tongue relative to the palate, and the length of the vowel, for example. The next section will describe these concepts and relate them to the categorization of vowels according to the IPA.

Tense–Lax, Close–Open, Long—Short

Vowels may also be classified according to parameters other than those we have previously discussed. Several classification systems were based on the premise that certain vowels are similar in their articulation; variations in

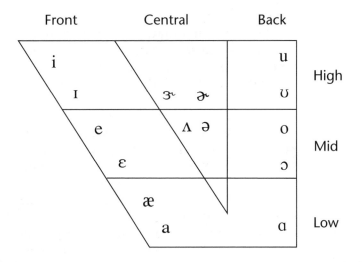

Vowel Symbol	Word Representing Vowel
/i/	heat
/ɪ/	hit
/e/	hate[1]
/ɛ/	head
/æ/	had
/a/	hot[2]
/u/	hoot
/ʊ/	hood
/o/	oat[1]
/ɔ/	hawed[2]
/ɑ/	hot
/ɝ/	heard
/ɚ/	fath<u>er</u>
/ʌ/	hut
/ə/	<u>a</u>way

[1]The given transcription represents these vowels as monophthongs. They are typically pronounced as diphthongs and would, therefore, have a slightly different transcription. See pages 84–87.

[2]Vowel sound may be dependent upon regional or individual pronunciations.

Figure 4.3 The Vowel Quadrilateral of the Vowels of General American English

production between these pairs of vowel cognates could be described relative to one specific dimension. Vowel oppositions such as those heard in the words h<u>ea</u>t–h<u>i</u>t, l<u>a</u>te–l<u>e</u>t, p<u>oo</u>l–p<u>u</u>ll, and c<u>oa</u>t–c<u>au</u>ght exemplify these vowel pairs.

First, the terms **tense vowels** and **lax vowels** have been used to describe variations in production (Heffner, 1975). *Tense* and *lax* indicate not only the tenseness and laxness of the tongue but of the entire articulatory mechanism (Sievers, 1901). However, other definitions exist for the tense and lax concept. For example, Shriberg and Kent (2003) and Garn-Nunn and Lynn (2004) state that the dimension of tenseness refers to the degree of muscular activity involved in the vowel articulation *and* the duration of the vowel. Thus, tense vowels have greater muscular activity and are longer in duration than lax vowels.

The second set of terms, **close vowels** and **open vowels**, refer to the vertical axis of vowel production. Thus, the terms *close* and *open* are defined according to the distance of the tongue from the palate. Close vowels are produced with the tongue closer to the palate while open vowels were articulated with the tongue farther away (Jones, 1932). The concept of close and open vowels was further developed to include four vowel positions. These four positions will be discussed in more detail in the next section, which examines how the International Phonetic Alphabet classifies vowels.

The last classification, long and short, represents the relative length of the vowel in question. Thus, **long vowels** were considered to be longer in duration than **short vowels**. Vowel duration is affected by several factors; however, the inherent length of some vowels appears to be longer than other vowels in similar contexts (Ladefoged, 2006). Therefore, the /i/ in "heed" is longer than /ɪ/ in "hid." Some authors (Shriberg & Kent, 2003; Small, 2005) relate the concepts long and short to the vowel's ability to function within the context of an open syllable. Thus, within one-syllable words, only long vowels can be present in open syllables (see, toe, new). While long vowels can be in closed syllables (heat, toad, moon), short vowels can only appear in closed syllables (hit, pet, put), not open syllables.

When we attempt to apply these classifications to the vowels of American English, certain guidelines should be kept in mind. First, all of these terms are relative. In this case, *relative* means that pairs of similar vowels should be compared under similar circumstances. When we look for similar vowel pairs, then we need to ask which two vowels are, for example, ee-type vowels or o-type vowels. (Note: For comparison purposes /e/ and /o/ are transcribed as single vowels in the following examples although they are typically pronounced as diphthongs. See page 85.) With this concept guiding our search, we will probably arrive at the following pairs:

ee-type vowels:	/i/ (e.g., "eat") and /ɪ/ (e.g., "it")
ay-type vowels:	/e/ (e.g., "mate") and /ɛ/ (e.g., "met")
oo-type vowels:	/u/ (e.g., "Luke") and /ʊ/ (e.g., "look")
ah-type vowels:	/o/ (e.g., "boat") and /ɔ/ (e.g., in some pronunciations of "bought")

Now comparing tense and lax of the vowel pairs becomes relatively easy. The first of the pair is tense, the second lax. Referring back to the vowel quadrilateral and comparing the tongue position relative to the palate for the pairs of vowels we will find that again, the first vowel of the pair is close, while the second one is relatively more open. By pronouncing each word of the pair listed above and listening to the vowel length, you should be able to hear that the first vowel in each pair is the long one, while the second is shorter in duration. However, it should be pointed out that there is some disagreement about whether /ɔ/ (the vowel in some pronunciations of "bought" or "law") is tense or lax. Some phoneticians call it a lax vowel (Chomsky & Halle, 1968; Heffner, 1975; Wise, 1957), while others have labeled it a tense one (Ladefoged, 2005; Shriberg & Kent, 2003). This goes back to the definition used to determine tense and lax and perhaps to

Although the concepts tense and lax were originally based on muscular tension, E. A. Meyer's (1910) experiments were probably the first to document that this is not always the case: Tense vowels do not necessarily demonstrate more muscular tension than lax ones. Later, Raphael and Bell-Berti (1975) reconfirmed this. The close–open distinction has also been questioned by several researchers (Ladefoged, DeClerk, Lindau, & Papcun, 1972; Meyer, 1910; Neary, 1978; Russell, 1928; Sweet, 1877). For example, Meyer (1910) reported that the vowel /ɪ/ is often articulated with the tongue closer to the palate than /e/. These findings suggest that the categorizations tense–lax, close–open, and long–short should be restricted to similar pairs of vowels. If this is done, the categorizations remain acceptable labels for vowels.

Concept Exercise **TENSE AND LAX**

To feel the difference between tense and lax vowels, place your first two fingers on your throat midway between the top of your larynx and your chin. Now pronounce /i/, the first vowel in "eat" and /ɪ/, the first vowel in "it." You should be able to feel more tension with /i/ while the throat should feel relatively more relaxed during the production of /ɪ/.

the vowel pairs that are compared. When you contrast /o/ to /ɔ/, it appears as if /ɔ/ would be considered lax. However, if /ɔ/ is compared to /ɑ/ (used in the typical Midwest pronunciation of "hot"), then the reverse seems to hold true—/ɔ/ feels tenser than /ɑ/. And if you are counting vowels, then you will find that /æ/, the vowel in "cat," is entirely left out of the discussion. On the whole, the labeling of the vowels with lower tongue positions seems to vary from source to source as to whether they are tense or lax. Wise (1957) wisely says that the difference in tension between vowels sharply distinguishes the high and mid vowels but "dwindles to negligibility with low vowels" (p. 61). Therefore, although some authors do summarize all the vowels of American English according to tense and lax, if you contrast pairs of vowels, the high and mid vowels lend themselves far easier to this classification. Table 4.2 lists the high and mid vowels of American English according to the dimensions tense–lax, close–open, and long–short.

FOCUS 3: *What is meant by tense–lax, close–open, and long–short in relationship to vowels?*

Table 4.2 High and Mid Vowels of General American English Categorized According to the Dimensions Tense–Lax, Close–Open, and Long–Short

Vowel Pairs	Word Example	Tense–Lax	Close–Open	Long–Short
/i/ vs. /ɪ/				
/i/	meet	tense	close	long
/ɪ/	mit	lax	open	short
/e/ vs. /ɛ/				
/e/	late	tense	close	long
/ɛ/	let	lax	open	short
/u/ vs. /ʊ/				
/u/	fool	tense	close	long
/ʊ/	full	lax	open	short
/o/ vs. /ɔ/				
/o/	coat	tense	close	long
/ɔ/	caught[1]	lax	open	short

[1]The production of this vowel in this word may depend on the pronunciation patterns or regional dialect of the speaker.

The International Phonetic Alphabet: A Different View of Vowel Categorization

Several sources (Abercrombie, 1967; Ball & Rahilly, 1999; International Phonetic Association, 1996) use a slightly different system for analyzing the vertical, up-and-down adjustments to the tongue during vowel articulation. Along the vertical plane, four degrees of tongue height are established: *close* (the tongue is closest to the roof of the mouth yet still within the vowel area), **close-mid, open-mid**, and *open* (the jaw is fully open, and so the tongue is low in the mouth). To establish these four degrees of tongue height, first, the tongue shape for the vowels that represent the highest and lowest vowels and those that are the most anterior versus posterior are plotted. Figure 4.4 illustrates this vowel area. In Figure 4.4, the outline of the tongue shape is noted for the four vowels that represent the extreme vowel positions: the tongue (1) high and toward the front of the mouth, /i/, (2) high and toward the back of the mouth, /u/, (3) low and toward the front, /a/, and 4) low and toward the back, /ɑ/.

Further reference vowels can now be defined: the two front vowels /e/ and /i/ and the two back vowels /ɔ/ and /o/ are placed between the extreme points so that the differences between each vowel and the next in the series are auditorily equal (International Phonetic Association, 1999). By definition, the use of auditory spacing means that the vowel descriptions are not based purely on articulation features. The terms *close, close-mid, open-mid,* and *open* can now be added to the quadrilateral representing equal points (as auditory and articulatory parameters) between the extreme vowel positions. Eight vowels are now added that correspond to each of these four divisions: four front vowels (one close, one close-mid, one open-mid, and one open) and four subsequent back vowels. This grid and the eight reference vowels are known as the **primary cardinal vowels**. In this sense, cardinal (= chief, fundamental, basic) refers to the points on

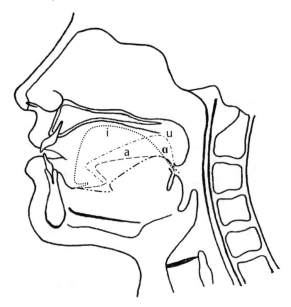

Figure 4.4 The Four Vowels of American English Representing the Extreme Vowel Positions

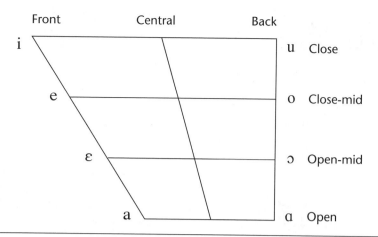

Figure 4.5   Vowel Quadrilateral with Cardinal Vowels

which the system hinges. This description of the primary cardinal vowels differs slightly from the original one proposed by Jones (1932), who first defined them. However, it is in agreement with those noted in the IPA (International Phonetic Association, 1996). Figure 4.5 is a schematic of the vowel quadrilateral with the eight cardinal vowels.

A second group of vowels, the **secondary cardinal vowels**, differ only in the lip rounding/unrounding when compared to their primary counterparts. Figure 4.6 is a vowel quadrilateral showing the vowels that are presented in the IPA chart. This includes the primary and secondary cardinal vowels as well as a few additional ones. In Figure 4.6, the vowel symbols that appear in pairs represent vowels that are articulated in a similar manner; however, the vowel on the right has lip rounding. Thus, /i/ and /y/ demonstrate comparable articulations; /y/ has lip rounding. (Thus, to produce /y/, hold the articulation of /i/ but now round your lips.)

FOCUS 4: *What are the divisions for categorizing vowels according to the IPA?*

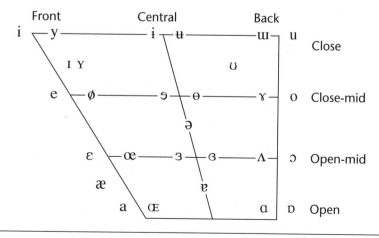

Figure 4.6   Vowel Quadrilateral with Primary Cardinal Vowels, Secondary Cardinal Vowels, and Other Vowels According to the IPA

Beginning Case Study

LORI, THE BILINGUAL TEACHER

Lori is trying to remember exactly about the vowels of Spanish. She knows that there is often a transfer between the speech sounds produced in the native language and the use of those sounds in the second language. Thus, there is a tendency to substitute similar speech sounds from the native language to the second language. After looking through her reference books, she finds that Spanish has five vowels. These five vowels are a portion of the cardinal vowel system and consist of /i/, /e/, /a/, /u/, and /o/. As Lori thinks about the vowels of American English, she is sure that there are far more vowels. This could be a portion of the vowel differences she is hearing in the speech of the Spanish adults. She would need to look in more depth at the vowels of American English and do some comparing.

Types of Vowels

This section will examine the different types of vowels of American English. First, there are two broad groupings: vowels that are considered monophthongs and those that are labeled as diphthongs. **Monophthongs** (*mono* = one, *phthong* = sound) are vowels that remain qualitatively the same throughout their entire production (Ladefoged, 2006). They are also called pure vowels (Abercrombie, 1967). On the other hand, **diphthongs** (*di* = two, *phthong* = sound) are vowels in which there is a change in quality during their production (Ladefoged, 2006).

Thus, diphthongs are composed of two distinct vowel elements; there is an audible change in vowel quality during their articulation. This is their distinction from the monophthongs, or pure vowels, in which the quality remains relatively constant.

There are several points of disagreement among phoneticians about the diphthongs. They disagree on (1) which sounds are actually labeled as diphthongs, (2) the exact IPA symbols that should be used to denote the various diphthongs, and (3) the notation that should be used to label the diphthongs. With this in mind, a system will be introduced that relies on the IPA symbols that were used in the *Handbook of the International Phonetic Association* (1999) and that reflect this author's pronunciation. The sounds that are labeled as diphthongs and their classification will be based on Shriberg and Kent (2003) and Bauman-Waengler (2008).

> The "ph" in both the words "monophthong" and "diphthong" is pronounced like the "ph" in "elephant," thus as [f]. Students will often pronounce it as a [p], which is incorrect.

Concept Exercise MONOPHTHONGS VERSUS DIPHTHONGS

You can hear the difference between a monophthong and a diphthong vowel if you slowly say the words "peep" and "pipe." The vowel quality in "peep" sounds the same throughout the production. It is considered a monophthong. The vowel in "pipe" is typically produced as a diphthong; there is a change in quality as the tongue glides from one articulatory position to another. Now try listening to the vowels as you say "moose" and "mouse." Which one is the diphthong?

Concept Exercise **ONGLIDE VERSUS OFFGLIDE**

The word "eye" consists of a diphthong in American English. Listen carefully as you prolong "eye" for 3 or 4 seconds. Do you notice that the vowel quality changes at the very end of the production? Now try the same type of prolongation with the exclamation "ow." Again, you will notice that the quality change occurs at the end of your production. For these two diphthongs in American English (and the others which will be introduced), the first portion, or onglide, is clearly longer and louder than the offglide.

Diphthongs may be classified according to several different parameters. First, the two vowel elements that compose the diphthong can be labeled. This results in an **onglide**, the first portion of the diphthong, and an **offglide**, which is the final portion. However, it is important to note that diphthongs are not two distinct vowels that are produced one after the other, but rather, there is a gliding transition from one vowel element to the next. Crystal (1987), for example, actually labels the diphthongs as vowel glides. In American English, during their production the onglide is more prominent; it is longer and more acoustically intense then the offglide (Ball & Rahilly, 1999; Garn-Nunn & Lynn, 2004; Shriberg & Kent, 2003).

Although two vowel symbols are used to represent diphthongs, they are considered to be one phonemic entity. Therefore, the words "boy," "pie," "cow," and "pay" all consist of two sounds: a consonant plus a diphthong. To denote this unity, several different types of transcriptions have been used (again a disagreement among phoneticians). For example, a connecting bar over the two vowel symbols /o͞ʊ/, a bow over the two vowel symbols /o͡ɪ/, or a bow below the two vowel symbols /ǫʊ/ can be seen in various texts. The author has chosen to use a common system that is used, for example, by Shriberg and Kent (2003). Thus, a bow will be placed over the two vowel symbols to exemplify their unity as a diphthong: /a͡ɪ/, for example. As mentioned earlier, there are various ways of transcribing the diphthongs. *Please check with your instructor to see which way he or she would like you to transcribe the diphthongs and which phonetic symbols should be used.* The following is offered as the system that will be used in this text:

Diphthong	*Words Commonly Pronounced with This Diphthong*
/e͡ɪ/	bake, ape, lane
/o͡ʊ/	boat, show, open
/a͡ɪ/	I, tie, line
/a͡ʊ/	house, out, shout
/ɔ͡ɪ/	boy, coil, point

Diphthongs are also categorized according to the type of articulatory movement from onglide to offglide. This categorization results in diphthongs being labeled *rising* or *falling*. A **rising diphthong** is one in which the gliding movement of the tongue moves from a lower to a higher articulatory position. If you think about the schematic of the vowel quadrilateral and draw a line from the onglide to the offglide portion of the diphthong, it would be a line that moves upward on the quadrilateral. A **falling diphthong** is one in which the gliding movement of the tongue moves from a higher to a lower articulatory position. Therefore, drawing a line from onglide to offglide on the vowel quadrilateral would result in

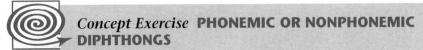

Try producing the following diphthongs in the given words first as a diphthong and then as a monophthong: in other words, articulating only the onglide. Which of the diphthongs are phonemic and which are nonphonemic?

Diphthong	Word with Diphthong	Contrast
/o͡ʊ/	boat	b [o͡ʊ] vs. b [o] t
/a͡ɪ/	file	f [a͡ɪ] l vs. f [a] l
/a͡ʊ/	gown	g [a͡ʊ] n vs. g [a] n

a downward-progressing line. If you try this with the five diphthongs that were just introduced, you will see that they are all rising diphthongs. This is shown in Figure 4.7.

Finally, diphthongs can be classified according to their linguistic function. This gives rise to the categorization of phonemic versus nonphonemic diphthongs. **Phonemic diphthongs** are those that have phoneme value; the production of these sounds as diphthongs (as opposed to their articulation as monophthongs) *can* change the meaning of a word. **Nonphonemic diphthongs** do not have phonemic value; the production of these sounds as diphthongs (as opposed to their articulation as monophthongs) *does not* change the meaning of a word. It is relatively easy to determine whether a diphthong is phonemic or nonphonemic. Could the meaning of the word change by reducing the diphthong to a monophthong? In other words, if *only the onglide portion of the diphthong is produced*, will that result in a word that we would recognize as a separate, distinctly different word? If we put this concept to the test with the diphthong /e͡ɪ/ (the vowel in "ate"), we arrive at the conclusion that /e͡ɪ/ is a nonphonemic diphthong. If the first sound in "ate" is produced as a monophthong [e] or as a diphthong /e͡ɪ/, the word will be identified in both cases as "ate." This diphthong does not have phonemic value. What about the diphthong /ɔ͡ɪ/ (the vowel in "coil")? Now, if we produce the first sound in "coil" as a diphthong /ɔ͡ɪ/ or

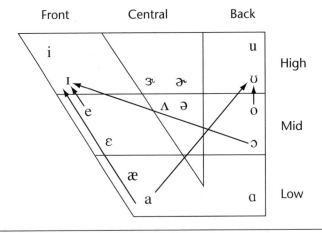

Figure 4.7 Vowel Quadrilateral with Rising Diphthongs

as a monophthong /ɔ/, we will find that it does change the meaning of the word from "coil" to "call." Therefore, /ɔɪ/ is a phonemic diphthong.

FOCUS 5: *What are diphthongs, and how are they categorized?*

The categories of monophthong and diphthong provide an easy way of classifying the vowels of American English. Let us begin with those vowels that are typically produced as monophthongs. For descriptive purposes, monophthongs are typically grouped into front, central, and back vowels. Typically, the order of the description for vowels is (1) the vowel articulation according to the vertical tongue dimension (high, mid, or low), (2) the vowel articulation according to the horizontal tongue dimension (front, central, or back), and (3) the degree of lip rounding or unrounding. For each of the vowels, the symbol noted in IPA will be introduced, a description will be given, and words that usually are pronounced with this vowel sound will be provided. In addition, the description according to the IPA Chart (page 55) will be added. Dialectal variations will also be noted.

Front Vowels

/i/

This is a vowel that is typically heard in the words "meet" or "eat." It is a high-front vowel. Therefore, the highest bulge of the tongue is relatively close to the palate and more forward in the mouth. The lips are unrounded when producing this vowel. If this vowel is produced in isolation, the lips are actually spread. Due to the high position of the tongue hump, the mandible is elevated.

/i/ = high-front, unrounded (spread) vowel

IPA description: Close, front vowel

Word examples: heat, eager, pea, she, keep

Dialectal variations (Vaux, 2005): In some words, /i/ and /ɪ/ can and are often interchanged. For example, the vowel in "been," the vowel in the second syllable of "cauliflower," the vowel in "creek," the last vowel in "handkerchief," the first vowel in "really," and the first vowel in "syrup" demonstrate this variation.

/ɪ/

This vowel is typically heard in the words "it" and "lip." It is considered a high-front vowel although the tongue position is not as high and as far forward as the production of /i/. If you say the vowel in "eat" and then the one in "it" you will notice that the tongue hump drops slightly. The lips are unrounded, perhaps even slightly spread for the production of this vowel. The mandible is elevated.

/ɪ/ = high-front, unrounded (spread) vowel

IPA description: Close, front vowel that is located midway between /i/ and /e/

Word examples: it, if, mit, kitten, big

Dialectal variations: See notes from /i/.

/e/ → For /e/, the tongue hump position has dropped to a mid-front position relative to /i/ and /ɪ/. For example, try producing the vowel in "it" and then the very first portion of the vowel in "ate." You should feel that the tongue hump moves farther away from the palate for "ate." The mandible is typically in a mid-open position, and the lips are unrounded. This vowel occurs typically as a diphthong in American English in words such as "day" and "train"; therefore, it will be covered in the section on diphthongs as well.

/e/ = mid-front, unrounded (spread) vowel

IPA description: Close-mid, front vowel

Since this vowel is commonly produced as a diphthong, word examples will be given in that section.

/ɛ/ → This vowel is typically heard in pronunciations of "red" and "bend." While still forward in the mouth, the bulge of the tongue has dropped to a lower mid-front position. The drop in the tongue position also affects the mandible, which is usually in a mid-open position during the production of this vowel. The lips are unrounded for /ɛ/.

/ɛ/ = mid-front, unrounded (spread) vowel

IPA description: Open-mid, front vowel

Word examples: end, effort, test, shed, rent

Dialectal variations (Vaux, 2005): The vowels /ɛ/ and /ɪ/ are often interchanged. This may be a portion of the one of the vowel shifts that is seen in the United States (see Chapter 6 on dialect). For example, the word "pen" may be pronounced as [pɪn] or "pencil" as [pɪnsəl]. Also noted in the Harvard survey (Vaux, 2005), the first vowel in "miracle" may be pronounced as [i], or [ɪ], or [ɛ].

/æ/ → This vowel is often heard in pronunciations of "cat" and "sand." When comparing productions of [ɛ] to [æ], you will find that the bulge of the tongue for [æ] drops still farther away from the palate. [æ] is considered a low-front vowel. The mandible is in a relatively open position for this vowel, and the lips are unrounded.

/æ/ = low-front, unrounded (spread) vowel

IPA description: Open-mid, front vowel that is located midway between /ɛ/ and /a/

Word examples: at, after, glad, sack, shadow

Dialectal variations (Vaux, 2005): This vowel may be used in variation with /ɑ/, for example, in the second vowel in "pajamas" or the vowel in the word "aunt."

/a/ → This vowel is not necessarily pronounced by every speaker of American English. Its use seems to vary depending on the region of the country you are in and the individual speaker's idiosyncrasies. However, the onglide portion of certain diphthongs can be pronounced with [a]; therefore, it will be discussed in the section on diphthongs as well. /a/ is considered a low-front vowel or, according to the IPA (2005), an open, front vowel: The tongue hump is farther from the palate than for the /æ/ vowel. For its production, the mandible is in a relatively open position, and the lips are unrounded.

/a/ = low-front, unrounded (spread) vowel

IPA description: Open, front vowel

Word examples: Depending upon the dialect, it can be heard in words such as r<u>a</u>ther, <u>a</u>sk, st<u>o</u>p, or l<u>o</u>ck.

Dialectal variations: In the New England dialect of the Northeast or in upstate New York, one might hear words such as "hot" and "farm" pronounced with [a] (Thomas, 1958).

See Figure 4.8 for a schematic of the tongue height of the front vowels.

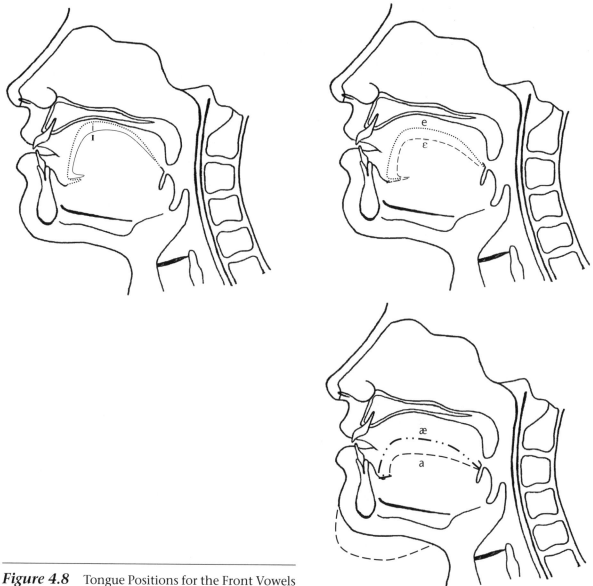

Figure 4.8 Tongue Positions for the Front Vowels

Reflect on This: Clinical Application

FRONT VOWELS—A DEVELOPMENTAL PERSPECTIVE

Several investigations (e.g., Davis & MacNeilage, 1990; Irwin, 1946; Irwin, 1948; Irwin & Chen, 1946; Kent & Bauer, 1985) found that front vowels predominated the vocalizations of very young babies, the babbling of infants, and the first words of children around 1 year of age. They noted a gradual decline in the percentage of front vowels after that time, with an increase in the relative proportion of back vowels.

Back Vowels

/u/

This vowel is often pronounced in "soup" or "tooth." It is a high-back vowel; the tongue's highest bulge is toward the back of the oral cavity and relatively close to the palate. The mandible is in a relatively closed position, and the lips are rounded.

/u/ = high-back, rounded vowel

IPA description: Close, back vowel

Word examples: s<u>oo</u>n, sh<u>oe</u>, b<u>oo</u>t, gl<u>ue</u>, fl<u>u</u>

Dialectal variations: The vowel in words such as "r<u>oo</u>f," "r<u>oo</u>m," "br<u>oo</u>m," and "r<u>oo</u>t" may be pronounced with [u] or [ʊ]. Also the vowel in "r<u>ou</u>te" may be pronounced as [u] or as the diphthong [a͡ʊ].

/ʊ/

This vowel can be heard in words such as "wood" or "should." It is considered a high-back vowel although the tongue hump has dropped when /ʊ/ is compared to /u/. The mandible is still relatively closed when producing this vowel, and the lips are rounded. However, if the lip rounding is contrasted between /u/ and /ʊ/, you will notice less lip rounding for /ʊ/.

/ʊ/ = high-back, rounded vowel

IPA description: Close, back vowel that is located midway between /u/ and /o/

Word examples: l<u>oo</u>k, p<u>u</u>ll, c<u>ou</u>ld, f<u>oo</u>t, st<u>oo</u>d

Dialectal variations: See those noted above with /u/.

/o/

This vowel is typically pronounced as a diphthong in American English and is treated in that section. However, it could be heard in words such as "boat," "soap," and "potat<u>o</u>." The bulge in the tongue is somewhat lower than for the /ʊ/ vowel; therefore, /o/ is considered to be a mid-back vowel. Lip rounding is present during the production of this vowel, and the mandible is usually in a mid-open position.

/o/ = mid-back rounded vowel

IPA description: Close-mid, back vowel with lip rounding

Word examples: Typically produced as a diphthong but could be heard as a monophthong in unstressed syllables such as "to'mat_o_" or "n_o_'bility."

/ɔ/ → Use of this vowel may be dependent upon regional dialect or on individual variations of a particular speaker. Some speakers differentiate between the pronunciations of "caught" and "cot," using [ɔ] in the first word and [ɑ] in "cot." These variations are a portion of an ongoing vowel merger that is occurring within several United States dialects. As a result of this merger in some parts of the United States, the distinctions between [ɔ] and [ɑ] are eliminated, with the result that [ɑ] is now consistently being used for both variations. This is discussed in detail in Chapter 6. However, this vowel can frequently be heard as the onglide of the diphthong in words such as "boy" or "coin." This vowel is a mid-back vowel. In comparison to /o/, the highest bulge in the tongue has moved farther from the palate. Lip rounding is present during the production of this vowel, and the mandible is in a mid-open position.

/ɔ/ = mid-back, rounded vowel

IPA description: Open-mid, back vowel

Word examples: Production of this vowel is highly dependent upon the speaker. It may be heard in l_aw_, f_a_ther, b_ou_ght, br_ou_ght, and t_au_ght.

Dialectal variations: Distinctions may be made between "cot" [kɑt] and "caught" [kɔt], for example. Also the first vowel in "Florida" may be pronounced as [o] or [ɔ].

/ɑ/ → This vowel can often be heard in words such as "hot" and "clock." It is a low-back vowel. The tongue's highest position has dropped; it is located a considerable distance from the palate, creating a vocal tract that is clearly open. The lips are unrounded (a differentiation that can clearly distinguish /ɑ/ from /ɔ/), and the mandible is in an open position. Use of this vowel varies according to the dialect and the speaker. However, it is a common vowel in the Midwest.

/ɑ/ = low-back, unrounded (spread) vowel

IPA description: Open, back vowel

Word examples: s_o_ck, st_o_p, kn_o_t, sh_o_p, t_o_ss

Dialectal variations: See notes above for /ɔ/.

/ɒ/ → The use of this vowel also depends on the speaker and the context. It is a low-front vowel very similar to /ɑ/ but with lip rounding. Heffner (1975) states that /ɒ/ is produced with a more retracted tongue than /ɑ/. In American English, the three vowels /ɑ/, /a/, and /ɒ/ are all allophonic variations of an ah-type vowel. In other words, one can interchange these vowels: They do not have phonemic value and, thus, do not create a difference in meaning. The lips are rounded, and the mandible is in an open position.

Use of this vowel varies according to the dialect and the speaker: however, it is heard in received pronunciation of British English.

/ɒ/ = low-back, rounded vowel

IPA description: Open, back vowel. It is distinct from /ɑ/ due to the lip rounding.

Word examples: s<u>o</u>ck, st<u>o</u>p, kn<u>o</u>t, sh<u>o</u>p, t<u>o</u>ss

Dialectal variations (Vaux, 2005): /ɒ/ may be used as the first vowel in "lawyer" as opposed to the often utilized diphthong /ɔɪ/. It is also a variation for the vowel in "caught" [kɒt].

See Figure 4.9 for a schematic of the tongue position for several of the back vowels.

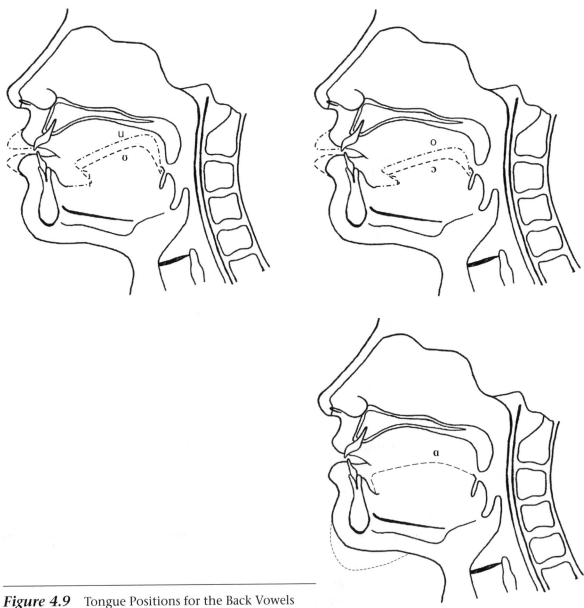

Figure 4.9 Tongue Positions for the Back Vowels

Reflect on This: Clinical Application

DO CHILDREN HAVE DIFFICULTIES PRODUCING VOWELS?

Vowel errors in children who are developing their sound systems in a normal manner are relatively uncommon. However, children with disordered articulation and/or phonology may show vowel difficulties. These difficulties seem to be basically of two types (Hargrove, 1982; Ingram, 1981; Khan, 1988; Leonard & Leonard, 1985; Pollock & Swanson, 1986; Stoel-Gammon & Herrington, 1990). First, the child may show a greatly reduced inventory of vowels. Therefore, the number of different vowels is far less than the inventory typical for American English. Second, the child may show vowel substitutions. In this case, the child replaces the vowel that is normally articulated in a word with a completely different vowel. Assessment of vowel quality should be a portion of every diagnostic protocol.

Central Vowels

/ɝ/ →

This vowel can often be heard in words such as "bird" and "sir." It is considered a mid-central vowel with r-coloring. Therefore, on the high-low dimension, these vowels are characterized by a tongue hump that is approximately halfway between the articulation of the high vowels, /i/ or /u/, for example, and the low vowels, /ɑ/ or /a/. On the front-back dimension, the tongue's highest position is again centrally located, neither too far forward nor back. There is considerable variation in the production of this vowel. First, there appear to be two variations of normal articulation. One variation, a so-called bunched production, results when the tongue body is retracted with a bulging of the tongue in its mid-portion. During this articulation, the front portion of the tongue is in a low, relatively flat position. The second type of /ɝ/ is labeled a retroflex in that the tip of the tongue curls back so that the underside is located under the front portion of the palate. There is typically some degree of lip rounding during the production of /ɝ/; however, this may vary from speaker to speaker and be dependent upon the context. There are two other features of this vowel that are important. First, /ɝ/ is considered a central vowel with **r-coloring.** Thus, this vowel has perceptual qualities that are similar to the r-sound, the first sound in "run" or "red." Second, this vowel is a stressed vowel. As such, its production is marked by more intensity, typically a somewhat higher fundamental frequency, and a longer duration when it is compared to a similar unstressed vowel (such as the following vowel to be discussed /ɚ/).

/ɝ/ = mid-central, rounded vowel with r-coloring

IPA description: Open-mid rounded central vowel with rhoticity. The /˞/ symbol attached to the /ɝ/ is the diacritic for rhoticity, or r-coloring. Therefore, the vowel on the IPA chart is actually the /ɜ/ vowel.

Word examples: w<u>or</u>d, p<u>ur</u>r, sh<u>ir</u>t, c<u>ur</u>b, f<u>er</u>n

Dialectal variations (Vaux, 2005): The vowel /ɜ/ is a dialectal variation of /ɝ/, which can be heard in New England or in some regions of the Southern United States. While similar in articulation to /ɝ/, this vowel does not have r-coloring due to a lower central position of the tongue (for the bunched production) or not as much tongue retroflexion (in the retroflexed articulation) (Ball & Rahilly, 1999). In these dialects, this loss of r-coloring may also occur for /ɚ/, resulting in /ə/.

/ɚ/ ➡ This vowel can often be heard as the final vowel in words such as "fath*er*" or "wond*er*." /ɚ/ is a mid-central vowel with r-coloring. Its articulation is similar to /ɝ/; however, the IPA designates /ɚ/ as a separate vowel with a tongue position that is slightly higher than /ɝ/. However, similar to /ɝ/, two production variations are possible, a bunched [ɚ] characterized by a retraction and a central bulging of the tongue hump and a retroflexed version in which the tongue tip is curled back. The notable difference between these two central vowels with r-coloring is that /ɚ/ is an unstressed vowel. As such, it is shorter in duration, not as intense, and typically has a lower fundamental frequency than [ɝ]. To note these differences, say the word "fu*rther*." The first vowel in this word is [ɝ], the second one [ɚ]. If the two vowels are compared, you can probably hear that the first vowel is longer, louder, and has a somewhat higher pitch than the second [ɚ] vowel. Due to its unstressed nature, /ɚ/ is typically unrounded, and the r-coloring may be described as being somewhat less than for /ɝ/ (Carrell & Tiffany, 1960). This vowel is often called the *schwar* vowel (schwa + r). See the explanation under /ə/.

/ɚ/ = mid-central, unrounded vowel with r-coloring

IPA description: Close-mid, central vowel with rhoticity, /ɚ/ is located midway between the close-mid, central vowel /ə/ and the open-mid, central vowel /ɜ/

Word examples: rath*er*, harb*or*, murm*ur*, bett*er*, strang*er*

Dialectal variations: Similar to those noted in /ɝ/.

/ʌ/ ➡ This vowel is typically heard in the words "nut" and "sun." It is a mid-central vowel that does not have r-coloring. Although several authors state that this vowel has a somewhat lower tongue position than the other central vowels (Carrell & Tiffany, 1960; Shriberg & Kent, 2003), some authors state that the tongue assumes a position very similar to [ɔ] but without the lip rounding (Heffner, 1975; IPA, 2005). See Figure 4.6 for the IPA's vowel quadrilateral with /ʌ/ located to the left of /ɔ/. These differences probably reflect the somewhat variable production possibilities of this vowel as well as dialectal variations in its realization. /ʌ/ is a stressed vowel. Its unstressed counterpart is the next vowel that will be discussed.

/ʌ/ = mid-central, unrounded vowel

IPA description: Open-mid, back vowel that is unrounded

Word examples: *u*nder, *u*p, l*u*ck, m*u*d, c*u*t

Dialectal variations (Vaux, 2005): This vowel may replace /ɝ/ in a word such as "flourish," thus [flʌ rɪʃ]. This has been noted in some sections of the East and the Southern states.

 /ə/

This vowel is typically heard as the first sound in the unstressed syllables of the words "ago" and "away." It is a mid-central vowel without r-coloring. The lips are unrounded during its production. X-ray tracings from Shriberg and Kent (2003) denote the tongue position to be somewhat higher during the articulation of [ə] when compared to [ʌ]. This is supported by the vowel quadrilateral from the IPA. As an unstressed vowel, its duration is relatively short. In multisyllabic words, the vowels in unstressed syllables are often produced as [ə]. This vowel is also called the schwa vowel. The word *schwa* comes from the Hebrew "shewa" meaning nothing, no vowel, designating a short vowel with an indistinct quality.

/ə/ = mid-central, unrounded vowel

IPA description: Close-mid, central vowel, /ə/ is located midway between the close-mid, central vowel /ə/ and the open-mid, central vowel /ɜ/.

Word examples: <u>a</u>round, <u>a</u>bove, <u>u</u>pon, Germ<u>a</u>n, judg<u>e</u>s

See Figure 4.10 for a schematic of the tongue position for the central vowels /ɝ/ and /ʌ/ and Table 4.3 for a summary of the production features of the American English vowels.

FOCUS 6: *How are each of the vowels of American English described according to the horizontal and vertical planes of the tongue as well as lip rounding?*

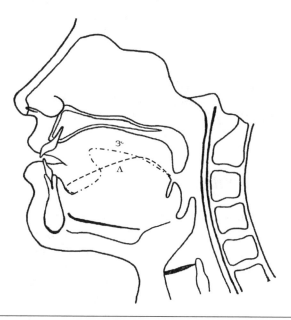

Figure 4.10 Tongue Positions for the Central Vowels

Table 4.3 Summary of the American English Vowels

Type	Vertical Up-Down Plane	Horizontal Front-Back Plane	Lip Position
Front			
/i/	high	front	unrounded
/ɪ/	high	front	unrounded
/e/	mid	front	unrounded
/ɛ/	mid	front	unrounded
/æ/	low	front	unrounded
/a/	low	front	unrounded
Back vowels			
/u/	high	back	rounded
/ʊ/	high	back	rounded
/o/	mid	back	rounded
/ɔ/	mid	back	rounded
/ɒ/	low	back	rounded
/ɑ/	low	back	unrounded
Central vowels			
/ɝ/	mid	central	rounded; r-coloring
/ɚ/	mid	central	unrounded; r-coloring
/ʌ/	mid	central	unrounded
/ə/	mid	central	unrounded

Reflect on This: Clinical Application

THE PROBLEM WITH CENTRAL VOWELS WITH R-COLORING

Central vowels with r-coloring are often produced in error by children with "r-problems." Children with r-problems often substitute "w" for "r" as in "wabbit" for "rabbit" or "wed" for "red." In addition, these difficulties with the r-quality extend to the vowels of American English that also demonstrate r-coloring. These children may produce the central vowels [ɝ] as [ɜ] and [ɚ] as [ə]. There are many articulatory similarities between the central vowels with r-coloring and r-consonants. Children with r-problems cannot achieve the necessary production features that signal this r-quality in both vowels and consonants.

Diphthongs

The following common diphthongs in General American English are categorized according to their (1) onglide and offglide vowels, (2) the type of articulatory movement, rising versus falling, and (3) the linguistic function, whether they are phonemic or nonphonemic diphthongs. Examples of words that are typically produced with the diphthong are also given.

 /eɪ/

For the onglide portion of this diphthong, /e/, the tongue hump has dropped to a mid-front position relative to /i/ and /ɪ/. For example, try producing the vowel in "it" and then the very first portion of the vowel in "ate." You should feel that the highest bulge of the tongue moves farther away from the palate for the onglide of "ate." The mandible is typically in a mid-open position, and the lips are unrounded. It should be noted that the diphthong /eɪ/ occurs most commonly in heavily stressed syllables and may be reduced to a monophthong /e/ in unstressed syllables (Shriberg & Kent, 2003).

/eɪ/ = onglide: mid-front, unrounded (spread) vowel;
offglide: high- front, unrounded (spread) vowel

Type of articulatory movement: rising

Linguistic function: Nonphonemic

Word examples: g<u>a</u>ze, h<u>ay</u>, sh<u>a</u>ke, <u>a</u>ble, m<u>ay</u>be

/oʊ/

For the onglide portion of this diphthong, /o/, is considered to be a mid-back vowel. Lip rounding is present during the production of this vowel, and the mandible is usually in a mid-open position. The offglide portion of this diphthong, /ʊ/, is a high-back vowel with lip rounding. It should be noted that the diphthong /oʊ/ occurs most commonly in heavily stressed syllables and may be reduced to a monophthong /o/ in unstressed syllables (Shriberg & Kent, 2003).

/oʊ/ = onglide: mid-back, rounded vowel;
offglide: high-back, rounded vowel

Type of articulatory movement: Rising

Linguistic function: Nonphonemic

Word examples: <u>oa</u>k, <u>ow</u>n, t<u>oa</u>d, <u>oa</u>tmeal, h<u>o</u>tel

/aɪ/

The onglide of this diphthong, [a], was discussed under front vowels; it is a low-front vowel that is unrounded. The onglide of this vowel may be produced as /ɑ/, depending on the regional dialect of the speaker. In this case, the onglide is a low, back unrounded vowel. The offglide /ɪ/ was also introduced in the section on front vowels. It is high-front vowel that is unrounded.

/aɪ/ = onglide: low-front, unrounded (spread) vowel;
offglide: high-front, unrounded (spread) vowel

Type of articulatory movement: Rising

Linguistic function: Phonemic

Word examples: <u>i</u>ce, sh<u>y</u>, m<u>i</u>ne, t<u>i</u>ger, ps<u>y</u>chic

Dialectal variations: The onglide [a] may be pronounced as [ɑ] in the Midwest and in New York state (Shriberg & Kent, 2003; Thomas, 1958). In the South, /aɪ/ is frequently reduced to /a:/ (Thomas, 1958).

/aʊ/

The onglide of this diphthong, /a/, is a low-front vowel that is unrounded. The onglide of this vowel may be produced as [ɑ], depending on the regional dialect of the speaker. The offglide of this diphthong, /ʊ/, is a high-back vowel with lip rounding.

/aʊ/ = onglide: low-front, unrounded (spread) vowel; offglide: high-back, rounded vowel

Type of articulatory movement: Rising

Linguistic function: Phonemic

Word examples: <u>ow</u>l, c<u>ow</u>, f<u>ou</u>nd, v<u>ow</u>el, ch<u>ow</u>der

Dialectal variations: The onglide /a/ may be pronounced as [ɑ] in the Midwest and Western Pennsylvania areas (Shriberg & Kent, 2003; Thomas, 1958). In the Eastern New England, New York City, and Mid-Atlantic areas, the /a/ as onglide is typically maintained (Thomas, 1958). A variant [æʊ] may be heard in eastern New England, New York City, and Mid-Atlantic and lowland Southern areas (Thomas, 1958).

/ɔɪ/ The onglide of this diphthong, /ɔ/, is a mid-back vowel with lip rounding, while the offglide of this diphthong, /ɪ/, is a high-front vowel that is unrounded.

/ɔɪ/ = onglide: mid-back, rounded vowel; offglide: high-front, unrounded (spread) vowel

Type of articulatory movement: Rising

Linguistic function: Phonemic

Word examples: ch<u>oi</u>ce, j<u>oi</u>n, t<u>oy</u>, m<u>oi</u>sture, l<u>oy</u>al

Dialectal variations: In the Mid-Atlantic areas, /ɔɪ/ is often changed to /oʊ/. In the lowland South, the /ɔɪ/ remains stable in the word-final position, such as in the word "boy" but is reduced to [ɔ:] before consonants. Thus, "boil" may be pronounced [bɔ:l] (Thomas, 1958).

Reflect on This: Clinical Application

VOWEL THERAPY

Clients from other countries who might be interested in accent reduction will often demonstrate vowels that are productionally different than those commonly noted in General American English. This can be a reflection of the vowel system of their native language. For example, the Japanese and Spanish vowel systems have only five vowels: /i/, /e/, /o/, /u/, and /a/. (To be more accurate, the Japanese /u/ vowel is unrounded; therefore, the IPA symbol would be /ɯ/). Therefore, to learn American English, several additional vowel qualities must be acquired as well as diphthongs and the central vowels with r-coloring. In addition, these speakers often have difficulty with the lengths of the vowels, producing longer vowels too short or shorter vowels too long. Our knowledge of the production features of the vowels of American English will be invaluable with these clients.

CENTERING DIPHTHONGS. **Centering diphthongs** are those diphthongs in which the offglide consists of a central vowel. In British English and in some dialects of American English, this may be a schwa vowel, /ə/. Thus, "far" would be pronounced as [fɑə] or [faə]. In this case, the onglide of the diphthong is /ɑ/ or /a/, while the schwa vowel represents the offglide. These are diphthongs with the same characteristics as the previously noted diphthongs; the onglide is acoustically louder and usually longer, while the offglide is typically not as loud and shorter. However, as diphthongs, both the onglide and offglide function as a single unity; a centering diphthong represents one vowel. There are also *centering diphthongs*, in which the offglide represents a central vowel with r-coloring. A better name for them perhaps is **rhotic diphthongs** (Lowe, 1994). Thus, the vowel nuclei in "cart," "barn," and "care" are all rhotic diphthongs. These rhotic diphthongs can be transcribed in two basic ways, as the vowel (as onglide) + /ɚ/ (as offglide) or the vowel (as onglide) + /r/ as the offglide. Thus, "cart" could be transcribed as [kɑɚt] or [kɑrt], "barn" as [bɑɚn] or [bɑrn], and "care" as [kɛɚ] or [kɛr]. The author has chosen the first transcription to use throughout this text to eliminate any confusion that the vowel + r-symbol could create. For example, Blockcolsky, Frazer, and Frazer (1987), in their book *40,000 Selected Words*, (an excellent source of single- and multisyllabic words ordered according to sound and sound combinations of American English), state that a word such as "cart" or "barn" has a final consonant cluster of /r/ + /t/ or /r/ + /n/ respectively. This is really not the case; it is not a consonant cluster but rather a rhotic diphthong consisting of a vowel plus a central vowel with r-coloring. However, *check with your instructor to see how he or she would like you to transcribe the rhotic diphthongs*. In General American English, certain centering diphthongs are more common than others. Thus, /ɪ/, /ɛ/, and /ɑ/, which can be heard in "dear" [dɪɚ], "bear" [bɛɚ], and "farm" [fɑɚm], are far more prevalent than /i/ or /u/.

One should also keep in mind when transcribing that not every vowel + /ɚ/ is a rhotic diphthong. For example, the words "fire" and "tower" would be transcribed [faɪɚ] and [taʊɚ], but typically in this case the words are pronounced as two syllables. (They can be said as one syllable but are more commonly said as two.) In this case, the vowel + /ɚ/ would not be a rhotic diphthong. That is probably the reason why some instructors teach the rhotic diphthongs as the vowel + /r/, that is, simply to avoid this confusion.

Beginning Case Study

LORI, THE BILINGUAL TEACHER, CONTINUED

As noted earlier, Spanish is a language with five vowels, all of which are long vowels. Therefore, the distinction between a long vowel such as [i] and a short vowel such as [ɪ] in American English will probably not be realized. It might be helpful to the Spanish speaker of American English to learn this long–short dichotomy. The tense–lax, close–open, long–short production features of American English will become valuable to reducing the Spanish accent. In addition, there are no central vowels in Spanish and no central vowels with r-coloring. The central vowels are often replaced by [a]; thus, the pronunciation of "cut" [kʌt] may sound like [kat], while those with r-coloring may be replaced by the trilled "r" of Spanish. By comparing the vowel system of Spanish to that of American English, many of the "accent" differences can be understood.

Allophonic Variations of Vowels

There are several allophonic variations that occur with vowels. One of the most common variations is **nasalization**. Normally, all the vowels in General American English are oral sounds; therefore, the velum is raised and the airflow is through the oral cavity. However, when English vowels are produced in the context of a nasal consonant (/m/, /n/, or /ŋ/), they become nasalized. This nasalization has to do with the function of the velopharyngeal mechanism. Vowels that are preceded by a nasal, such as in the word "me," are nasalized as the velopharyngeal opening for the nasal consonant continues through the vowel. However, vowels that are followed by a nasal, such as in the word "I'm," also become somewhat nasalized. In this case, the velopharyngeal port begins to open in anticipation of the upcoming nasal (Shriberg & Kent, 2003). If a vowel is preceded and followed by a nasal, such as in "men," the vowel will again be nasalized. This allophonic variation is considered to be in complementary distribution, as nasalized vowels occur only in the context of a nasal consonant. The nasalization of these vowels can be marked using a diacritic. Thus, "men" could be transcribed as [mɛ̃n] to demonstrate this nasalization.

A second type of allophonic variation involves **monophthongization** or **diphthongization**. In this case, monophthong vowels can become diphthongs, and vowels that are typically produced as diphthongs are articulated as monophthongs. Monophthong vowels can be produced as diphthongs in certain dialects, such as in the South. For example, Shriberg and Kent (2003) note that "cat" [kæt] is articulated as [keæ͡t]. The opposite trend is noted by Hartman (1985), in which diphthongs become monophthongs in the South Midland area. For example, "oil" [ɔi͡l] becomes [ɔl]. In addition, as previously mentioned, the diphthongs /ei͡/ and /ou͡/ are often produced as monophthongs in unstressed syllables.

The third type of allophonic variation is labeled **reduction**. Reduction occurs as the rate of speaking increases or as the stress on a vowel is decreased. In these cases, the length is reduced and the vowel becomes centralized; the vowels typically are reduced to a schwa vowel (Shriberg & Kent, 2003). For example, in "furniture," the [ɪ] ([fɝnɪtʃɚ]) becomes [fɝnət̪ʃɚ].

Case Study

Eric had just turned 4 years old when his parents brought him into the clinic. Eric demonstrated many consonant problems as well as vowel errors. The following is a transcription of a few words he articulated.

Word	Target	Child's Production
1. pillow	[pɪloʊ͡]	[baloʊ͡]
2. eight	[eɪ͡t]	[aɪ͡t]
3. red	[rɛd]	[wɑd]
4. cat	[kæt]	[taɪ͡t]
5. wagon	[wægən]	[wɔɪ͡dən]
6. foot	[fʊt]	[fɔt]
7. duck	[dʌk]	[dɑ]
8. cow	[kaʊ]	[tɑ]
9. toy	[tɔɪ͡]	[dʌ]
10. rock	[rɑk]	[waɪ͡]

The following vowel changes occurred:

1. High-front vowel is changed to a low-back vowel.
2. Onglide portion of diphthong is changed; mid-front vowel is changed to a low-front vowel.
3. Mid-front vowel is changed to a low-back vowel.
4. Monophthong is changed to a diphthong; low-front monophthong is changed to a diphthong with a low-front onglide and a high-front offglide.
5. Monophthong is changed to a diphthong; low-front monophthong is changed to a diphthong with a mid-back onglide and a high-front offglide.

Can you describe the other vowel changes noted in numbers 6 through 10?

Summary

FOCUS 1: *What are the productional and functional differences between vowels and consonants?*

Vowels are characterized by the following: (1) no constriction of the vocal tract during their production, thus, open sounds; (2) sagittal midline of the vocal tract remains open; (3) are voiced sounds, (4) are acoustically more intense, thus, demonstrate more sonority. Consonants are characterized by the following: (1) significant constriction of the vocal tract during their production, thus, constricted sounds; (2) constriction occurs primarily along sagittal midline of vocal tract; (3) are voiced or voiceless sounds; (4) are acoustically less intense, thus, demonstrate less sonority.

The functional difference between vowels and consonants relate to their ability to function as syllable nuclei, as the center of the syllable. Vowels are typically the center of syllables; only certain consonants (syllabics) can function as syllable nuclei.

FOCUS 2: *What are the three dimensions used to describe vowel articulation?*

The highest point of the bulge or hump of the tongue is referenced according to the following dimensions:

1. *The tongue's position relative to the palate*, i.e., closer or farther away from the palate, which provides the references of *high, mid,* or *low.* According to this dimension, vowels are *high,* indicating the tongue hump is fairly close to the palate, *mid,* farther away from the palate, or *low.* The position of the mandible, or lower jaw, is also sometimes described relative to specific vowel productions. However, whether the angle of the jaw is relatively open or closed follows from the tongue height relative to the palate. High vowels demonstrate a relatively closed jaw position while low vowels have a relatively low or open jaw position.

2. *The anterior/posterior dimensions of the tongue*, which provide the references of *front, central,* or *back.* Vowels are labeled *front, back,* or *central* depending upon which part of the hump of the tongue is elevated. For the front vowels, the most observable characteristic is the heightened hump of the tongue at the front portion of the tongue. For the back vowels, the hump of the tongue is posterior, creating a narrow channel in the upper pharynx. The central vowels are characterized by a centralized positioning of the bulge of the tongue. When contrasted to the front or the back vowels, the central vowels have a more neutral tongue position.

3. The *degree of lip rounding or unrounding.* Unrounded, or spread vowels are produced either with the muscles of the lips quite inactive or neutral or with the contraction of specific muscles that draw back the corners of the lips. Rounded vowels are produced when the mouth opening is reduced by contraction of the muscles of the lips.

FOCUS 3: *What is meant by tense–lax, close–open, and long–short in relationship to vowels?*

The terms *tense* and *lax* are associated with more muscular activity (tense) versus less muscular activity (lax), not only of the tongue but of the entire articulatory mechanism.

The terms *close* and *open* refer to the vertical axis of vowel production, i.e., the distance of the tongue from the palate. Close vowels are produced with the highest bulge of the tongue closer to the palate, while open vowels are articulated with the bulge of the tongue farther away from the palate.

The last classifications, *long* and *short*, represent the relative length of the vowel in question. Thus, long vowels were considered to be longer in duration than short vowels. Some authors relate the concepts long and short to the vowel's ability to function within the context of an open syllable. Thus, within one-syllable words, only long vowels can be present in open syllables (see, toe, new), while short vowels cannot—they can only appear in closed syllables (hit, pet, put).

FOCUS 4: *What are the divisions for categorizing vowels according to the IPA?*

The IPA describes vowels somewhat differently in relationship to the vertical, up-and-down plane. Four degrees of tongue height are established: close (the bulge of the tongue is closest to the roof of the mouth), close-mid, open-mid, and open (the jaw is fully open, and the tongue is low in the mouth). To establish these four degrees of tongue height, first, the tongue shape for the vowels that represent the highest and lowest vowels and those that are the most anterior and posterior are plotted. The four vowels that represent the extreme vowel positions are (1) the tongue high and toward the front of the mouth (i), (2) the tongue high and toward the back of the mouth (u), (3) the tongue the low and toward the front (a), and (4) the tongue low and toward the back (ɑ). Further reference vowels can now be defined: The two front vowels, /e/ and /ɛ/, and the two back vowels, /ɔ/ and /o/, are placed between the extreme points so that the differences between each vowel and the next in the series are auditorily equal. The use of auditory spacing means that the vowel descriptions are not based purely on articulation features. The terms *close, close-mid, open-mid,* and *open* represent equal points (as auditory and articulatory parameters) between the extreme vowel positions.

FOCUS 5: *What are diphthongs, and how are they categorized?*

Diphthongs (di = two, phthong = sound) are vowels in which there is a change in quality during their duration. Thus, diphthongs are composed of two distinct vowel elements; there is an audible change in vowel quality during their articulation. This is their distinction from the monophthongs, or pure vowels, in which the quality remains relatively constant throughout the production. It is important to note that diphthongs are not two distinct vowels that are produced one after the other, but that rather there is a gliding transition from one vowel element to the next.

Diphthongs may be classified according to several different parameters. First, the two vowel elements that compose the diphthong can be labeled. This results in an onglide, the first portion of the diphthong, and an offglide, which is the final portion.

Second, diphthongs are also categorized according to the type of articulatory movement from onglide to offglide. This categorization results in diphthongs being labeled *rising* or *falling*. A rising diphthong is one in which the gliding movement of the tongue moves from a lower to a higher articulatory position. The diphthongs of American English are considered rising diphthongs.

Third, diphthongs can be classified according to their linguistic function. This gives rise to the categorization of phonemic versus nonphonemic diphthongs. Phonemic diphthongs are those that have phoneme value as diphthongs. The production of these sounds as diphthongs (as opposed to their articulation as monophthongs) changes the meaning of a word. Nonphonemic diphthongs do not have phonemic value; the production of these sounds as diphthongs (as opposed to their articulation as monophthongs) does not change the meaning of a word.

In addition, certain diphthongs are referred to as centering diphthongs. In this case the offglide, or less prominent element of the diphthong, is a central vowel. In General American English, certain centering diphthongs are more common than others. Thus, /ɪ/, /ɛ/, and /ɑ/, which can be heard in "dear" [dɪɚ], "bear" [bɛɚ], or "farm" [fɑɚm], are far more prevalent than /i/ or /u/. Several authors refer to the diphthongs that are paired with /ɚ/ as rhotic diphthongs.

 FOCUS 6: *How are each of the vowels of American English described according to the horizontal and vertical planes of the tongue as well as lip rounding?*

Front Vowels

/i/ high-front vowel that is unrounded

/ɪ/ high-front vowel that is unrounded

/e/ a mid-front vowel that is unrounded, the onglide of the diphthong /eɪ/

/ɛ/ mid-front vowel that is unrounded

/æ/ low-front vowel that is unrounded

/a/ low-front vowel that is unrounded

Back Vowels

/u/ high-back vowel that is rounded

/ʊ/ high-back vowel that is rounded

/o/ the onglide of the diphthong /oʊ/ is a mid-back vowel that is rounded

/ɔ/ mid-back vowel that is rounded

/ɒ/ low-back vowel that is rounded

/ɑ/ low-back vowel that is unrounded

Central Vowels

/ɝ/ mid-central vowel that is rounded and has r-coloring

/ɚ/ mid-central vowel that is unrounded and has r-coloring

/ʌ/ mid-central vowel that is unrounded

/ə/ mid-central vowel that is unrounded

Further Readings

Ball, M., & Gibbon, F. (2002). *Vowel disorders*. Boston: Butterworth-Heinemann.

Ball, M., & Rahilly, J. (1999). *Phonetics: The science of speech*. New York: Oxford University Press.

Ladefoged, P. (2005). *Vowels and consonants*. Oxford, UK: Blackwell.

Ladefoged, P. (2006). *A course in phonetics* (5th ed.). Boston: Thomson Wadsworth.

Key Terms

back vowels p. 76
centering diphthongs p. 99
central vowels p. 76
close vowels p. 80
close-mid vowels p. 82
cognates p. 74
diphthongization p. 100
diphthongs p. 84
falling diphthong p. 85
front vowels p. 76
high vowels p. 75
lax vowels p. 79
lip retraction p. 77
lip spreading p. 77
long vowels p. 80
low vowels p. 75
mid vowels p. 75
monophthongization p. 100
monophthongs p. 84
nasalization p. 100

nonphonemic diphthongs p. 86
nucleus p. 73
offglide p. 85
onglide p. 85
open vowels p. 80
open-mid vowels p. 82
phonemic diphthongs p. 86
primary cardinal vowels p. 82
r-coloring p. 93
reduction p. 100
rhotic diphthong p. 99
rising diphthong p. 85
rounded vowels p. 77
sagittal midline p. 73
secondary cardinal vowels p. 83
short vowels p. 80
sonority p. 74
tense vowels p. 79
unrounded vowels p. 77

Think Critically

1. The diphthongs /aɪ/, /aʊ/, and /ɔɪ/ were classified as phonemic diphthongs. What does that mean? For each of these diphthongs, provide a pair of words that demonstrates that they are phonemic diphthongs.

2. Why would children who have r-problems (such as "wabbit" for "rabbit") have difficulty with the central vowels with r-coloring?

3. What is meant by the term *centering diphthong*? Can you find three words that contain centering diphthongs?

4. Find words that contain the following vowels: /i/, /ɪ/, /ɛ/, /æ/, /u/, /ʊ/, /ɝ/, /ʌ/.

5. There were four variations of ah-type vowels: /a/, /ɑ/, /ɒ/, and /ɔ/. Which of these variations do you use in your speech? Do you differentiate between the production of [ɑ] and [ɔ] in some words, such as "caught" and "cot"?

Test Yourself

1. Which one of the following is a high-front vowel that is unrounded?
   a. [u]
   b. [ɪ]

c. [a]

d. [ɛ]

2. Which one of the following is a mid-back vowel that is rounded?

   a. /u/

   b. /ɑ/

   c. /a/

   d. /ɔ/

3. Which one of the following vowels is a low-back vowel that is rounded?

   a. /ɑ/

   b. /a/

   c. /æ/

   d. /ɒ/

4. Within an unstressed syllable, vowel reduction can occur. The reduced vowel commonly assumes which quality?

   a. a vowel that has a lower articulation

   b. a diphthong quality

   c. the schwa vowel, /ə/

   d. it is completely reduced, the vowel is not articulated at all

5. Which one of the following is not a characteristic of a vowel?

   a. open sounds

   b. constriction occurs along sagittal midline

   c. acoustically more intense

   d. demonstrates more sonority

6. Which one of the following is considered a tense vowel?

   a. /i/

   b. /ɛ/

   c. /ʊ/

   d. /ɪ/

7. Which one of the following is a rhotic diphthong?

   a. /ɝ/

   b. /i͡ɚ/

   c. /r/

   d. /ɚ/

8. Which one of the following is not a dimension used to describe vowels in American English?

   a. the rounding or unrounding of the lips

   b. voicing or lack of voicing

   c. the extent to which the tongue is raised in the direction of the palate

   d. the anterior-posterior dimensions of the tongue relative to that portion of the tongue that is raised

9. The diphthongs of American English are
   a. rising diphthongs.
   b. falling diphthongs.
   c. all phonemic diphthongs.
   d. unrounded.
10. Which one of the following vowels has r-coloring?
   a. /ʌ/
   b. /ə/
   c. /ɚ/
   d. /ɒ/

Answers: 1.b 2.d 3.d 4.c 5.b 6.a 7.b 8.b 9.a 10. c

For additional information, go to www.phonologicaldisorders.com

Articulatory Phonetics

PRODUCTION FEATURES
OF CONSONANTS

Chapter Highlights

- What is meant by *active articulator*? Which terms are used to reference these points?
- What is meant by *passive articulator*? Which terms are used to reference these points?
- What are the characteristics of stop-plosive productions?
- What are the characteristics of nasal productions?
- What are the characteristics of fricative productions?
- What are the characteristics of affricate productions?
- What are the characteristics of approximant productions?

Chapter Application: Case Study

Keith was an audiologist who had just started working at a university clinic. One of his jobs was starting an aural rehabilitation program. There were several children who had hearing impairments and two children who had just received cochlear implants. All of these children had problems with consonant productions. One child with a significant hearing loss, Hallie, had just been fitted with hearing aids at age 4. Another child, Melissa, who was also 4 years old, had just received bilateral cochlear implants. Keith knew a lot about the diagnostic end of audiology. He had worked for several years testing hearing and fitting hearing aids, but he had to admit that aural rehabilitation was an area that he had received training in but really had not done anything practical with since his graduate program. Now he was confronted with several children and graduate clinicians who needed his assistance to set up aural rehabilitation programs for these children. All of the children needed work with consonant production, and Keith began to think about how the different consonants are produced. What kind of feedback could he provide to get the various consonants articulated in a way that would result in, for example, a normal-sounding /k/?

Note: A cochlear implant is a small, complex electronic device that can help to provide a sense of sound to a person who is profoundly deaf or severely hard-of-hearing. The implant works by directly stimulating any functioning auditory nerves inside the cochlea with electrical impulses. It is surgically implanted in the inner ear and activated by a device worn outside the ear. A cochlear implant is very different from a hearing aid. Hearing aids amplify sounds so they may be detected by damaged ears. Cochlear implants bypass damaged portions of the ear and directly stimulate the auditory nerve. Signals generated by the implant are sent by way of the auditory nerve to the brain, which recognizes the signals as sound. An implant does not restore or create normal hearing. Instead, under the appropriate conditions, it can give a deaf person a useful auditory understanding of the environment and help her or him to understand speech; post-implantation therapy may be required (Spencer & Marschark, 2003).

Consonants are important speech sounds within any language system. Many languages do not have a large number of different vowels within their inventory but may have twenty or more consonants. For example, both Spanish and Japanese have only five different vowels that are used as meaning-distinguishing phonemes (Iglesias & Goldstein, 1998; Ladefoged, 2005). On the other hand, both languages contain close to twenty different consonants (Goldstein and Washington, 2001; Okada, 1999). Although American English has over a dozen contrastive vowels, it still has far more consonants. When examining disordered speech, we also find that it is characterized, for the most part, by aberrant articulation of consonants, not typically vowels. Therefore, consonants, specifically their production features, become very important in our work as speech-language pathologists with children and adults with speech impairments.

The way that we describe the production of consonants is different from the noted vowel features provided in the previous chapter. If we go back to the definition of consonants versus vowels, then it will be clear that other articulatory features will need to be emphasized. Vowels were defined as relatively open productions that are without significant articulatory constriction, whereas consonants are typically produced *with* significant articulatory constriction. These oppositions lead to a different system of classifying consonants.

Historically, the production features of consonants have been described in slightly different ways reflecting varying degrees of detail and contrasting categorizations. The system that is used in this textbook draws heavily on the updated classification of the IPA 2005. In addition, the description

Concept Exercise **VOWELS VS. CONSONANTS**

Say the vowel /ɑ/ as in "h*o*p," and then try the first sound in "*p*ea" (/p/) or "*t*ea" (/t/). Note the openness of the vowel production as opposed to how the lips come together for /p/ and the tongue touches the roof of the mouth for /t/. These production differences lead to different descriptions for consonants than for vowels.

presented emphasizes detailed and specific production features. For anyone interested in speech sound production, such as individuals working with children or adults with speech impairments, those interested in radio or television broadcasting, or actors who are working with speech variations in the theater, this detail will be important if not necessary. Therefore, the first goal of this chapter is to describe in detail the production features of consonants according to four dimensions: the active articulator, the passive articulator, the manner of production, and the voicing characteristics of each consonant of American English. Several consonants will also be discussed that are not a portion of the American English inventory. These consonants might be used to describe normal articulatory variations as well as those presented by children or adults with misarticulations.

Active Articulator, Passive Articulator, Manner of Articulation, and Voicing

Four phonetic categories will be used to describe the production features of consonants: (1) the active articulator, the anatomical structure that actually moves during the generation of speech sounds; (2) the passive articulator, the immovable portion of the vocal tract that is paired with the active articulator; (3) the manner, the type of constriction the active and passive articulators produce for the realization of a particular consonant, or the way in which the airstream is modified as a result of the interaction of the articulators; and (4) voicing, the presence or absence of vocal fold vibration.

There are several ways to describe the articulation of consonants. In several texts, place, manner, and voicing are used (Edwards, 2003; Shriberg & Kent, 2003; Small, 2005). However, "place" of articulation is not used consistently. Often it is used to reference two articulators, such as the term *labio-dental*, which refers to an articulation that involves the lips (*labio*) and the teeth (*dental*), or the term *lingua-alveolar*, indicating an articulation involving the tongue (*lingual*) and the alveolar ridge (*alveolar*). However, in other examples, only one descriptor is used for "place," such as *palatal* (referencing some point along the hard palate) or *lingual* (referencing some point of the tongue). This is problematic for two reasons. First, for students beginning their study of phonetics, this lack of consistency may be confusing. Second, this type of categorization does not provide enough detail when students actually begin to work with children and adults with speech disorders. Historically, many authors have emphasized the importance of the active articulator (e.g., Gorecka, 1989; Halle, 1983; Sagey, 1986;). However, Ladefoged (1997) makes a strong case for using this type of classification system, because it provides a better way to organize phonetic features. Although his argument is more linguistically oriented, the reasoning is clear. By describing the active articulator, more satisfactory statements can be made about important articulatory features. Therefore, for the purpose at hand, both the active and passive articulators will be discussed. It should always be kept in mind that these descriptions are based upon somewhat standard pronunciations. Slight variations in production will, of course, be evidenced by individual speakers.

Active Articulator

The **active articulator** refers to the anatomical structure that actually moves during the generation of speech sounds. If you say /t/ or /l/, then you will notice that the tongue is moving toward the roof of the mouth. Therefore, specific portions of the tongue are considered to be active articulators. Also, if you produce /f/ or /v/, you will find that the lower lip is moving to a position in which it comes into contact with the front teeth. Thus, the lower lip is also considered an active articulator. The tongue and lower lip are given specific names to denote their status as active articulators. When the bottom lip is used as an active articulator, the term **labial** is used as a descriptor. For the previous examples, /f/ and /v/ are considered labial sounds. The tongue, on the other hand, is divided into several areas to further specify which portion is directly involved in the articulation of a given speech sound. Note the different parts of the tongue that are involved in the production of /d/ versus /g/, for example. For /d/, the front of the tongue briefly touches the roof of the mouth, while /g/ is characterized by the back of the tongue making contact with the very back of the palate (actually the soft palate or velum). The divisions of the tongue include the following:

1. **apical**: The tip of the tongue or apex of the tongue, as active articulator.
2. **coronal**: The front and lateral edges of the tongue (including the apex).
3. **predorsal**: The anterior one-third of the tongue.
4. **mediodorsal**: The middle one-third of the tongue.
5. **postdorsal**: The posterior one-third of the tongue.

(This classification system draws from sources such as Bauman-Waengler, 2008; von Essen, 1979; and Waengler, 1983) These divisions are exemplified in Figure 5.1.

Some authors use the term *dorsal* or *dorsum* to refer to the posterior portion of the tongue. For the purposes at hand, *dorsal* and *dorsum* will reference the body of the tongue. In addition, the term *blade* is used for that part of the tongue that lies below the alveolar ridge when the tongue is at rest (Ladefoged, 1997). This text will use the term *predorsal* for that descriptor.

These labels can be clarified by introducing some examples. Sounds that are typically produced with just the very tip of the tongue, such as the voiceless and voiced "th" sounds (/θ/, /ð/) are referred to as apical productions when denoting the active articulator. A coronal sound would involve using more than just the tip of the tongue; the lateral edges would also be actively involved in the articulation: /n/ is an example of a coronal sound. The term *mediodorsal* as active articulator references the central portion of the tongue and is typically used to describe the first sound in "you," /j/. Examples of postdorsal sounds, in which the posterior portion of the tongue is active during a production, would include /k/ and /g/. The consonants of American English are summarized according to the active articulator in Table 5.1.

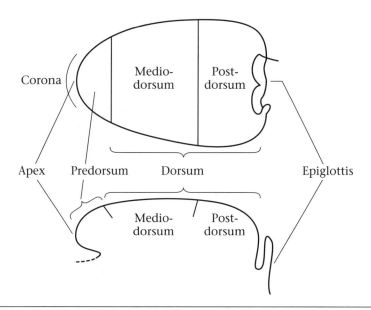

Figure 5.1 Divisions of the Tongue

Source: From *Articulatory and Phonological Impairments: A Clinical Focus* (3rd ed., p. 23), by J. Bauman-Waengler, 2008, Boston: Allyn and Bacon. Reproduced with permission.

Table 5.1 Phonetic Description: Active Articulator

Active Articulator	Phonetic Descriptor	Examples
Lower lip	Labial	/p/ "pie," /b/ "boy" /m/ "me" /f/ "fig," /v/ "van" /w/ "win," /ʍ/[1] "when"
Tip of tongue	Apical	/s/ "sun," /z/[2] "zoo" /θ/ "thin," /ð/ "the" /r/[2] "run" /l/ "lamp"
Lateral rims of tongue	Coronal	/t/ "toe," /d/ "do" /n/ "no" /ʃ/ "shoe," /ʒ/ "beige"
Surface of tongue	Dorsum	
Anterior portion	Predorsal	/s/ "soup," /z/ "zip"
Central portion	Mediodorsal	/j/ "yes," /r/ "rose"
Posterior portion	Postdorsal	/k/ "cat," /g/ "go" /ŋ/ "sing"

[1]Historically, the /ʍ/ was used in "wh" words such as "where" or "when" and was a voiceless sound. It has now merged with /w/ throughout much of the United States (Wolfram & Schilling-Estes, 2006).

[2]/s/, /z/, and /r/ appear in two places, as two different articulations of these sounds exist. This will be discussed in more detail later in the chapter.

FOCUS 1: *What is meant by* **active articulator?** *Which terms are used to reference these points?*

The active and passive articulators are interrelated. During the articulation of speech sounds, the active, movable articulator approximates or actually touches a specific area of the vocal tract. The passive articulator, the second element of our phonetic description, involves those specific structures that the active articulator touches or moves closer to.

Passive Articulator

The **passive articulator** denotes the immovable portion of the vocal tract that is paired with the active articulator. The passive articulator consists of those structures that do not or cannot move during the production of speech sounds. During the production of American English consonants, the passive articulators are the upper lip, the front teeth, the hard palate, and the soft palate or velum. The palate or hard palate is the bony part of the roof of the mouth, while the soft palate or velum is the muscular part. The velum is the posterior two-fifths of the roof of the mouth (MacKay, 1987).

The phonetic terms that are used to indicate the various passive articulators include the following:

1. **labial**: The upper lip.
2. **dental**: The upper teeth are the passive articulators.
3. **alveolar**: The alveolar ridge (a protuberance formed by the alveolar process, which is a thickened portion of the maxilla housing the teeth).
4. **prepalatal**, **mediopalatal**, and **postpalatal**: Approximately the first third, the second third, and the posterior third of the hard palate.
5. **velar**: If the velum is the passive articulator.
6. **glottal**: There is narrowing of the **glottis**, the space between the vocal folds.

Labial sounds include /m/ or /b/, where both lips come together for the articulation. Both /f/ and /v/ are considered dental sounds; the lip as active articulator approximates the upper teeth. /t/ and /d/ are considered alveolar sounds, the tongue making contact with the alveolar ridge, while "sh" (/ʃ/), is considered a prepalatal articulation.

A mediopalatal articulation corresponds to the typical production of the first sound in "yes," /j/. In General American English, a postpalatal articulation does not normally occur; however, a velar articulation is exemplified by /k/ and /g/. See Table 5.2 for a summary of the consonants of

Concept Exercise **"S" AND "SH"**

Note the difference in tongue placement between /s/ and "sh," /ʃ/. The tongue moves slightly back for the production of /ʃ/, corresponding to the difference between an alveolar articulation for /s/ and /z/ and a prepalatal one for /ʃ/ and /ʒ/.

Table 5.2 Phonetic Description: Passive Articulator

Passive Articulator	Phonetic Descriptor	Examples
Upper lip	Labial	/p/ "<u>p</u>ot", /b/ "<u>b</u>ed" /m/ "<u>m</u>ore"
Upper teeth	Dental	/f/ "<u>f</u>an," /v/ "<u>v</u>ote" /θ/ "<u>th</u>ought," /ð/ "<u>th</u>en"
Alveolar ridge	Alveolar	/t/ "<u>t</u>oad," /d/ "<u>d</u>oor" /n/ "<u>n</u>ice" /s/ "<u>s</u>ee," /z/ "<u>z</u>ebra" /l/ "<u>l</u>ick"
	Postalveolar	/ʃ/ "<u>sh</u>op," /ʒ/[1] "rou<u>g</u>e" /r/[1] "<u>r</u>ice"
Surface of hard palate Anterior portion	Prepalatal	/ʃ/ "<u>sh</u>ip," /ʒ/ "<u>l</u>acque" /r/ "<u>r</u>ope"
	Mediopalatal	/j/ "<u>y</u>awn" /r/ "<u>r</u>abbit"
	Postpalatal	Does not normally exist in General American English
Soft palate	Velar	/k/ "<u>k</u>ite," /g/ "<u>g</u>ate" /ŋ/ "thi<u>ng</u>" /w/ "<u>w</u>est," /ʍ/[2] "<u>wh</u>ere"
Glottis	Glottal	/h/ "<u>h</u>ot"

[1] /ʃ/, /ʒ/ and /r/ appear in two places, as two different articulations of these sounds exist. This will be discussed in more detail later in the chapter.
[2] Historically, the /ʍ/ was used in "wh" words such as "where" or "when" and was a voiceless sound. It has now merged with /w/ throughout much of the United States (Wolfram & Schilling-Estes, 2006).

> When used as the active articulator, the term *labial* becomes "labio" and *apical* becomes "apico." On the other hand, although "coronal" is the label used for the active articulator denoting the edges of the tongue, "corona" is the plural form.

American English according to the passive articulators. Figure 5.2 represents the specific structures of the oral cavity as active and passive articulators.

In a phonetic description of consonants, the active and passive articulators are typically paired. Thus, the active articulator for /m/ is the bottom lip (labial) while the passive articulator is the top lip (labial). Now one could put the two together and state that /m/ is a labio-labial sound; however, it is much simpler to state that it is a bilabial articulation. If we examine /f/, the active articulator is the bottom lip (labial), which approximates the upper teeth (dental). Thus, the description for /f/ is labio-dental.

In another example, /d/, the edges of the tongue (corona) as active articulator come in contact with the alveolar ridge (alveolar) as the passive articulator, resulting in a coronal-alveolar consonant. It should be kept in mind that these descriptions reflect typical, standard productions of the consonants. Individual minor variations from speaker to speaker, of course, exist.

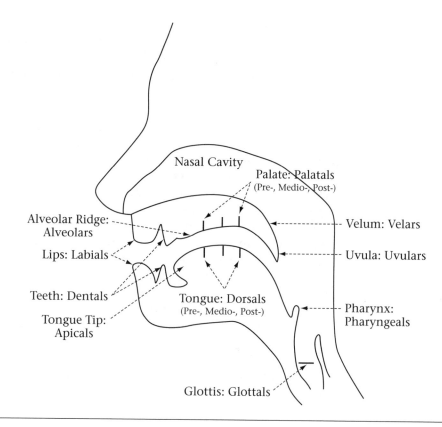

Figure 5.2 Structures of the Oral Cavity as Active and Passive Articulators

Source: From *Articulatory and Phonological Impairments: A Clinical Focus* (3rd ed., p. 24), by J. Bauman-Waengler, 2008, Boston: Allyn and Bacon. Reproduced with permission.

 FOCUS 2: *What is meant by* **passive articulator?** *Which terms are used to reference these points?*

Active and passive articulators represent two parts of the total phonetic classification system. The third element, manner of articulation, examines the interaction between these active and passive articulators.

Manner of Articulation

This term refers to the type of constriction the active and passive articulators produce for the realization of a particular consonant. Or, stated another way, **manner of articulation** refers to the way in which the airstream is modified as a result of the interaction of the articulators. There are various manners of articulation. One manner of articulation consists of consonants that are produced when a complete occlusion between the active and passive articulators occurs. For another manner of articulation, the articulators come very close to one another; thus, a narrow opening between the active and passive articulators exemplifies these types of consonants. For still other consonants, there is a relatively wide distance between the articulators. Several variables play a role in describing the manner of articulation. For example, the action of the velum as well as the release phase of the articulation will characterize specific manners of articulation. The following manners of articulation are used to describe the consonants of General American English: stop-plosives, nasals, fricatives, affricates, glides, laterals, and rhotics. According to the classification system of the IPA, the glides, laterals, and rhotics are termed *approximants*; they will be discussed in more detail in the following paragraphs.

STOP-PLOSIVES

Some textbooks refer to these consonants as *stops* (Shriberg & Kent, 2003; Small, 2005), while others use the term *plosives* to denote this specific manner of articulation (Ball & Rahilly, 1999; MacKay, 1987). The two terms *stop* and *plosive* actually refer to different phases of this consonant's production: *stop* draws attention to the second closure phase, while the term *plosive* emphasizes the release portion and the characteristic sound that is associated with these consonants. It is also true that in American English these consonants can be unreleased, i.e., the plosive portion does not take place. This typically happens at the end of a word or utterance.

In American English, the consonants associated with this manner of articulation are /p/, /b/, /t/, /d/, /k/, and /g/. The first sounds in the following words exemplify these sounds: pot, bought, tot, dot, cot, and got. **Stop-plosives** are defined by complete blockage of the oral cavity. In other words, the articulators actually come together creating a closure in the oral cavity to block off the airflow, which results in a build-up of air pressure behind this occlusion. This pressure is released suddenly, which creates the characteristic "explosive" sound of these consonants. The velum is raised, blocking off air flow to the nasal cavity. Although different terms are used to describe the production stages of this consonant class, it is generally agreed that there are three phases: (1) the shutting or approach phase, (2) the closure or stop phase, and (3) the release stage (Ball & Rahilly, 1999; MacKay, 1987). The first phase, the **shutting** or **approach phase**, is characterized by the articulators moving from a previous open state to a closed state. For the **closure** or **stop phase**, the articulators are held closed for a period of time (40–150 ms), during which there is a build-up of air pressure behind the closure (Ball & Rahilly, 1999). The **release phase** consists of a sudden separation of the articulators, that then allows for the burst of air that gives these sounds their characteristic quality.

When produced in isolation, the stop-plosives are characterized by these three phases. However, when influenced by surrounding sounds in connected speech, these phases may be reduced to a closure (stop) portion that is released into a following sound or just a stop with no compression or release. These differences are considered allophonic variations of that particular sound.

Stop-plosives may also vary in the amount of pressure that is built up behind the occlusion when the articulators come in contact during the stop portion and then are released. In American English, as well as in many other languages, the voiceless stop-plosives, in this case /p/, /t/, and /k/, are produced with greater pressure than the voiced stop-plosives /b/, /d/, and /g/. In other words, the build-up of air pressure within the oral cavity (intraoral air pressure) is considerably more for voiceless stop-plosives than for voiced. While this is not the case in all contexts, it does occur at the beginning of a stressed syllable, as in "pillow," "teacher," and "kennel." The release of this increased air pressure creates a puff of air called **aspiration**. Voiceless stop-plosives are aspirated at the beginning of stressed syllables regardless if that occurs word-initially (such as in "pan" or "tuna") or within a word (such as in "upon" or "attack"). However, voiceless stop-plosives are not aspirated following /s/ as in "stew" or "spoon" (Small, 2005).

The stop-plosives that have clearly more intraoral pressure, which translates into a stronger puff of air (aspirated stop-plosives), are often called **fortis consonants**, from the Latin word for "strong." On the other hand, those stop-plosives that have considerably less intraoral pressure (unaspirated stop-plosives) are termed **lenis consonants**, derived from the Latin word for "weak." As previously noted, in American English, voiced stop-plosives are lenis; however, not all voiceless stop-plosives are fortis. Only those with aspiration are considered fortis productions.

Beginning Case Study

KEITH, THE AUDIOLOGIST

One of the children in the aural rehabilitation program had trouble differentiating voiceless and voiced stop-plosives. Keith thought it might be a good idea to emphasize the fortis and lenis production qualities of these sounds. Therefore, he used the stronger puff of air associated with the voiceless, aspirated stop-plosives to differentiate between the two productions. When the child spoke word pairs such as "pen"–"Ben," "toe"–"doe," and "came"–"game," he placed a small feather in front of the child's lip so that she could visually see the extra air pressure that occurred during the production of the voiceless stop-plosives. This visual feedback helped her to begin to understand the production differences between the voiceless, aspirated fortis and the voiced lenis productions.

NASALS

FOCUS 3: *What are the characteristics of stop-plosive productions?*

In American English, the consonants associated with this manner of articulation are /m/, /n/, and /ŋ/. The last sounds in the following words exemplify these sounds: su<u>m</u>, su<u>n</u>, su<u>ng</u>. **Nasals** are defined by a complete blockage of the oral cavity, similar to the stop-plosives that were previously discussed. Therefore, the articulators come together, creating a closure in the oral cavity. However, for the nasal consonants, the velum is lowered so that there is not a build-up of intraoral air pressure; rather, the airstream is directed through the nasal cavities. The characteristic quality of these sounds is achieved by two factors that are related to resonance properties. First, the velum is lowered (relaxed), allowing air to flow through the nasal cavities; therefore, nasal resonance contributes to the distinguishing quality of these sounds. Second, the placement of the oral blockage creates cul-de-sac resonance properties within the oral cavity, which are coupled to those created by the airflow through the nasal cavities. *Cul-de-sac* refers in this case to a tube open at one end and closed at the other end. The blockage within the oral cavity is the closed end of the tube, while the opening at the nostrils is the open end. For the nasal consonant /m/, the oral occlusion is forward in the mouth at the lips. For /n/, the oral blockage occurs more centrally at the alveolar ridge, while for /ŋ/ this oral closure is farther back in the oral cavity at the level of the velum. These specific oral occlusions between active and passive articulators are used when classifying the nasals consonants. In American English all nasal consonants are voiced; that is, during their production there is simultaneous vocal fold vibration. There is direct comparability between the stop-plosives and the nasals in relationship to active and passive articulators. Both /p/ and /b/ are produced with the articulators making contact at the lips: They are considered to be bilabial consonants. This is also the case with the nasal consonant /m/. Active and passive articulators for the stop-plosives /t/ and /d/ are the same as the nasal /n/; these consonants are produced with the edges of the tongue (corona) making contact with the alveolar ridge (alveolar). The back of the tongue (postdorsal) as active articulator and the velum (velar) as the passive articulator define the stop-plosives /k/ and /g/ as well as the nasal /ŋ/. If voicing is considered, then /b/ and /m/, /d/ and /n/, and /g/ and /ŋ/ are identical with the exception of the velar activity. For the stop-plosive consonants, the velum is elevated (tensed), closing off the oral cavity from the nasal cavity. On the other hand, the velum is lowered (relaxed), allowing passage of airflow through the nasal cavity for the nasal consonants.

FOCUS 4: *What are the characteristics of nasal productions?*

FRICATIVES →

In American English, the consonants associated with this manner of articulation are /f/, /v/, /s/, /z/, /ʃ/, /ʒ/, /θ/, /ð/, and /h/. The first sounds in the following words exemplify these sounds: <u>f</u>an, <u>v</u>an, <u>s</u>ip, <u>z</u>ip, <u>sh</u>ock, <u>J</u>acques, <u>th</u>igh, <u>th</u>y, and <u>h</u>igh. Although /h/ is included in this group, its production is somewhat different from the other fricatives and will be discussed at the end of this section. **Fricatives** result when the active and passive articulators approximate each other so closely that the air is forced with considerable pressure through the constriction that is formed. As the air is pressed through this narrow passageway, its flow creates an audible noise, a frictionlike quality called *frication*, which gives these consonants their name.

The articulators that create this close approximation can be at various places in the oral cavity. For /f/ and /v/, a constriction is created between the inner edge of the lower lip (labial) and the edges of the upper incisors (dental). A more anterior constriction can also be noted for the th-sounds, /θ/ and /ð/, which are produced with a narrow passageway between the tongue tip and the upper incisors. For /s/ and /z/ and for the sh-sounds, /ʃ/ and /ʒ/, the constriction is farther back in the mouth; a narrow opening is created between the front portion of the tongue and the alveolar ridge.

Fricatives can also be classified according to the shape of the opening through which the airflow is forced. Ball & Rahilly (1999) refer to this as the channel shape, which is referenced by an imaginary cross-section, from left to right, of the speaker's face. A **grooved channel fricative** is one in which the channel for the airflow is extremely narrow. Both /s/ and /z/

Reflect on This: Clinical Application

USING THE NASAL /ŋ/ TO ACHIEVE /g/

A fairly common substitution for younger children is using /t/ and /d/ to replace /k/ and /g/ sounds. Therefore, the child might say "tat" for "cat" and "date" for "gate." If the child can say an accurate /ŋ/, then this could be used to aid in the production of /g/. Have the child prolong /ŋ/ while occluding the nostrils. Next direct the child to allow the air to go through the mouth. While the resulting sound with the pinched nostrils will not be a normal-sounding /g/, it can be used to demonstrate the placement of /g/ as well as the oral airflow.

Concept Exercise **LIP ROUNDING**

In addition to the positioning of articulators for /ʃ/ and /ʒ/, these sounds are produced with varying degrees of lip rounding. Say the words "shop," "should," and "sheep" and note how the lip rounding changes somewhat depending on the vowel following "sh." Some children may demonstrate sh-productions that are auditorily conspicuous: They sound "off." The tongue placement for these sounds may be accurate; the child simply lacks the necessary lip rounding that gives this speech sound its characteristic quality. Try producing each of the above words again with and without lip rounding and note the qualitative change that occurs in the sh-sound.

are considered grooved fricatives, as the air flows through a narrow opening that is created by a sagittal (front to back), v-shaped furrow of the tongue. A fricative with a wider and flatter channel shape is called a **slit fricative**. The widening and flattening of the channel is known as a **wide slit channel** with, for example, the th-sounds, /θ/ and /ð/, and a **narrow slit channel** for the sh- productions, /ʃ/ and /ʒ/. For the th-productions, the tongue shape is somewhat flat, and the airflow extends over a broader surface. On the other hand, for /ʃ/ and /ʒ/ the tongue is slightly grooved, though not nearly as much as for /s/ and /z/. The fricative channel shapes are exemplified in Figure 5.3.

There is also a special group of fricatives known as the sibilants. **Sibilant** fricatives are those with greater acoustic energy and more high-frequency components than other fricatives. In other words, these fricatives are louder and contain higher frequencies in their acoustic display. The fricatives that belong to this group include /s/, /z/, /ʃ/, and /ʒ/.

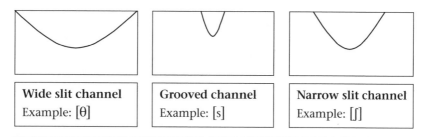

Wide slit channel
Example: [θ]

Grooved channel
Example: [s]

Narrow slit channel
Example: [ʃ]

Figure 5.3 Channel Shapes for Fricative Consonants

Reflect on This: Clinical Application

FRICATIVES AND SPEECH DISORDERS

Fricatives seem to be difficult for children, as a rather narrow opening between the articulators must be maintained over a longer period of time. For example, one of the most common speech sound errors in children is the aberrant production of /s/ (McDonald, 1964; Weiss, 1980). Most children at some point in their development have trouble with this sound. Other fricatives, such as the th-sounds, /θ/ and /ð/, are among the latest sounds to develop. For example, the data from Smit (1993a) show that most children do not produce this sound correctly until age 6 or 7.

Beginning Case Study

KEITH, THE AUDIOLOGIST

Children with high-frequency hearing losses often have difficulty with the sibilant sounds. Due to their hearing losses, they cannot hear the higher frequencies and/or the intensity differences between these higher frequencies and, therefore, have trouble distinguishing between these sounds. The result may be that these sounds are distorted. In addition, Keith noticed that Hallie did not use lip rounding on her sh-productions. He thought that, by being shown the lip rounding and providing visual feedback with a mirror, she could easily learn the lip rounding associated with this sound. Her sh-productions sounded clearly far better with the lip rounding. He was still having trouble with her s-sounds. The distortions sounded like a "th." He would have to look a little bit more into the characteristics of /s/ productions.

THE CASE OF /h/

There seem to be some differences when discussing the classification of the /h/ consonant of American English. According to the International Phonetic Alphabet (2005), /h/ is classified as a glottal fricative. Glottal (sometimes called laryngeal) fricatives are produced by a constriction of the airstream between the vocal folds or by a narrowing of the ventricular bands above the vocal folds or by both sets of bands functioning together to narrow the opening (Heffner, 1975). In other languages, such as Syrian Arabic or Dutch, this seems to be the case. The Dutch "h" is considered to be a moderately strong glottal fricative with friction produced at the margins of the vocal folds as they approximate one another (Vandeputte, Vincent, & Hermans, 1986). If one looks across languages, there seems to be a wide variation in /h/ production from those that are articulated with constriction and resulting friction noise to those with little constriction and consequently little or no friction quality. The American English /h/ seems to be one of the latter. "The usual *h* sounds of English and German, to take the most accessible examples of a very widespread phenomenon, can hardly be said to be glottal or laryngeal fricatives at all, since no audible sound is produced by the air as it passes through the larynx" (Heffner, 1975, p. 150). Ladefoged (2005) also states that, although /h/ is usually dis-

---

Concept Exercise SIBILANTS

Listen to the difference in loudness as you say at a comfortable loudness /s/, /ʃ/, /f/, and /θ/, the first sounds in "sigh," "shy," "five," and "thigh." You will notice that under comparable circumstances /s/ and /ʃ/ sound clearly louder than /f/ and /θ/. In many circumstances, such as over a telephone or in a crowded room with background noise, the fricative noise for /f/ and /θ/ is inaudible, their distinction resulting only in the formant movements from the consonant to the following vowel production (Ladefoged, 2005). Due to their relatively low intensity and similarity in acoustic properties, /f/ and /θ/, as well as /v/ and /ð/, are not reliably distinguishable from each other. Already, decades ago, Miller and Nicely (1955) found /v/ and /ð/ to be the sounds that were confused most often when noise was added to the stimuli.

---

cussed in the context of fricatives, it is not really a voiceless fricative, because the source of the noise is not air being forced through a narrow gap. Instead, the sound source is the turbulence that results as the air passes across the edges of the open vocal folds and other surfaces of the vocal tract. Therefore, the resonances of the whole vocal tract will be more prominent and "the sound is more like that of a noisy vowel" (Ladefoged, 2001, p. 58).

/h/ has also been classified as a glide. However, MacKay (1987) states that this is a phonological classification and not a phonetic one. It is phonological in that the distribution and behavior of the sound are the primary criteria; /h/ behaves like a glide. It occurs at the beginning of a syllable but not at the end, for example. This distribution is comparable to the glides /w/ and /j/.

It appears as if the vowel following /h/ does have an impact on this sound's production. Since the movement of the tongue plays no role in the articulation of /h/, the tongue is often brought into the required position for the following vowel. This may lead to coarticulatory effects, the following vowel influencing /h/ so completely that the resonance of the vowel is more prominent than the glottal friction. "What once was a voiceless glottal fricative /h/ is replaced by a voiceless vowel preceding the voiced vowel" (Heffner, 1975, p. 151). Indeed, some authors have classified /h/ as a voiceless vowel (Borden, Harris, & Raphael, 2003), a vowel onset or attack (Heffner, 1975), or a breathed (devoiced) vowel (Jones, 1932). Whichever classification you might decide on, it should be kept in mind that /h/ does not neatly fit the definition of fricative that was previously given. However, in an attempt to adhere to the classification system provided by the International Phonetic Alphabet, the phonetic description of /h/ as a voiceless glottal fricative will be used.

FOCUS 5: *What are the characteristics of fricative productions?*

AFFRICATES ➔

In American English, the consonants associated with this manner of articulation are /tʃ/ and /dʒ/. The first sounds in the following words exemplify these sounds: <u>ch</u>ug, <u>j</u>ug. An **affricate** is defined as a stop-plosive portion releasing to a homorganic (*hom* = same, *organic* = active articulator) fricative portion. The stop-plosive and fricative are articulated in one movement and are functionally (phonemically) considered one unit. Production characteristics consist of a complete closure between the active and passive articulators. The velum is raised, which results in the build-up of expiratory air pressure behind the occlusion, which is then *slowly* released resulting in a fricative portion of the speech sound. This slow release, as opposed to the sudden expulsion of air that is normally noted in stop-plosive productions, characterizes the affricates.

The affricates should not be considered merely a stop-plosive + fricative combination for several reasons. First, the phonetic production characteristics are unique for this manner of articulation. The active articulator must be similar for both the stop-plosive and the fricative portion. When examining the affricates /tʃ/ and /dʒ/, we see that this is the case. The active articulator for the stop-plosives /t/ and /d/, as well as the fricatives /ʃ/ and /ʒ/ consists of the edges of the tongue (coronal). If we look at other stop-plosive + fricative combinations, such as /ks/ in "licks" or /ps/ in "lips," we find that this is not the case. The active articulator for /k/ is the back, postdorsal section of the tongue, while for /s/ the coronal edges of the tongue serve this function. In /ps/, the active articulator for /p/ is the lower lip (labial), which is distinctly different from the front edges of the tongue for /s/.

Second, affricates are unique in that the stop-plosive + fricative combination functions as a unit, in this case as a single phoneme. Word oppositions such as "cheese" /tʃiz/ and "tease" /tiz/ attest to this fact.

Due to their phonetic transcription—/tʃ/ (t + ʃ) and /dʒ/ (d + ʒ)—it is easy to visualize that the affricate productions are merely the stop-plosives /t/ and /d/ followed by the fricatives /ʃ/ and /ʒ/. However, this is not entirely accurate. For example, Kantner and West (1960) note that, first, the initial stop portion of /t/ is articulated closer to the articulatory position for /ʃ/; therefore, it is produced more posteriorly than is normally the case with an isolated /t/. Second, movement from the stop to the fricative portion of the affricate is characterized by the front of the tongue dropping relatively slowly, creating momentarily a constriction that is typical for the /ʃ/ sound. This is different from the release of an isolated /t/ in which the tongue drops suddenly to a neutral position. The lip rounding that was noted previously for /ʃ/ and /ʒ/ is speaker and context dependent for the affricates /tʃ/ and /dʒ/.

FOCUS 6: *What are the characteristics of affricate productions?*

APPROXIMANTS

According to the IPA, the approximants consist of what have typically been labeled the liquids and glides. Thus, in American English the consonants associated with this manner of articulation are the liquids /l/ and /r/ and the glides /w/ and /j/. The first sounds in the following words exemplify these sounds: lip, rip, wish, and yes. **Approximant** as manner of articulation refers to those consonants in which the articulators come close to one another (approximate), but not nearly as close as the constriction that creates the fricative speech sounds. Therefore, the distance between active and passive articulators is wider; there is a much broader passage of air. The airflow for voiced approximants remains smooth, as opposed to the turbulent airflow for fricatives. Due to this smooth airflow and relatively wide opening, the term *frictionless continuant* has also been used to classify these sounds. Continuants are those sounds in which the primary constriction does not block the flow of air. Vowels, fricatives, nasals, and the approximants are considered continuants.

These speech sounds can be further divided into semivowel, central, and lateral approximants: the semivowel approximants include /w/ and /j/, whereas /r/ is considered a central approximant and /l/ a lateral approximant.

The **semivowel approximants** have often been named **glides** due to the movement of the articulators during their production; there is a gliding movement of the active articulator from a partly constricted position into a more open position. This group of consonants is considered the most open type of approximant, thus the name *semivowel*. According to their production, the semivowels are nearly as open and as resonant as the vowels; their acoustic formants are also similar to vowels. However, they are classified as consonants due to their phonemic function within American English. In other words, the semivowel approximants act like consonants; they do not serve as syllable nuclei but only as the onset or a portion of the onset of syllables. For example, "we" (/wi/), "queen" (/kwin/), "yawn" (/jɑn/), and "cute" (/kjut/) demonstrate these semivowel approximants as single sounds or within consonant clusters at the beginning of a syllable.

The **central approximant** of American English is /r/ and is often referred to as a liquid or rhotic consonant. The production qualities include a central airflow in which the articulators come close to one another but not close enough to create turbulent airflow or friction. The term *rhotic* indicates an r-like quality, or having an "r" timbre. There are several different "r" productions, which will be discussed later in the chapter.

The **lateral approximant** /l/ is produced with closure between the tongue and the roof of the mouth with the air escaping smoothly on one or both sides of the tongue. Thus, a lateral approximant consists of the air passing *laterally* over the sides of the tongue while the tongue blocks the center of the oral cavity. There are some noticeable differences between the /l/ productions when they occur in initial as opposed to final-word position. These differences will be described in detail in the section on individual consonant production.

The various manners of articulation are summarized in Table 5.3.

Table 5.3 Phonetic Description: Manner of Articulation

Manner of Articulation	Phonetic Descriptor	Examples
Complete blockage between the active and passive articulators Velum is raised	Stop-plosive	/p/, /b/ /t/, /d/ /k/, /g/
Complete blockage between the active and passive articulators Velum is lowered	Nasal	/m/ /n/ /ŋ/
Air is forced through a narrow constriction between the articulators	Fricative	/f/, /v/ /s/, /z/ /ʃ/, /ʒ/ /θ/, /ð/ /h/
Stop-plosive releasing to a homorganic fricative portion	Affricate	/tʃ/, /dʒ/
The articulators approximate one another but not enough to create friction	Approximate	/w/, /ʍ/ /j/ /r/ /l/

FOCUS 7: *What are the characteristics of approximant productions?*

Voicing

The fourth phonetic category that can be used to describe the production features of consonants is voicing. **Voicing** is the term used to denote the presence or absence of simultaneous vocal fold vibration resulting in voiced or voiceless consonants. The stop-plosives, fricatives, and affricates have pairs of voiceless-voiced cognates such as /p/ and /b/. Both sounds are produced with a similar articulation, but one is voiceless (/p/) and one is voiced (/b/). The nasals and approximants (with the exception of /ʍ/) are voiced; they are produced with vocal fold vibration. The voiced and voiceless consonants of General American English are summarized in Table 5.4.

Types of Consonants

Consonants are typically divided into various groupings based on their articulatory features, their acoustic characteristics, or their functional role as phonemes. First, if articulatory features are examined, consonants can be labeled either continuants or noncontinuants. **Continuant** sounds are those in which the vocal tract is not completely blocked, but rather a continuous flow of air is achieved. On the other hand, **noncontinuants** are those in which there is complete obstruction of the flow of air. In American English, the noncontinuants are the stop-plosives and affricates; the continuants are the other consonant types. The dichotomy of obstruent

Table 5.4 Phonetic Description: Voicing

Voicing	Phonetic Descriptor	Examples
With vocal fold vibration	Voiced	/b/, /d/, /g/ /v/, /z/, /ʒ/, /ð/ /dʒ/ /m/, /n/, /ŋ/ /w/, /r/, /l/, /j/
Without vocal fold vibration	Voiceless	/p/, /t/, /k/ /f/, /s/, /ʃ/, /θ/, /h/ /tʃ/ /ʍ/

versus sonorant is based on both articulatory and acoustic characteristics. **Obstruents** are those sounds that are produced with a complete or narrow constriction at some point in the vocal tract. **Sonorants** refer to the resonant quality of sounds produced with a relatively open vocal tract. Sonority is a quality attributed to a sound on the basis of its fullness or largeness and is highly correlated to the audibility of the voice (Heffner, 1975). Thus, sonorants are those sounds that have more acoustic energy, that are louder.

As was noted in the Chapter 4, vowels are considered to be sonorants. However, there is a group of consonants that are also considered sonorants: Nasals and approximants are also considered to be within this category. For nasals, the resonant quality is a result of airflow through the nasal cavity; for the approximants, it is due to the relatively wide opening between the articulators. This resonant quality of certain consonants has also led to the terms **resonant consonants** versus **nonresonant consonants**; nasals and approximants are considered to be resonant consonants, while all the other consonants of American English are nonresonant consonants. The final categorizations have to do with the function of the sound within a syllable. If a speech sound can function as the nucleus of a syllable, then it is considered to be a **syllabic sound**. Vowels are syllabics, but also some consonants can serve as syllable nuclei. For example, nasals and the lateral approximant /l/ can, under certain circumstances, be the nucleus of the syllable. If you say the word "button" casually or quickly, then /n/ could be the nucleus of the second syllable, thus [bʌtn̩]. A similar possibility can be noted with the word "little," [lɪtl̩]. A small line is placed under the consonant to indicate its function as the syllable nucleus. The last label semivowel seems to be used in two ways. In the older literature (Forchhammer, 1940; Heffner, 1975), *semivowel* referred to those consonants that could function as both syllabics and nonsyllabics. Therefore, the previously noted examples of the nasals and lateral approximant would be considered semivowels. Other authors (Ball & Rahilly, 1999; Shriberg & Kent, 2003) use the term *semivowel* to refer to the glides /w/ and /j/. **Semivowel** is used to denote the similarity between the articulation of the glides and other vowels. For the purpose at hand, the glides /w/ and /j/ will be considered semivowels. Table 5.5 summarizes the consonants according to these categories.

Table 5.5   Consonant Types

Category	Stop-Plosives	Nasals	Fricatives	Affricates	Approximants
Continuant		X	X		X
Noncontinuant	X			X	
Obstruent	X		X	X	
Sonorant		X			X
Resonant		X			X
Nonresonant	X		X	X	
Syllabic		X			lateral /l/
Nonsyllabic	X		X	X	/w/, /j/, /r/
Semivowel					/w/ and /j/

Individual Consonants

Stop-Plosives

/p/ - /b/

Word examples: p̲ig–b̲ig, rap̲id–rab̲id, tap̲–tab̲

Phonetic description: /p/ = voiceless bilabial stop-plosive,
/b/ = voiced bilabial stop-plosive

The closure or stop portion is achieved by the bottom lip (labial) coming into contact with the top lip. Air pressure is created behind this bilabial occlusion due to the fact that the velum is elevated, closing off the oral from the nasal cavity. There is simultaneous vocal fold vibration during the production of /b/. The voiceless bilabial stop-plosive /p/ can be aspirated during its production.

/t/ - /d/

Word examples: t̲oe–d̲oe, lit̲er–lead̲er, hit̲–hid̲

Phonetic description: /t/ = voiceless coronal-alveolar stop-plosive,
/d/ = voiced coronal-alveolar stop-plosive

The closure or stop portion is achieved by the edges of the tongue (corona) coming into contact with the alveolar ridge (alveolar). Air pressure is created behind this occlusion; the velum is elevated closing off the oral from the nasal cavity. There is simultaneous vocal fold vibration during the production of /d/. The voiceless coronal-alveolar stop-plosive /t/ can be aspirated during its production. See Figure 5.4 for a schematic of the tongue position.

ALLOPHONIC VARIATIONS OF /t/ AND /d/. A frequent allophonic variation of /t/ and /d/ is what is known as the flap, tap, or one-tap trill, /ɾ/.

/ɾ/

Word examples: Can be heard in words such as "lad̲d̲er," "but̲t̲er," and "cit̲y" when these stop-plosives are preceded and followed by vowels.

Phonetic description: /ɾ/ = voiced coronal-alveolar tap, flap, or one-tap trill

Concept Exercise **ALLOPHONIC VARIATIONS**

Produce the word "ladder," slowly and consciously feeling the build-up of air pressure and the release for /d/. Now try a casual production of the same word with the tongue briefly touching the alveolar ridge producing /ɾ/. Note the differences in how the two articulations feel and, importantly, how they sound.

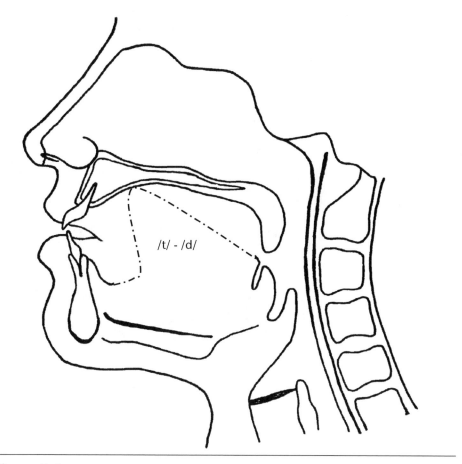

Figure 5.4 Tongue Position for /t/ and /d/: Coronal-Alveolar Articulation

This sound involves a single rapid contact between the active and passive articulators. The contact is very brief; there is not a build-up of air pressure. Instead, it is a rapid and relaxed movement toward the alveolar ridge in which the tongue tends to "bounce off" and produce a much briefer occlusion. The velum is elevated during the production, and there is simultaneous vocal fold vibration.

/k/ - /g/

Word examples: <u>c</u>ap–<u>g</u>ap, ba<u>ck</u>er–ba<u>gg</u>er, sa<u>ck</u>–sa<u>g</u>

Phonetic description: /k/ = voiceless postdorsal-velar stop-plosive, /g/ = voiced postdorsal-velar stop plosive

The closure, or stop, portion is achieved by the posterior body of the tongue (postdorsal) coming into contact with the soft palate or velum (velar). Air pressure is created behind this occlusion; the velum is elevated closing off the oral from the nasal cavity. There is simultaneous vocal fold vibration during the production of /g/. The voiceless postdorsal-velar stop-plosive /k/ can be aspirated. See Figure 5.5 for a schematic of the tongue position for /k/ and /g/.

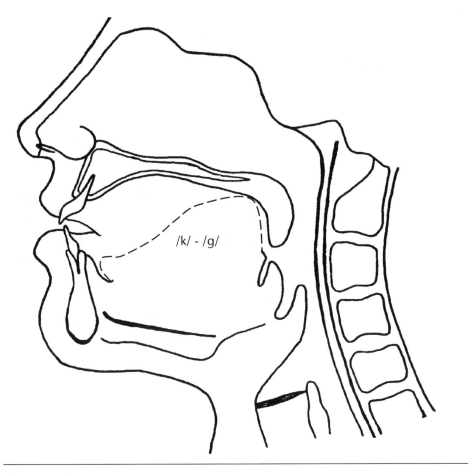

Figure 5.5 Tongue Position for /k/ and /g/: Postdorsal-Velar Production

Nasals

/m/

Word examples: <u>m</u>op, ha<u>mm</u>er, tri<u>m</u>

Phonetic description: /m/ = voiced bilabial nasal

For /m/, there is a complete occlusion between the lower lip (labial) as active articulator and the upper lip (labial) as the passive articulator. The velum is lowered; therefore, there is no build-up of air pressure, but rather the air flows freely through the nasal cavity. There is simultaneous vocal fold vibration.

/n/

Word examples: <u>n</u>o, po<u>n</u>y, to<u>n</u>

Phonetic description: /n/ = voiced coronal-alveolar nasal

For /n/, there is a complete occlusion between the edges of the tongue (corona) and the alveolar ridge (alveolar). There is no build up of air pressure behind this closure, because the velum is lowered, allowing air to flow freely through the nasal cavity. There is simultaneous vocal fold vibration.

Reflect on This: Clinical Application

IPA SYMBOLS THAT MIGHT BE USED FOR SOUND SUBSTITUTIONS FOR /k/ AND /g/.

These consonants are not a portion of the American English inventory but might be heard as sound substitutions for /k/ and /g/.

/q/ - /ɢ/

Phonetic description: /q/ = voiceless postdorsal—uvular stop-plosive, /ɢ/ = voiced postdorsal—uvular stop-plosive

These sounds are produced by occlusion of the posterior portion of the tongue (postdorsal) with the very back portion of the soft palate or velum ending in the uvula (uvular). These consonants are sometimes classified as postvelar stop-plosives. The velum is elevated during this production, and there is simultaneous vocal fold vibration during /ɢ/. For children who possibly misarticulate /k/ and /g/, this articulation would show evidence of a correct manner of articulation but one in which the active and passive articulators are moved posteriorly.

The glottal stop is considered an allophonic variation of some stop-plosive productions and can serve to release vowels in stressed syllables (Edwards, 2003) or separate successive vowels between words (Wise, 1958).

/ʔ/

Word examples: "Oh" [ʔoʊ] releasing a vowel or "Anna asks" [ænəʔæsks] often demonstrate the glottal stop separating the successive vowels.

Phonetic description: /ʔ/ = voiceless glottal stop

If the vocal folds are brought together and suddenly released after a build-up of subglottal air pressure, a slight popping noise is created. This resulting sound is a glottal stop. The glottis refers to the space between the vocal folds, thus, in this situation *glottis* (glottal) is the term used to designate the active and passive articulators. The velum is elevated during its production, and it is considered a voiceless, unaspirated consonant. Some children with misarticulations use the glottal stop as a sound substitution.

/ŋ/

Word examples: si<u>ng</u>er, ri<u>ng</u> (/ŋ/ does not occur initiating a syllable)

Phonetic description: /ŋ/ = voiced postdorsal-velar nasal

For /ŋ/ there is a complete occlusion between the back portion of the dorsum of the tongue (postdorsal) and the soft palate or velum (velar). There is no build-up of air pressure behind this closure, because the velum is lowered, allowing air to flow freely through the nasal cavity. There is simultaneous vocal fold vibration.

Fricatives

/f/ - /v/

Word examples: <u>f</u>an–<u>v</u>an, o<u>ff</u>er–o<u>v</u>er, lea<u>f</u>–lea<u>v</u>e

Phonetic description: /f/ = voiceless labiodental fricative, /v/ = voiced labiodental fricative

A narrow constriction is created between the inner edge of the lower lip (labio) and the edges of the upper incisors (dental). The velum is elevated. There is simultaneous vocal fold vibration for /v/.

/θ/ – /ð/

Word examples: <u>th</u>in (/θ/)–<u>th</u>an (/ð/), ba<u>th</u>tub (/θ/)—ba<u>th</u>ing (/ð/) brea<u>th</u> (/θ/)—brea<u>the</u> (/ð/)

Phonetic description: /θ/ = voiceless interdental or apico-dental fricative, /ð/ = voiced interdental or apico-dental fricative

There are two types of th-productions. The first type of articulation occurs if the tongue tip is protruded slightly between the upper and lower incisors; thus, the air is being channeled over the tongue tip and the edge of the upper incisors. This is labeled an interdental production (*inter* = between, *dental* = teeth). A second type of production results when the tongue is moved slightly posterior, resulting in the tongue tip (apico) approximating the inner surface of the front incisors (dental). Both /θ/ and /ð/ are wide slit channel fricatives indicating that the tongue is flat and the airflow extends over a broader surface of the tongue. The velum is elevated for these sounds, and /ð/ is produced with simultaneous vocal fold vibration. See Figure 5.6 for a schematic of the tongue positions for the two types of productions /θ/ and /ð/.

/s/ – /z/

Word examples: <u>s</u>ip–<u>z</u>ip, bu<u>ss</u>ing–bu<u>zz</u>ing, pea<u>ce</u>–pea<u>s</u>

Phonetic description: /s/ = voiceless apico-alveolar or predorsal-alveolar fricative, /z/ = voiced apico-alveolar or predorsal-alveolar fricative

Articulation of /s/ and /z/ can be accomplished in two different ways. The apico-alveolar production is realized with the tongue tip up: There is a narrow channel created by sagittal grooving of the tongue (the s-sounds are grooved channel fricatives). The air is forced over this narrow opening between the tongue tip (apico) and the alveolar ridge (alveolar). For the predorsal-alveolar production, the tongue tip is down behind the lower incisors. The tongue arches toward the alveolar ridge; however, due to the positioning of the tongue tip, the narrow channel is now between the front portion of the tongue (predorsal) and the alveolar ridge (alveolar). For all s-productions, the velum is elevated. For /z/, there is simultaneous vocal fold vibration. See Figure 5.7 for a schematic of the two types of s-productions.

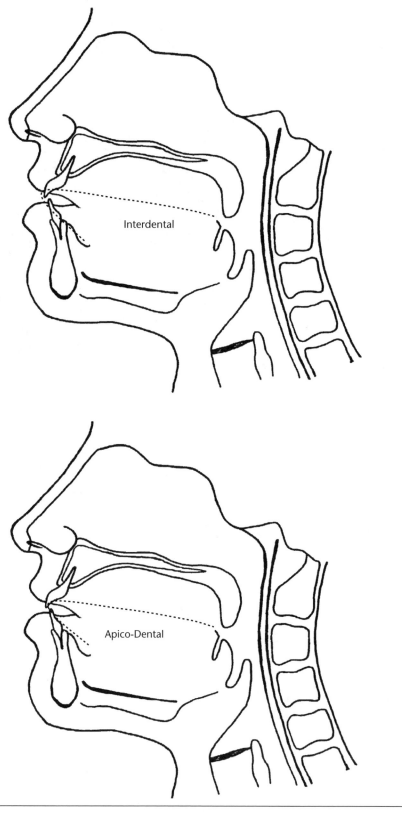

Figure 5.6 Tongue Positions for /θ/ and /ð/: Interdental and Apico-Dental Productions

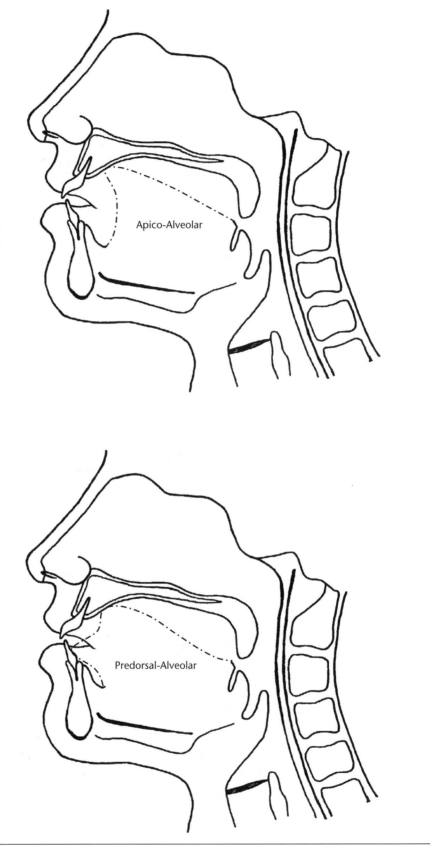

Figure 5.7 Two Types of /s/ Productions: Apico-Alveolar and Predorsal-Alveolar

Concept Exercise TWO TYPES OF S-PRODUCTIONS

Most, but not all, individuals use the tongue-tip-up apico-alveolar /s/ and /z/ articulations. Say two or three s-words, such as "sum," "sob," and "sap" and see which type of s-articulation you normally use. Now try making the other type of s-sound. You will probably find that it is not very easy. Practice going through the production characteristics of a predorsal-alveolar production and see if you can achieve an /s/ that sounds within normal limits. What type of adjustments did you have to make to your tongue position to finally get a good sounding /s/? Do you think that you could tell a child how to make those adjustments?

Reflect on This: Clinical Application

USING TWO DIFFERENT S-PRODUCTIONS IN THERAPY

Although most individuals utilize the apico-alveolar s-production in normal conversational speech, many clinicians use the predorsal-alveolar as their model when attempting to correct a faulty s-sound. Why? For the apico-alveolar /s/, the tongue tip is approximating the alveolar ridge; it is, so to speak, hovering below the alveolar ridge. This position must be precisely maintained for the entire duration of the sound. For many children, especially those who use a "th" for "s" substitution, this is a difficult task. If the tongue tip moves slightly forward, which can very easily happen, the "old" faulty articulation results. On the other hand, for the predorsal-alveolar production, the tongue tip is resting behind the lower incisors. First, this provides the child with an easily identifiable spot for the tongue tip; it gives the child something to "hold onto." Second, in this position the child cannot move the tongue tip forward and easily revert to the old articulation. Third, this "new" articulation is something quite different from the faulty production. It is often easier for a child to accomplish a completely different production task than to make minor adjustments to a previously learned one.

Beginning Case Study

KEITH, THE AUDIOLOGIST

Keith noted that Hallie distorted her /s/ productions. They sounded far more like th-sounds. They had tried to get a "tongue-tip-up" apico-alveolar production but found that Hallie could not differentiate this production from her s-distortion. Keith thought maybe that he and the clinicians could try a "tongue-tip-down" predorsal placement. It made sense to him that this type of s-production, with the child's tongue placed behind the lower teeth, might be a better choice for Hallie. With this type of production the clinician could provide visual feedback, first with a mirror to support the initial placement and then with the some type of acoustic display as feedback to help support the auditory signal that she could not hear due to her hearing loss.

/ʃ/ – /ʒ/

Word examples: <u>sh</u>ock–<u>J</u>acques, wa<u>sh</u>er–plea<u>s</u>ure, bru<u>sh</u>–bei<u>g</u>e

Phonetic description: /ʃ/ = voiceless coronal-prepalatal or coronal-postalveolar fricative, /ʒ/ = voiced coronal-prepalatal or coronal-postalveolar fricative

These fricatives are produced with sagittal grooving of the tongue; however, the channel that is created is wider and flatter than noted for /s/ and /z/. The differences in the two phonetic descriptions for /ʃ/ and /ʒ/ reflect minimal production variations; for the coronal-prepalatal articulation the edges of the tongue (corona) approximate the anterior area of the palate directly behind the alveolar ridge (prepalatal). The coronal-postalveolar version is generated by a slightly more anterior placement of the tongue. Here the edges of the tongue (corona) come very close to an area that is just posterior to the highest point of the alveolar ridge (postalveolar). There is one additional feature of /ʃ/ and /ʒ/: lip rounding. Both /ʃ/ and /ʒ/ demonstrate lip rounding; however, the degree of lip rounding depends on the surrounding context. The velum is raised during the articulation of these fricatives, and /ʒ/ is produced with simultaneous vocal fold vibration. See Figure 5.8 for a schematic of the two types of tongue positions for /ʃ/ and /ʒ/.

/h/

Word examples: <u>h</u>ead, a<u>h</u>ead

Phonetic description: /h/ = voiceless glottal fricative

The production characteristics of /h/ were discussed in detail on pages 120–121. As noted earlier, the typical /h/ of American English does not neatly fit the given categorization of a fricative. The sound source for /h/ appears to be the result of air passing over the edges of the open vocal folds as well as other portions of the vocal tract. This sound is influenced by the following vowel and has been labeled a voiceless vowel or vowel onset preceding a voiced vowel. The velum is raised during the production of /h/, and there is no vocal fold vibration during its articulation.

Reflect on This: Clinical Application

USING A TONGUE-TIP-DOWN PLACEMENT FOR /ʃ/

Some children may have difficulties with both the s- and sh-sounds. For example, children who demonstrate a tongue position that is too far forward for /s/ may also use this anterior tongue positioning for /ʃ/. Typically, the tongue shape is also somewhat flat; there is not enough sagittal grooving. The resulting productions may approximate th-sounds. If the clinician decides to use the tongue-tip-down, predorsal-alveolar /s/ placement, /ʃ/ may also be achieved with the tongue tip down behind the lower incisors. The resulting /ʃ/ articulation could phonetically be described as a predorsal-postalveolar fricative. Therefore, the tongue tip and edges are behind the lower incisors; the predorsal section of the tongue is now approximating the posterior portion of the alveolar ridge.

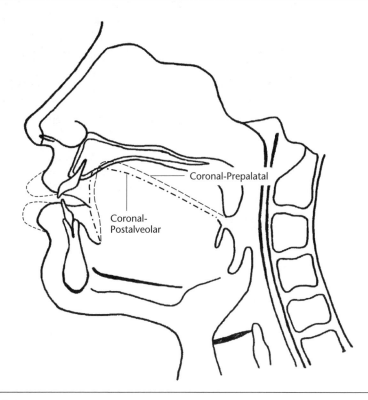

Figure 5.8 Two Tongue Positions for /ʃ/ and /ʒ/: Coronal-Prepalatal and Coronal-Postalveolar

Reflect on This: Clinical Application

FRICATIVES THAT MIGHT BE USED AS SOUND SUBSTITUTIONS IN ABERRANT SPEECH

Several other fricatives could be heard as sound substitutions for various consonants that are produced in error by children or adults with speech disorders. The following are a few of the more familiar ones.

/ɸ/ - /β/

These consonants do not occur in American English but they are speech sounds in other languages, such as Japanese (/ɸ/) and Spanish (/β/). They can be used as sound substitutions in aberrant speech; for example, a child could substitute these sounds for /f/ and /v/—the manner remains the same, but the passive articulator is moved anteriorly.

Phonetic description: /ɸ/ = voiceless bilabial fricative, /β/ = voiced bilabial fricative

(continues)

FRICATIVES THAT MIGHT BE USED AS SOUND SUBSTITUTIONS IN ABERRANT SPEECH (*continued*)

These sounds are produced by bringing the lips together so that a horizontally long but vertically narrow passageway is left between them for the breath stream to pass. To pronounce this sound, spread the lips in a smile with a narrow gap between the lips while acting as if you are blowing out a candle (MacKay, 1987). The velum is elevated during the production of these sounds, and /β/ is produced with simultaneous vocal fold vibration.

/ç/ - /ʝ/ → These sounds do not typically occur in American English but are speech sounds, for example, in German (/ç/) and Swedish (/ʝ/). They can occur as sound substitutions, such as for /ʃ/ or /ʒ/. Here the fricative manner of production remains the same; however, the active and passive articulators are positioned too far back.

Phonetic description: /ç/ = voiceless mediodorsal-mediopalatal fricative, /ʝ/ = voiced mediodorsal-mediopalatal fricative. (These sounds are often simply labeled dorsal-palatal.)

These sounds are produced with a narrow opening between the middle of the tongue (mediodorsal) and the middle of the palate (mediopalatal). In American English, /j/ is also a voiced mediodorsal-mediopalatal sound. The only difference between /j/ and /ʝ/ is the degree of constriction; /ʝ/ demonstrates a far narrower opening between the active and passive articulator. The velum is elevated during the production of these sounds, and /ʝ/ has simultaneous vocal fold vibration.

Reflect on This: Clinical Application

SYMBOLS FOR POSSIBLE /k/ AND /g/ SUBSTITUTIONS

/x/ - /ɣ/ → These sounds do not typically occur in American English, but they are speech sounds, for example, in German (/x/) and Turkish (/ɣ/). These sounds may be used as substitutions by children who are attempting to produce /k/ and /g/. If the tongue is not raised enough to produce a stop-plosive occlusion, then these fricatives could result.

Phonetic description: /x/ = voiceless postdorsal-velar fricative, /ɣ/ = voiced postdorsal-velar fricative

These sounds are produced when a narrow opening is created between the posterior portion of the tongue (postdorsal) and the soft palate or velum (velar). The velum is tensed during the production of these sounds, and there is simultaneous vocal fold vibration for /ɣ/.

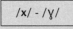

Concept Exercise A NEW SOUND

Prolong /j/, for example, the first sound in "yes." Now try to make the constriction between the middle of the tongue and the middle of the palate narrower. This should be /ʝ/. If /ʝ/ is whispered, (a voiceless production) /ç/, results.

Concept Exercise THE /x/

As you slowly release /k/, maintain airflow. If you lower the tongue slowly, a narrow opening between the articulators results in a frictionlike sound. This is the /x/ production.

Reflect on This: Clinical Application

LATERAL S-PRODUCTIONS

/ɬ/ - /ɮ/

These sounds do not typically occur in American English but are speech sounds in languages such as Welsh (/ɬ/) and Zulu (/ɮ/). They are, however, fairly common substitutions for /s/ and /z/ misarticulations. If a child produces a lateral "s," for example, the tip of the tongue is in contact with the alveolar ridge, and the lateral edges of the tongue are lowered.

Phonetic description: /ɬ/ = voiceless apico-alveolar lateral fricative or approximant, /ɮ/ = voiced apico-alveolar lateral fricative or approximant

For production of this sound, the tip of the tongue (apex) is in direct contact with the alveolar ridge (alveolar). There is no sagittal grooving of the tongue, rather, the lateral edges of the tongue are flattened. The air flows freely over the lateral edges of the tongue and into the cheeks.

Affricates

/tʃ/ - /dʒ/

Word examples: <u>ch</u>ug–<u>j</u>ug, la<u>tch</u>ing–lo<u>dg</u>ing, ba<u>tch</u>–ba<u>dge</u>

Phonetic description: /tʃ/ = voiceless coronal-alveolar (postalveolar) stop-plosive phase followed by a voiceless coronal-postalveolar fricative portion, /dʒ/ = voiced coronal-alveolar (postalveolar) stop-plosive phase followed by a voiced coronal-postalveolar fricative portion

The affricates /tʃ/ and /dʒ/ are characterized by a stop-plosive portion that releases to a homorganic fricative portion. Due to the articulation of the fricative portion of this sound, the articulation for the stop-plosive phase is slightly more posterior than is typically the case with /t/ and /d/. The velum is elevated during the production, and there is simultaneous vocal fold vibration for /dʒ/.

Approximants/Glides

/ʍ/ - /w/

Word examples: <u>wh</u>en–<u>w</u>in, no<u>wh</u>ere–a<u>w</u>ay. It should be remembered that throughout the United States the /ʍ/ has been merged with /w/. Therefore, the voiceless /ʍ/ may not occur in any productions. However, it will be covered in this section so that the reader will be familiar with the production and the phonetic symbol used for this voiceless production.

Phonetic description: /ʍ/ = voiceless labio-velar fricative, /w/ = voiced labio-velar approximant or glide

One major articulation characteristic of both /ʍ/ and /w/ is lip rounding, giving these sounds the phonetic description of bilabial. In addition, the tip of the tongue is low behind the incisors; the body of the tongue is raised toward the velum, similar to the production of the vowel /u/. This elevation of the back of the tongue toward the velum adds the descriptor *velar*. The velum is elevated during the articulation of these sounds, and /w/ has simultaneous vocal fold vibration. See Figure 5.9 for a schematic of the tongue positon for /w/ and /ʍ/.

Although these sounds are paired, voiceless /ʍ/ and voiced /w/, their production characteristics have been described somewhat differently. As noted earlier, the International Phonetic Alphabet labels /ʍ/ as a voiceless

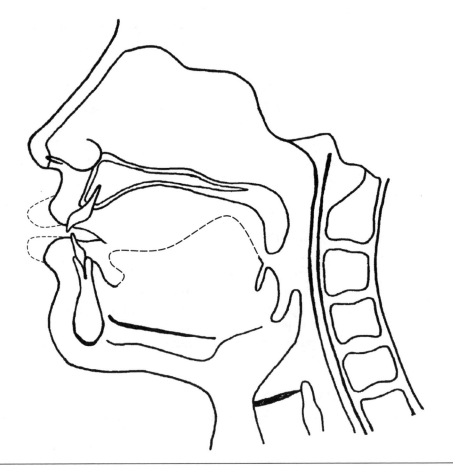

Figure 5.9 Tongue Position for /w/ and /ʍ/

labio-velar *fricative*, while /w/ is classified as an *approximant*. This is due to the friction noise and the degree of turbulent airflow that many speakers exhibit during /ʍ/.

Although textbooks typically give "wh" word examples for /ʍ/, such as "where," "when," or "whale," it should be remembered that many speakers do not actually use /ʍ/; its appearance in Standard American English has declined (Edwards, 2003) or even disappeared (Wolfram & Schilling-Estes, 2006). Therefore, pronunciation differences for "which–witch" or "while–wile" may not exist. The /ʍ/ should be seen as an allophonic variation of /w/ that historically was linked to the orthography of words, namely those spelled with "wh." /ʍ/ is not a separate phoneme of American English.

/j/

Word examples: yellow, onion

Phonetic description: /j/ = voiced mediodorsal-mediopalatal approximant or glide (rather than repeating medio- for both descriptions, /j/ is often referred to as a dorso-palatal approximant or glide)

For the production of /j/, the body of the tongue is flat rather than grooved; the airstream is forced through a broad opening. The middle portion of the tongue (mediodorsal) is in a position approximating /i/, but it is flattened slightly more toward the midsection of the palate (mediopalatal). There is a quick gliding transition between /j/ and the following vowel. The velum is elevated during this sound articulation, and there is simultaneous vocal fold vibration. See Figure 5.10 for a schematic of the tongue position for /j/.

/r/

Word examples: run, arrow

Phonetic description: /r/ = voiced mediodorsal-mediopalatal central approximant (bunched production), or voiced apico-postalveolar central approximant (tongue tip raised), or voiced apico-prepalatal central approximant (retroflex)

As mentioned in an earlier section, there are many variations of r-productions. A common articulation is the so-called *bunched* /r/. The middle of the tongue is raised (mediodorsal) toward the middle of the palate (mediopalatal); the tongue tip is relatively low, near and behind the front lower incisors. In addition, the tongue is retracted into a compact "bunched" form, giving this articulation its characteristic name. For the *tongue-tip-raised* version, the tip of the tongue (apico) is elevated and points directly toward the rear of the alveolar ridge (postalveolar). For the third type of /r/, the *retroflex* articulation, the body of the tongue is hollowed and the

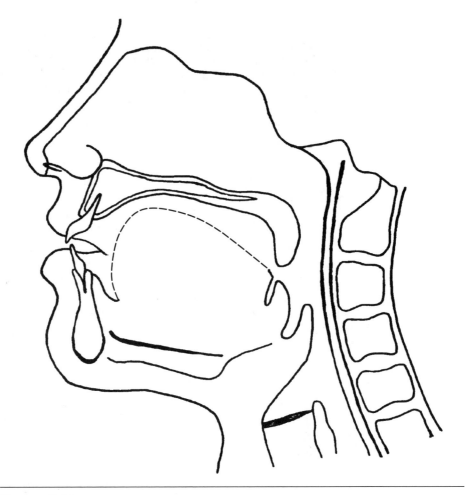

Figure 5.10 Tongue Position for /j/.

tongue is bent backwards in a more retroflexed position. Here the term *apico* refers to the underside of the tongue as it curls backward approximating the front portion of the palatal area (prepalatal). Lip rounding may be present but is variable depending on the context and the speaker. The velum is elevated, and there is simultaneous vocal fold vibration. It should be kept in mind that, although the symbol /r/ will be used in this text to represent all three r-productions, officially, according to the IPA notation system, the bunched production does not have a representative phonetic symbol, the tongue-tip-raised version is /ɹ/, and the symbol /ɻ/ is used for the retroflex central approximant. Laver (1994) suggested the symbol [Ψ] for the bunched-r, but this has not been accepted by the International Phonetic Alphabet classification system. See Figure 5.11 for a schematic of the tongue positions for the two types of r-productions, bunched and refroflexed.

/l/ →

Word examples: <u>l</u>eap, ye<u>ll</u>ow, ye<u>ll</u>

Phonetic description: /l/ = voiced apico-alveolar lateral approximant

For the production of /l/, there is contact between the tip of the tongue (apico) and the alveolar ridge (alveolar). The edges of the tongue are flat (as opposed to raised), allowing the air to escape laterally over the sides of the

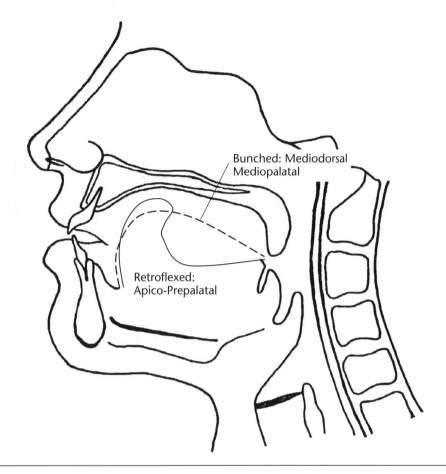

Figure 5.11 Tongue Positions for the Two Types of /r/ Productions: Bunched and Retroflexed

tongue. The velum is elevated, and there is simultaneous vocal fold vibration during the /l/ articulation.

In American English, there are two types of l-articulations, a so-called "light" (or "clear") and a "dark" version. These two l-sounds are allophonic variations: They each appear in certain contexts; however, they are not two different phonemes—they do not establish phonemic contrasts. The light l-sound (which is transcribed /l/) typically occurs before a vowel, such as at the beginning of a word such as *light* or a syllable such as *yellow*. The exception to this is possibly when /l/ occurs before the high back vowels /u/ (*loop*) or /ʊ/ (*look*), but this may vary from speaker to speaker. The dark l-sound occurs after vowels, such as in *pull* or *shawl*. There are characteristic production differences between the light and dark l-articulations. The light l-sound has been described as having an /ɪ/ quality that results from a convex shape of the tongue (*convex* = surface that is curved or rounded outward, as the exterior surface of a sphere), especially its frontal portion near the palatal or prepalatal area. The dark "l" has an /ʊ/ or /o/ quality that is caused by an elevation of the tongue's posterior portion. This high-back elevation produces a concave upper surface of the tongue behind the alveolar occlusion (*concave* = surface that is hollow, as the interior surface of a sphere). Officially, a dark "l" is transcribed [ɫ]. See Figure 5.12 for a schematic of the light and dark /l/ productions.

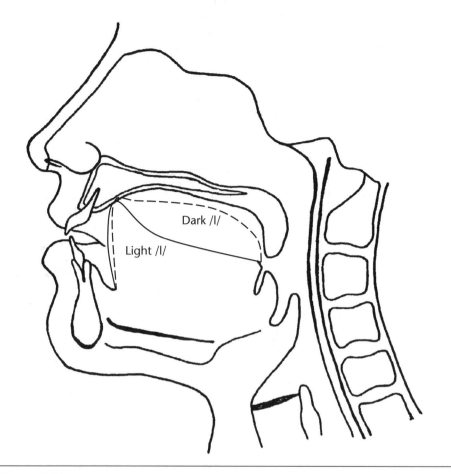

Figure 5.12 Light and Dark /l/ Productions

Reflect on This: Clinical Application

POSSIBLE R-SUBSTITUTIONS

/ʊ/

This is not a speech sound in American English but can be heard in Sindhi (the Indic language spoken in Pakistan) or Slovene (the language spoken in the Republic of Slovenia), for example. This sound may also be used by children as a substitution for /r/. Although Shriberg and Kent (2003) note that a derhotacized /r/ is one that "lacks the expected /r/ quality" (p. 118) (somewhere between an /r/ and a /w/), Gibbon (2002) states (based on intuition and not clinical data) that most typically developing children pass through a stage where /w/ is replaced by /ʊ/. On the other hand, children with r-problems may stick with /ʊ/ longer, and some use this substitution until adulthood. Therefore, this substitution and the phonetic symbol are important when documenting r-problems.

Phonetic description: /ʊ/ = voiced labiodental approximant

This sound is produced by creating a rather wide opening between the lower lip (labio) and the upper incisors (dental). The velum is elevated during the production, and there is simultaneous vocal fold vibration.

Concept Exercise LABIODENTAL APPROXIMANT

Prolong /v/ and then, while maintaining the voicing, attempt to create a somewhat wider opening between the articulators. In other words, move the bottom lip slightly away from the upper incisors. The resulting sound is /ʋ/.

This concludes the section on the consonants of American English and the more common sound substitutions that a clinician might encounter. Of course, other production modifications may occur that might result in speech sounds noted on the chart from the IPA in Chapter 3. In addition, certain symbols can be added to the basic notation to demonstrate articulatory changes in the original speech sounds. These symbols are called diacritics and will be discussed in more detail in Chapter 7.

Case Study

Amanda was a 4-year-old child who was having difficulty in preschool. She wasn't able to do the tasks that the other 4-year-old children could do, and she was difficult to understand. Here are a few words that the speech-language therapist transcribed from Amanda's speech.

Example	Word	Target	Child's Production
1.	swing	[swɪŋ]	[θwɪŋ]
2.	shovel	[ʃʌvəl]	[tʌbəl]
3.	frog	[frɑg]	[fwɑg]
4.	thumb	[θʌm]	[fʌm]
5.	knot	[nɑt]	[dɑt]
6.	coat	[koʊt]	[toʊt]
7.	fishing	[fɪʃɪŋ]	[fɪtɪŋ]
8.	lamp	[læmp]	[wæmp]
9.	zoo	[zu]	[du]
10.	three	[θri]	[twi]

Amanda had trouble with s-sounds. She substituted a [θ] for [s]. In "shovel" she used a [t] instead of [ʃ] and a [b] instead of a [v]. Can you pick out the other errors that Amanda has?

Summary

FOCUS 1: *What is meant by* active articulator? *Which terms are used to reference these points?*

Active articulator refers to the anatomical structure that actually moves during the generation of speech sounds. The tongue and lower lip are given specific names to denote their status as active articulators: (1) When the bottom lip is used, *labial* is the designated term; (2) the tip of the tongue or apex of the tongue, *apical*; (3) the front and lateral edges of the tongue (including the apex), *coronal*; and (4) the anterior one-third of the tongue, *predorsal*, the middle one-third of the tongue, *mediodorsal*, and the posterior one-third of the tongue, *postdorsal*.

FOCUS 2: *What is meant by* passive articulator*? Which terms are used to reference these points?*

Passive articulator denotes the immovable portion of the vocal tract that is paired with the active articulator. The passive articulator consists of those structures that do not or cannot move during the production of speech sounds. The phonetic terms that are used to indicate the various passive articulators include the following: (1) the upper lip, *labial*; (2) the upper teeth, *dental*; (3) the alveolar ridge, *alveolar*; (4) the palate is divided into *pre-*, *medio-*, and *postpalatal* areas; and (5) the velum, the term *velar* is used.

FOCUS 3: *What are the characteristics of stop-plosive productions?*

The stop-plosive production is characterized by complete blockage within the oral cavity: The articulators actually come in contact with one another (shutting or approach phase). As a result of the closed velum, intraoral air pressure builds up behind this occlusion (closure or stop phase). This pressure is suddenly released, which creates the characteristic stop-plosive sound (release phase). In American English, voiceless stop-plosives can be produced with more forceful air pressure resulting in aspirated, fortis productions. Voiced stop-plosives, and in some contexts, voiceless ones have typically less intraoral air pressure and are considered to be unaspirated, lenis productions.

FOCUS 4: *What are the characteristics of nasal productions?*

The manner of articulation that is associated with nasal productions is characterized by complete blockage within the oral cavity: The articulators come in contact with one another, as with the stop-plosives. However, the nasal consonants, as their name implies, are defined by an open velopharyngeal passage with air subsequently flowing through the nasal cavity.

FOCUS 5: *What are the characteristics of fricative productions?*

Fricative consonants are characterized by the active and passive articulators approximating each other so closely that the air is forced with considerable pressure through the constriction that is formed. As the air is pressed through this narrow passageway, its flow creates an audible noise, a friction-like quality called frication, which gives these consonants their name.

Fricatives can also be classified according to the shape of the opening through which the airflow is forced. A grooved fricative is one where the channel for the airflow is extremely narrow. Both /s/ and /z/ are considered grooved fricatives because the air flows through a narrow opening that is created by a sagittal (front to back), v-shaped furrow of the tongue. Fricatives with a wider and flatter channel shape are termed *slit fricatives*. The widening and flattening of the channel varies from sound to sound, giving rise to what is known as a wide slit channel, as with the th-sounds, /θ/ and /ð/, and a narrow slit channel for the sh-productions, /ʃ/ and /ʒ/. For the th-productions, the tongue shape is somewhat flat, and the airflow extends over a broader surface. On the other hand, for /ʃ/ and /ʒ/ the tongue is slightly grooved, though not nearly as much as for /s/ and /z/.

FOCUS 6: *What are the characteristics of affricate productions?*

Affricates are characterized by a productional unit that has two parts: (1) a stop-plosive followed by a (2) homorganic fricative portion. For the stop-plosive component, a complete closure is formed between the active and passive articulators that is slightly farther back in the mouth than for a typical /t/ or /d/ production. The velum is raised, resulting in the build-up of expiratory air pressure behind this occlusion. The fricative element is established by a slow release of this constriction that demonstrates productional qualities that are similar to /ʃ/ or /ʒ/. Although the affricates are composed of these two production portions, they function as one unit. Thus, [tʃ] and [dʒ] are single phonemic entities, not consonant clusters or blends.

FOCUS 7: *What are the characteristics of approximant productions?*

Approximants demonstrate a wider distance between the articulators than noted for the fricative productions. In addition, the airflow for voiced approximants remains smooth, as opposed to the turbulent airflow for fricatives. There are several different classifications of approximants. First, semivowel approximants or glides (/w/ and /j/) are characterized by a gliding movement of the articulators from a partly constricted position into a more open position. Second, the central approximant (/r/) has a central airflow in which the articulators come close to one another, but not close enough to create turbulent airflow or friction. There are several production variations of this speech sound. Third, the lateral approximant /l/ is produced with closure between the tongue and the roof of the mouth, with the air escaping smoothly on one or both sides of the tongue. The central /r/ and the lateral /l/ approximants are collectively also termed *liquids*.

Further Readings

Ball, M., & Müller, N. (2005). *Phonetics for communication disorders*. London: Routledge.

Catford, J.C. (2002). *A practical introduction to phonetics*. Cambridge, UK: Cambridge University Press.

Heffner, R. (1975). *General phonetics*. Madison: University of Wisconsin Press.

Roach, P. (2000). *English phonetics and phonology: A practical course* (3rd ed.). Cambridge, UK: Cambridge University Press.

Key Concepts

active articulator p. 111
affricate p. 121
alveolar p. 113
apical p. 111
approach phase p. 116
approximant p. 122
aspiration p. 116
central approximant p. 123
closure phase p. 116
continuant p. 124
coronal p. 111
dental p. 113
fortis consonants p. 116
fricatives p. 118
glides p. 123
glottal p. 113
glottis p. 113
grooved channel fricative p. 118
labial pp. 111, 113
lateral approximant p. 123
lenis consonants p. 116
manner of articulation p. 115
mediodorsal p. 111
mediopalatal p. 113

nasals p. 117
narrow slit channel fricative p. 119
noncontinuants p. 124
nonresonant consonants p. 125
obstruents p. 125
passive articulator p. 113
postdorsal p. 111
postpalatal p. 113
predorsal p. 111
prepalatal p. 113
release phase p. 116
resonant consonants p. 125
semivowel approximants p. 123
semivowel p. 125
shutting phase p. 116
sibilant p. 119
slit fricative p. 119
sonorants p. 125
stop phase p. 116
stop-plosives p. 116
syllabic sound p. 125
velar p. 113
voicing p. 124
wide slit channel fricative p. 119

Think Critically

1. Some younger children have trouble producing /k/ and /g/; they substitute /t/ and /d/ for these sounds. Thus the word "key" would be pronounced [ti] and "go" as [dou]. Both of the target sounds and the substitutions are stop-plosives. Compare the two articulations and see if you might be able to describe to a child what they would have to do to change the articulation from /t/ to /k/ and from /d/ to /g/.

2. There were three variations of /r/ described: bunched, tongue tip raised, and retroflexed. Describe the differences between each of these productions. Which one of the r-productions do you use in the following words: run, grow, tree, reel, rouge, brown?

3. Describe the difference between the light /l/ and the dark /l/. Find four words in which the light /l/ is used and four words in which the dark /l/ is used.

4. Describe the differences between the "tongue-tip-up" s-production and the "tongue-tip-down" production. How would you describe to a child the articulation placement of the two s-productions?

5. Children often have trouble with the lip rounding associated with the sh-sounds (/ʃ/ and /ʒ/). Which type of vowel contexts would promote lip rounding? Can you find five words which you could use to assist the lip rounding of /ʃ/ or /ʒ/?

1. Which one of the following is a lateral approximant?
   a. /r/
   b. /l/
   c. /j/
   d. /w/

2. Which one of the following is a voiced postdorsal-velar nasal?
   a. /g/
   b. /n/
   c. /ŋ/
   d. /h/

3. Which manner of articulation is characterized by air being forced through a narrow opening between the active and passive articulator, creating a turbulent friction quality?
   a. stop-plosives
   b. affricates
   c. approximants
   d. fricatives

4. One of the active articulators is the coronal edges of the tongue. Which one of the following sounds is produced with this active articulator?
   a. /r/
   b. /g/
   c. /t/
   d. /w/

5. Which one of the following is not an approximant?
   a. /w/
   b. /h/
   c. /j/
   d. /r/

6. /w/ is considered a labio-velar sound. The passive articulator label of "velar" describes that
   a. the velum is not elevated.
   b. the back portion of the tongue is elevated toward the velum.
   c. the lips (labio) and the velum (velar) come in close contact with one another.
   d. the velum vibrates.

7. The phonetic description for the "bunched" /r/ is a
   a. a voiced mediodorsal-mediopalatal central approximant.
   b. a voiced apico-alveolar central approximant.
   c. a voiced mediodorsal-mediopalatal obstruents.
   d. a voiced apico-postalveolar central approximant.

8. /h/ is described as a
    a. voiceless glottal fricative.
    b. voiceless vowel onset preceding a voiced vowel.
    c. voiceless glide.
    d. all of the above.
9. Which one of the following manners of articulation is considered a noncontinuant?
    a. nasal
    b. approximant
    c. stop-plosive
    d. fricative
10. Which one of the approximants can serve as a syllabic consonant?
    a. /l/
    b. /w/
    c. /ɹ/
    d. /j/

Answers: 1. b   2. c   3. d   4. c   5. b   6. b   7. a   8. d   9. c   10. a

For additional information, go to www.phonologicaldisorders.com

Dialect and Language Variations

Chapter Highlights

- What is the difference between Standard English and vernacular dialects?
- What are the main types of dialects?
- What are the three variables that seem to have an overall effect on the regional dialects? Explain these three variables.
- Which four regional areas were defined?
- Why is it difficult to define social dialects?
- What is African American Vernacular English? What features are unique to this dialect?
- What are limited English proficient students?

Chapter Application: Case Study

 Julie was a kindergarten teacher who had recently moved from a small town in California to Mobile, Alabama. She had grown up in the Midwest in the middle of the cornfields of Iowa, moving to California after she had graduated from college with her teaching credentials. After just getting married in the summer, her husband had accepted a wonderful job in Mobile. Her first day of class was fun and exciting. The children complained about her "Northern" dialect, and here she was thinking that everyone else had the dialect. And many of the children in her class had what she thought was a Southern dialect while others spoke African American English. She knew that there were specific differences between these dialects and General American English but she had never worked with children with a Southern dialect or with those who spoke African American English. She was a bit concerned about speech sound differences that she heard in many of the children. She knew from experience that there were always children in her kindergarten class who still were struggling with "s," "r," or "th" sounds, but she was unfamiliar with the sound changes that might occur in these two specific dialects. In addition, she wondered about the influence of the sound differences in Southern dialect and African American English in relationship to teaching beginning reading. She needed some more information about the Southern dialect of the Mobile, Alabama, area and African American English.

We are all very adept analyzers of the speech and language characteristics of individuals within our society. We can immediately tell if we are talking to someone from a geographic region other than our own based primarily on his or her pronunciation, on speech characteristics. And we are certainly aware of foreign accents, recognizing them as distinct from any regional or ethnic dialects that we may know. In a society that is composed of a wide range of geographical, ethnic, and social as well as cultural possibilities, speech and language differences seem unavoidable. These distinctions in speech and language that exist between groups of individuals within a society are referred to as dialects. **Dialect** is a neutral label that refers to any variety of a language that is shared by a group of speakers. Although this chapter focuses on the variations in speech sounds represented by a dialect, it should be kept in mind that dialects are systematic, highly regular, and cross all linguistic parameters such as vocabulary, word forms, plural endings, sentence structure, pragmatics, and melodic patterns (American Speech-Language-Hearing Association, 2003).

The purpose of this chapter is, first, to define dialect and to compare and contrast the popular conceptions versus the technical, professional viewpoints concerning this term. This will also include a differentiation between what has been labeled General American English or Standard English as opposed to Vernacular English. The second portion of this chapter will examine regional dialects, i.e., those variations that are primarily due to geographical circumstances. The focus will be on distinguishing the typical sound changes that occur relative to the various geographical regions of the United States. The next portion of the chapter defines the social and ethnic diversities that distinguish dialects. Phonological characteristics of African American Vernacular English will be provided to illustrate one dialect within the United States that has received a considerable amount of attention and has been widely researched.

The last portion of this chapter will focus on foreign dialects. In one of the more recent reports, it was estimated that over 4.5 million children speaking more than 460 different languages begin school with limited English proficiency (Office of English Language Acquisition, 2002). These numbers demonstrate the challenge facing both teachers and speech-language specialists as they address dialect issues in a truly multicultural society. Consonant and vowel inventories of the most prevalent foreign languages within the United States will be examined as well as the clinical implications that these differences present.

Dialect: Popular Versus Professional Usage

There are many different dialects of American English that are shared by a specific group of speakers. To speak a language is to speak some dialect of that language. The technical use of "dialect" as a neutral term implies no particular social or attitudinal evaluations; that is, there are no "good" or "bad" dialects. Dialects are simply those language variations that typify a group of speakers within a language. The factors that may correlate with a particular dialect usage may be as simple as geographical status or as complex as a notion of cultural identity. It is important to keep in mind that socially acceptable or "standard" versions of a language constitute dialects as much as those varieties that are considered socially isolated or stigmatized language differences.

There is often a difference in viewpoints between what dialects represent when one examines the popular viewpoint versus the professional usage. The following examples demonstrate some commonly held beliefs about dialect (Wolfram & Schilling-Estes, 2006).

1. I worked in southern Alabama and the people there most certainly have quite a dialect.
2. A graduate student in northwestern Pennsylvania said in class, "I'm from Chicago, I talk differently; I guess I have a real dialect."
3. Those children really don't speak English; they speak a dialect.

One popular use of the term *dialect* refers to those individuals who speak differently from the local, native community (statement 1). If we travel from the Midwest to Philadelphia, Texas, or the Deep South, then the native individuals sound differently. We have a tendency to label this as dialect. Being a native Midwesterner, the author was also made very aware that this is a two-way street when teaching in south Alabama and having students complain about not being able to understand my "Northern dialect." That only other people speak a dialect is ethnocentric; what one group of speakers considers the "norm" is another group's dialect. Professionally, *dialect* is a label that refers to any variety of a language that is shared by a group of speakers.

A second common use of the term *dialect* is to refer to those varieties of English that have become recognized, for one reason or another, throughout our society (statement 2). We are all aware of what a Southern drawl sounds like, or a Boston accent. New Yorkers or Chicagoans accept their speech as being different due to the widespread consensus that they speak a dialect; the characteristic speech patterns of these regions have become popularized through the media. The same level of awareness is not present if we speak of a Denver or a Cedar Falls dialect. Reported variations in dialect follow this same pattern; there is a lot more information available on certain dialects, such as those on the East Coast, as opposed to those in the Midwestern states. However, every area of the United States can be represented by a dialect. Every area of the United States has its dialect; however, some dialects appear to be more popularized than others.

The third statement is an extreme use of the term *dialect*. Here *dialect* refers to a type of deficient, inadequate use of English. In this case, dialect is perceived as an unsatisfactory attempt to speak "correct" English that results in a deficit form of English. Professionally, dialects are not considered deviant or substandard versions of American English; in fact, they are *different* language patterns. These language patterns are often complex and demonstrate a rich use of language forms and functions; they are most certainly not simplifications or errors. This can be exemplified by citing some of the variations noted in African American Vernacular English (AAVE). It has often been quoted that in AAVE the plural-s form is deleted, for example, "one car," "three car." This is only the case when the quantifier, in this case "three," is present. If the sentence would be ambiguous without the plural ending, such as "Grab my book," versus "Grab my books," then the plural is added. Or perfect tense is expressed by *been* to denote action

It is the position of the American Speech-Language-Hearing Association (ASHA) that no dialectal variety of American English is a disorder or pathological form of speech or language. Each dialect is a functional and effective variety of American English. Each serves a communicative and social-solidarity function that helps maintain communicative and social network for the community of speakers who use it. Each dialect is a symbolic representation of the geographic, historical, social, and cultural background of its speakers (American Speech-Language-Hearing Association, 2003).

Some examples of playing the dozens:

"Your mother looks so ugly, she look like nine miles of bad road with a detour at the end" (Smitherman, 1994, p. 11).

"You're so ugly; you went into a haunted house and came out with a job application" (Morgan, 1998, p. 268).

completed a long time ago that is still relevant ("I been known him a long time") versus use of the uninflected *be* to indicate a habitual state ("She be working at McDonald" indicating that she is working at McDonald's now) (Rickford, 1999). In addition, there is a rich tradition of witty, sarcastic dialogue that goes on between two participants. This is known as signifying, playing the dozens, snapping, and sounding to mention just a few of the terms. The idea of the game is to say something really funny, humorous, and exaggerated about a person or your mother. One of the basic rules of playing the dozens is that what you say cannot be literally true (Smitherman, 1996). These word plays demonstrate a highly developed sense of dialogue and humor.

To summarize, first, dialects are language variations that reflect intricate language patterns and very often a rich cultural history. They are by no means substandard variations of language. Second, everyone who speaks a language speaks some dialect; it is not possible to speak a language without speaking a dialect of the language. And third, the professional notion of dialect exists apart from the social status of the language variety; in other words, dialects should not be negatively or positively valued.

However, one *does* refer to Standard English. Does this mean "proper English"? Or "correct English"? The next section examines Standard English and its relationship to dialect or so-called vernaculars.

Standard English and Vernacular English

Many languages have what are referred to as "standards." Some standards provide a language form that serves as a bridge between dialects. For example, in some countries, such as France, Spain, and Germany, the language variations that are referred to as dialects are so different that one speaker may not understand another dialect speaker. To establish a common language that can be used to effectively communicate, "standards" are established. While this is not the case in American English, there is a language form that is referred to as Standard English.

There appear to be two sets of representations of Standard English, a formal and an informal version. **Formal Standard English**, which is applied primarily to written language and the most formal spoken language situations, tends to be based on the written language and is exemplified in guides of usage or grammar texts. When there is a question as to whether a form is considered Standard English, then these grammar texts are consulted. An informal definition of Standard English is more difficult to define. **Informal Standard English** takes into account the assessment of the members of the American English speaking community as they judge the "standardness" of other speakers. This notion exists on a continuum ranging from standard to nonstandard speakers of American English (Wolfram & Schilling-Estes, 2006). It relies far more heavily on grammatical structure than pronunciation patterns. In other words, listeners will accept a range of regional variations in pronunciation but will not accept the use of socially stigmatized grammatical structures. For example, a rather pronounced Boston or New York regional dialect is accepted, but structures such as "double negatives" would not be considered Standard English. On the other hand, **vernacular dialects** refer to those varieties of spoken American English that are considered to be outside the continuum of informal Standard English (Wolfram & Schilling-Estes, 2006). Vernacular dialects are signaled by the presence of certain structures. Therefore, a set of nonstandard English structures mark them as being vernacular. For example, the presence of double negation, lack of subject–verb agreement, and using variations from standard verb forms would be features that would label the speaker as utilizing a vernacular dialect. Although there may be a core of features that exemplify a particular vernacular dialect, not all speakers display the entire set of structures described. Therefore, differing patterns of usage exist among speakers of one particular vernacular dialect.

FOCUS 1: *What is the difference between Standard English and vernacular dialects?*

Dialectal Variations and Change

Before we begin our description of the various regional and social dialects that exist within the United States, it is important to consider some parameters relative to the study of dialect. First, the speech and language parameters of American English are not static; they are dynamic entities that change constantly. As you read this text, the dialect features within the United States are in the process of alteration. What is recognized today as contemporary knowledge regarding dialect features will not be the same tomorrow. For example, Standard English had a somewhat different form in the past and will be altered in the future. There are many reasons for this change. One obvious reason is that young people become slowly older and replace older individuals. These youngsters are in turn replaced by still younger speakers of American English. New terms, expressions, and pronunciation patterns slowly evolve from this aging process. Many of the extensive dialect studies were based on surveys that were conducted in the 1930s and 1940s. More recent information has demonstrated that, relative to certain features, dialects may not have changed greatly, while there is evidence that in other respects some dialect areas are losing the distinctiveness they possessed.

Wolfram (1991) notes four sociocultural changes that have impacted dialect: (1) new patterns of migration within the United States, (2) changing relationships among cultural groups, (3) redefinition of cultural centers, and (4) improved means of transportation and communication to formerly remote areas. As new immigrants continue to move into America, foreign languages continue to affect American English. For example, Hispanic English has become very widespread in certain states, producing such variations as a merger of such phonemes as /ʃ/ and /tʃ/, producing "wash" as "watch," and the reduction of word-final consonants, resulting in a pronunciation of [lɛf] for "left." Changing relationships among cultural groups includes the desegregation of ethnic communities and the adoption and variation of certain features from other ethnic groups. This would include the large influence of African American music, fashion, and speech patterns on the youth culture. Adolescents all over the nation can

Gullah is a dialect (officially a creole) that is spoken on the Sea Islands and coastal regions of South Carolina, Georgia, and northeastern Florida. This distinction was maintained for many years due primarily to the geographic isolation of the community. Creoles will be discussed later in the chapter.

be heard using terms and phrases that are a portion of African American English. A third type of sociocultural change is the shifting of cultural centers. In the early 1900s, many Americans left rural areas for the economic advantage of larger cities. This created a transplant of certain dialect features that characterized rural speech. The current trend is just the opposite; the move continues from the inner cities to the suburbs, shifting the focus of linguistic change. For example, Eckert (1988) demonstrated that suburban Detroit, as opposed to inner-city Detroit, served as the center of dialect change for adolescent teenagers in that area. Finally, we find that the improvement of transportation and communication to previously remote areas has influenced language variations. This has often resulted in a phenomenon known as dialect endangerment. As certain areas such as the Outer Banks and the Sea Islands (home of the Gullah speech community) become more accessible to tourists, the distinctive variations that were fostered in relative isolation and spoken by relatively few people are quickly becoming extinct.

What Are the Defining Boundaries of a Dialect?

Dialects may vary along several parameters. First, one can describe a dialect according to its hypothesized causative agent. In this way, two main categories are formed: (1) those dialects corresponding to various geographical locations that are considered **regional dialects** and (2) those that are in general related to socioeconomic status and/or ethnic background, labeled as **social** or **ethnic dialects**. In addition, dialects are classified according to their linguistic features. This would include the phonological, morphosyntactical, semantic, and pragmatic differences that are distinctive when that dialect is compared to informal Standard English. It appears that regional dialects typically demonstrate phonological and semantic features that are unique. On the other hand, social and ethnic dialects may vary along *all* of the previously stated linguistic features.

This chapter will examine regional, social, and ethnic dialects, with the primary focus on phonological aspects of these differences. However, it should always be kept in mind that dialects do demonstrate other language variations as well. Phonological variations within a dialect can be very obvious, such as the pronunciation patterns of a pronounced Southern dialect, or quite subtle, existing somehow below the conscious level as they set apart groups of speakers.

These phonological variations may incorporate four dimensions: substitution processes, phonotactic processes, consonant cluster variations, and prosodic variability. **Substitution processes** occur when a sound in one dialect corresponds to a different sound in another dialect. For example, certain dialects distinguish between the productions of the vowels [ɔ] and [ɑ], using [ɔ] in "caught" and [ɑ] in "cot." Other dialects do not realize this difference, resulting in the same pronunciation for both words. **Phonotactic processes** are those variations in which phonemes are added or deleted when compared to informal Standard English. For example, "l" and "r" are absent in a number of dialects, resulting in the pronunciation of [wʊf] for "wolf" and [kɑd] for "card." A specific type of phonotactic process, **consonant cluster variations**, are those phonological differences that affect strings of consonants. One important consonant cluster variation that impacts dialects of American English relates to the sequences of consonants at the end of words. Words such as "west," "find," "act," and "cold" may be reduced to [wɛs], [faɪn], [æk], and [koʊd]. Although this kind of cluster reduction is found in the informal speaking styles of practically all speakers of Standard English, it is typically restricted to those instances in which the word following the cluster begins with a consonant (e.g., "ac' cool" or "col' feet"). On the other hand, speakers of vernacular dialects may reduce the cluster in other situations as well (e.g., "wes' end", "I's col' out"). The fourth area, **prosodic variability**, refers to noted differences in intonational contours of sentences, the timing of sounds and syllables, and stress patterns of words that may distinguish a particular dialect. Thus, whether the words "Ju-ly," "ho-tel," and "the-a-ter" are stressed on the first or second syllable are predictive of specific dialects.

It is of interest to note that phonological variations within a dialect are typically socially significant only when they apply to consonant variations; vowel differences are seen as interesting but unimportant (Wolfram, 1991). Therefore, the diphthongization of certain vowels heard in the South or the characteristic changes in the e, a, ɒ vowels noted in the Boston area are not valued socially nor are they stigmatized. On the other hand, changes in consonant productions are more apt to be considered as socially significant, even to the point of stereotyping the speaker (Wolfram & Schilling-Estes, 2006). For example, if a speaker says [bæf] for "bath," [diz] for "these," or [fʌm] for "thumb," this would be far more significant than changes in the vowel qualities. The next section on regional dialects will examine both the vowel and consonant variations that seem to delineate the main regional areas of the United States. We will find that dialects are changing, and this change is creating a new mapping of regional dialects within the United States.

FOCUS 2: *What are the main types of dialects?*

Regional Dialects

One initial question posed about the regional dialects of American English references the number of separate dialects: How many regional dialects exist within the United States? A large corpus of information has been collected, extending from small microcultures of dialect to general trends that can be applied to the United States as a whole. The fact still remains that discrete boundaries between dialects are often difficult to determine, and the differences that are unique to one particular dialect are not always easy to establish. As a result, the answer depends on how detailed you would like to be. Therefore, an answer to our original question would probably be somewhere between two and 200. A second complication when trying to map out regional dialect areas is the fact that many of the earlier mappings were more lexically oriented. In other words, primarily differences in vocabulary were used to differentiate between regional dialect areas. However, since our main focus is phonology, these types of mappings may not be the best way to look at regional dialects. A third variable is related to the relatively rapid changes in dialect that have been observed. Although a great amount of data has been collected over the last years, the shifts in U.S. dialects during this century have been rapid enough to outpace the data collection. With these difficulties in mind, this section on regional dialects will first provide a general overview of the three variables that seem to have an overall effect on the regional dialects: (1) the Northern Cities and South vowel shifts, (2) the merging of specific vowels, and (3) the variations of r-productions.

Northern Cities and South Vowel Shifts

The Northern Cities and South vowel shifts are examples of chain shifts. **Chain shifts** are systematic changes in vowel systems in which the vowels shift in respect to their articulatory features. The articulatory features may change according to tongue height, tongue position (fronting or backing of the tongue), or rounding of the lips. Also, sets of features can change together, such as shortening or lengthening of vowels, deletion, epenthesis (the insertion of a sound segment in a word, typically the /ə/ vowel, e.g., /sənoʊ/ for "snow"), and metathesis (the transposition of sounds, e.g., /æks/ for "ask") (Labov, 1991).

Chain shifts demonstrate the tendency of sound systems to maintain specific phonemic distinctions. They do this by the fact that surrounding vowels also change, so there is a rotation of the *entire* vowel system. Thus, as one vowel changes its production features, other vowels shift to accommodate this change. For example, if the tongue height of one vowel is somewhat lowered, the neighboring vowel will also shift to a lower articulatory position. This maintains articulatory distance between the vowels. If the entire system did not change, but only the articulatory features of one or two vowels, then the productions of certain vowels might become so close that we could perceive them as one and the same vowel. When we say "Northern Cities," we are referring to the northern tier of the United States from the White Mountains of New Hampshire across Western New England, New York state, northern Pennsylvania, Ohio, Indiana, Illinois, Michigan, and Wisconsin. It is most strongly advanced in the largest cities: Syracuse, Rochester, Buffalo, Cleveland, Toledo, Detroit, Flint, Gary, Chicago, and Rockford (Carpenter, 2003; Labov, 1991). On the other hand, the Southern vowel shift is found throughout the Southern states, the South Midland and the Southern mountain states. The Northern Cities shift and the Southern shift rotate the vowels in opposite directions (Labov, Yaeger, & Steiner, 1972; Labov, 1994). This, in effect, moves the pronunciation patterns of these two dialects of American English farther away from each other.

The Northern Cities shift is characterized by the movement of the articulatory positions of several vowels. The shift begins when [æ], the vowel in "cad," begins to sound like the [iə] of "idea." Since a shift has occurred, the vowel [ɑ] in "cod" then shifts forward to fill the space that has opened up, so that it sounds somewhat like [æ] in "cad" to speakers and listeners of other dialects. The next closest vowel, [ɔ] in "cawed," moves downward to the position formerly occupied by [ɑ], while the [ʌ] in "cud" now moves forward to fill the spot left by [ɔ.] Finally, the vowel [ɛ] in "ked" moves into the direction of [ʌ]. The [ɪ] vowel in "kid" moves

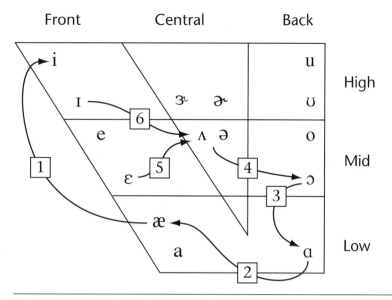

Figure 6.1 The Northern Cities Vowel Shift

downward and backward to a more centralized production. Although this sounds complicated and confusing, if one is able to use the vowel quadrilateral and the shifts around this quadrilateral as a reference point, then the Northern Cities shift is fairly easy to understand. This rotation is shown in Figure 6.1.

A few examples will probably better illustrate this shift. It should be remembered that the vowels are not being replaced by other vowels in this chain reaction, but rather are sounding more like the noted vowels in the rotation process.

1. Start of vowel shift: the tongue position for [æ] moves upward and forward in the direction of [i͡ə].

   "How <u>sad</u>" [ha͡ʊ <u>sæd</u>] starts to sound like [ha͡ʊ <u>si͡əd</u>]

2. The tongue position for [ɑ] moves upward and forward in the direction of [æ] to fill the space as the articulation of [æ] moves.

   "<u>Stop</u> it" [<u>stɑp</u> ɪt] starts to sound like [<u>stæp</u> ɪt]

3. The tongue position for [ɔ] moves downward to fill the space previously occupied by [ɑ].

   "He <u>caught</u> a cod" [hi <u>kɔt</u> ə kɑd] starts to sound like [hi <u>kɑt</u> ə kɑd]

4. The tongue position for [ʌ] moves downward and backward to fill the space previously occupied by [ɔ].

   "He's <u>shut</u> in" [hiz <u>ʃʌt</u> ɪn] starts to sound like [hiz <u>ʃɔt</u> ɪn]

5. The tongue position for [ɛ] moves back in the mouth to fill in the space previously occupied by [ʌ].

   "<u>Let's</u> go" [<u>lɛts</u> go͡ʊ] starts to sound like [<u>lʌts</u> go͡ʊ]

6. The tongue position for [ɪ] becomes more centralized, moving into the [ʌ] direction.

   "He <u>will</u> go" [hi <u>wɪl</u> go͡ʊ] starts to sound like [hi <u>wʌl</u> go͡ʊ]

The vowel rotation for the Southern vowel shift moves in an opposite direction from the Northern Cities shift. How does this look practically? It begins when [ɑɪ] becomes a monophthong and its articulation shifts slightly more forward. The onglide of the diphthong [eɪ] drops until it becomes the lowest vowel in the system. Therefore, [eɪ] in "cake" ([keɪk]) sounds somewhat like [kaɪk]. The [i] vowel (which is described as a diphthong [iə] in this example) follows a similar path as the [e] vowel; thus, the position moves somewhat back and downward. The short front vowels [ɪ] and [ɛ] shift forward and upward until they reach the positions formerly occupied by [i] and [eɪ]. Thus, "tin" ([tɪn]) might sound somewhat like [tin] and "ten" ([tɛn]) like [teɪn]. The [æ] vowel also moves in a parallel direction with [ɪ] and [ɛ], namely forward and upward. The back vowels [u] and [o] move forward and become more centralized. Next, the vowel [ɔ], as in "cord" [kɔɚd], moves into the [oɚ] position, often becoming merged with [o] so that "cord" and "code" sound as if the vowel quality is the same. Finally, the [ɑɚ] vowel, as in "card," shifts up and back to the position vacated by [ɔɚ]. The Southern vowel shift is illustrated in Figure 6.2. Unlike the Northern Cities vowel shift, the Southern shift is more advanced in rural areas of the South than metropolitan areas.

This could be further exemplified by the following:

1. [ɑɪ] becomes a monophthong [ɑ], and its articulation shifts slightly forward.

   "How nice" [haʊ naɪs] sounds more like [haʊ nɑs], the [ɑ] sounding a bit more centralized, in the direction of [ʌ]

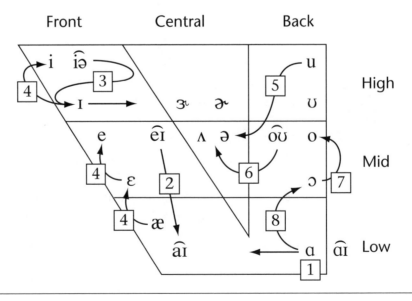

Figure 6.2 Southern Vowel Shift

2. The onglide of [eɪ] drops becoming a low front vowel approximating [a], thus [aɪ].

   "Way to go" [weɪ tu goʊ] sounds more like [waɪ tu goʊ]

3. [i] moves somewhat down and back.

   "She's so bad" [ʃiəz soʊ bæd] sounds more like [ʃɪz soʊ bæd] (the [ɪ] may even sound a bit centralized)

4. The vowels [ɪ], [æ], and [ɛ] shift forward and upward to [i] and [e].

   "Let him go" [lɛt hɪm goʊ] sounds more like [let him goʊ]

   The vowel [æ] moves forward and upward.

   "I can't" [aɪ kænt] sounds more like [aɪ kent]

5. [u] becomes more centralized.

   "Hey you" [heɪ ju] sounds more like [heɪ jʌ]

6. [oʊ] becomes more centralized.

   "Oh no" [oʊ noʊ] sounds more like [ʌ nʌ]

7. [ɔɚ] moves into the [oɚ] position.

   "It's torn" [ɪts tɔɚn] sounds like [ɪts toɚn]

8. [ɑɚ] moves into the [ɔɚ] position.

   "How hard" [haʊ hɑɚd] sounds more like [haʊ hɔɚd]

Mergers

As noted above, chain shifts rotate features yet preserve phonemic distinctions by maintaining articulatory distance between the two vowels. On the other hand, **mergers** neutralize features, and phonemic distinctions are lost. Thus, two sounds, in this case two vowels, tend to become more like each other. The phonemic boundary between the two becomes indistinct, and one vowel may emerge as the prevalent pronunciation. There are basically two types of mergers: (1) unconditioned mergers, which affect the phonemes wherever they appear, and (2) conditioned mergers, which occur in a specific phonemic environment. The only unconditioned merger in the vowel system of General American English is the collapse of the distinction between [ɑ]/[a] and [ɔ].

The distinction between [ɑ]/[a] and [ɔ] is one that often distinguishes words such as "cot" and "caught," "hock" and "hawk," and "Don" and "dawn." In approximately half of the United States these word pairs are pronounced the same, i.e., the distinct vowel quality between the words has become merged. There are distinct areas where this merger predominates: Northeastern New England, including Maine, New Hampshire, Vermont, and the northeastern portion of Massachusetts, stopping a bit south of the Boston area, Western Pennsylvania (which extends northward to

Concept Exercise **SOUTHERN VOWEL SHIFT**

   Can you come up with some more examples that might fit the Southern chain shift? Even if you are not from the South, you might be able to come up with some words or phrases that could exemplify this process.

include Erie), Virginia, northern Kentucky, a southward extension of the Canadian merger, and the American West. Some variation is noted in certain large cities such as Los Angeles, the Bay area, and Denver. This merger continues to expand and is stronger in younger speakers. See area 2 on Figure 6.3. There are certain geographical areas in which this merger is not occurring. The Inland North, most of the South, and the mid-Atlantic states show considerable resistance to the spread of this merger. See area 1 on Figure 6.3.

A second merger, in this case a conditioned merger, is the distinction between [ɪ] and [ɛ] before [m] and [n]. This would be represented in words such as "pin" and "pen" or "him" and "hem." Results of this merger demonstrate that a high front vowel is used so that "pin" and "pen" sound like "pin" to speakers of other dialects. As a result distinctions are used by speakers such as "ink pen" and "safety pin" to dichotomize the two words, which sound similar in this merger process (Labov, 1996). This merger has been known to exist for a longer period of time within Southern dialects. Its continued expansion in these areas has been documented by Brown

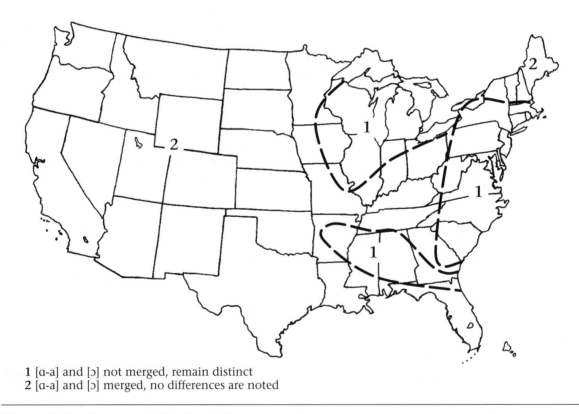

1 [ɑ-a] and [ɔ] not merged, remain distinct
2 [ɑ-a] and [ɔ] merged, no differences are noted

Figure 6.3 The Merger of [ɑ-a] and [ɔ]
Source: Adapted from Labov (1996).

(1990) and Bailey and Ross (1992). It is also widespread throughout the South Midland (southern Ohio, central Indiana, Illinois, Missouri, and Kansas), Texas, and a scattering of points in the West. The areas where the pen–pin distinction is solidly maintained include the inland and a portion of the South Midland, all of Pennsylvania, and the middle Atlantic states. On the other hand, the merger does seem to be extending northward and westward from its base in the South. Figure 6.4 demonstrates this merger: (1) notes areas where a distinction between [ɪ] and [ɛ] before nasals is maintained while (2) notes areas where there is no distinction.

Variations of R-Productions

Another major variable in American English dialects is the regional use of "r." In this instance, we are referring to the centering rhotic diphthongs such as [ɑ͡ɚ] in "car," [ɛ͡ɚ] in "bear," and the central vowel with r-coloring [ɝ] in "bird," which were discussed in Chapter 5. Several production

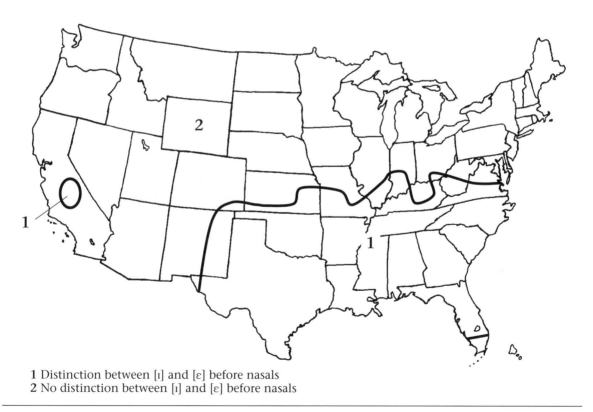

1 Distinction between [ɪ] and [ɛ] before nasals
2 No distinction between [ɪ] and [ɛ] before nasals

Figure 6.4 The Merger of [ɪ] and [ɛ] Before Nasals

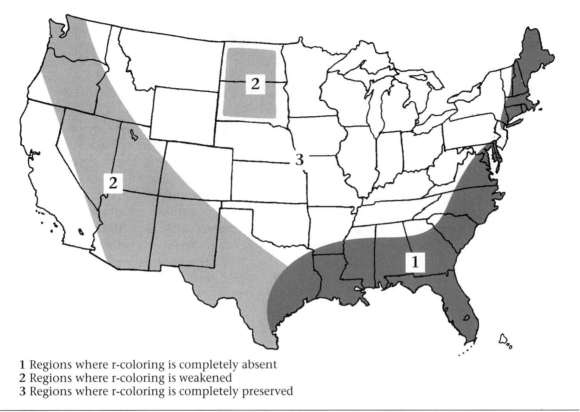

1 Regions where r-coloring is completely absent
2 Regions where r-coloring is weakened
3 Regions where r-coloring is completely preserved

Figure 6.5 Variations of r-Lessness

Source: Hartman (1985).

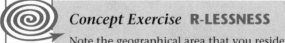

Concept Exercise **R-LESSNESS**

Note the geographical area that you reside in. Do you fit the pattern described for producing rhotic vowels?

possibilities may occur with these r-sounds. First, the r-coloring is completely absent. For example, "bird" would be pronounced [bɜd] and "car" as [kɑə]. The second possibility is that the characteristic r-quality has been weakened, often attributed to less retroflexion of the tongue (Hartman, 1985). Finally, this r-sound may be totally preserved, which is the case in many regions of the United States. Figure 6.5 is a map of the regional distribution of "r" variations. The area marked 1 represents regions where the r-coloring is completely absent. The region marked 2 is where the r-quality has been weakened. The unmarked area represents those portions of the United States where the r-quality is completely preserved.

FOCUS 3: *What are the three variables that seem to have an overall effect on the regional dialects? Explain these three variables.*

Phonological Geography of the Mainland United States

There are some differing viewpoints on how to divide up the United States into distinct regional dialect areas. A traditional view listed three dialect groups in the United States: Northern, Midland, and Southern. More recently a simple North–South distinction has been suggested, but significant differences in the boundaries of each proposed area were noted. On the other hand, many researchers believe that there are no discrete dialect boundaries and no clear-cut dialect divisions within American English. However, data from the Telsur Project show clear and distinct dialect boundaries with a high degree of similarity within each dialect. The Telsur Project of the Linguistics Laboratory of the University of Pennsylvania is one of the largest and most extensive ongoing collections of data related to the dialect regions of the United States. The data consist of phonetic transcriptions and acoustic analyses of vowel systems of informants. These data have been recently compiled in the *Atlas of North American English* (Labov, Ash, & Boberg, 2005) and represent the active processes of change and diversification that the authors have been tracing since 1968 (Labov, 1991, 1994, 1996; Labov, Yaeger, & Steiner, 1972). Their results document four major dialect regions: the North, the South, the West, and the Midland. The first three demonstrate a relatively uniform development of the sound shifts of American English, each moving in somewhat different directions. The fourth region, the Midland, has considerably more diversity, and most of the individual cities have developed dialect patterns of their own. The following is given as a brief summary of these four major dialect regions based on Labov, Ash, and Boberg (2005). Figure 6.6 demonstrates the dialect areas of the United States based on the results of the Telsur Project.

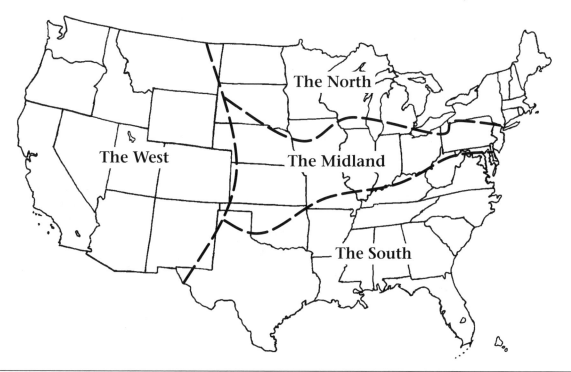

Figure 6.6 Dialect Areas of the United States Based on the Results of the Telsur Project
Source: Labov, Ash, & Boberg (1997).

NORTH. The area marked "North" is divided into the North Central region, the Inland North, Eastern New England, New York City, and Western New England. For the short vowels /ɪ/, /ɛ/, /æ/, /ʊ/, /ʌ/, and /ɑ-a-ɔ/, these areas all evidence the Northern Cities vowel shift, which was discussed previously. For the long vowels, which include the diphthongs, the North Central and the Inland North regions maintain a long high position, which is typical of the vowel quadrilateral that has been presented in this text. The r-coloring of postvocalic r-productions (rhotic diphthongs) such as in "farm" [fɑɚm] is also maintained in these areas.

On the other hand, the Eastern New England area demonstrates r-lessness in which (1) rhotic diphthongs, such as those noted in "farm" ([fɑɚm]) and "care" ([kɛɚ]), could be produced without the r-coloring, as in [fɑəm] or [fɑm] for "farm," ([kɛə]) or [kɛ] for "care"; (2) stressed central vowels with r-coloring, such as in "bird" ([bɝd]) and "shirt" ([ʃɝt]), could be produced as [bɜd] for "bird" and [ʃɜt] for "shirt"; and (3) unstressed central vowels with r-coloring, such as in "mother" ([mʌðɚ]) and "over" ([oʊvɚ]), will lose the r-coloring, resulting in possible pronunciations such as [mʌðə] for "mother" and [oʊvə] for "over." In addition, [ɑ] and [ɔ] are merged into an intermediate vowel, typically [ɑ] or more frequently [a]. Thus, distinct pronunciations for words such as [kɔt] for "caught" and [kɑt] for "cot" are not realized. Instead, one similar vowel is used for both words. The exception to this appears to be the town of Providence, which has the characteristic r-lessness but does not merge the [ɑ] and [ɔ] vowels.

New York City appears to have a unique dialect that is not reproduced farther west and, therefore, cannot fit neatly into any larger regional groupings. The long vowels maintain a high position that is similar to that noted for the North Central and Inland North areas. There is consistent r-lessness of postvocalic "r" *except for* the central vowel with r-coloring [ɝ] (the vowel sound heard in "bird") and when final "r" is followed by a vowel in the next word, such as "the car is here," [ðə kɑɚ ɪz hɪə]. In addition, the [æ] vowel splits into a lax and tense form, and the production differences between [ɑ] and [ɔ] are maximal, the [ɔ] vowel being raised to a mid-high position. No clear patterns of sound change seem to be occurring in Western New England. The Northern Cities shift seems to be transitional in this area.

SOUTH. The South demonstrates the Southern shift, which was noted earlier beginning with the monophthongization of [ɑɪ] and the subsequent shifts that occurred. However, a small area of the Southeast is distinct from the rest of the South, and includes the two cities of Charleston and Savannah. In these cities, there is a low level of monophthongization, and subsequently the Southern shift is not fully recognized. Another characteristic of the Southern region is the [ɑ] – [ɔ] distinction. With the exception of the margins of the South—west Texas, Kentucky, Virginia, and the city of Charleston—this distinction is marked not by a change in the vowel quality but by a back upglide for [ɔ]. Thus, acoustically the nuclei of the vowels are very similar; however, [ɔ] is productionally signaled by a back upgliding movement of the tongue, something close to the production of [ɔʊ].

Beginning Case Study

JULIE, THE KINDERGARTEN TEACHER

Julie realized that many of the vowel changes that she was hearing were due to the influence of the Southern vowel shift and the Southern regional dialect. She would have to be careful with her pronunciation and try to predict the pronunciation patterns of the vowels as she began to teach sound–letter correspondence for the vowel sounds. She wondered about the similarities and differences between the Southern dialect and African American Vernacular English. It seemed that many of the vowel dialect features were similar; however, there were some differences that she also could hear. She decided to get some more information on African American Vernacular English.

MIDLAND. Speakers in the Midland area do not seem to participate in either the Northern Cities shift or the Southern shift. They are distinct from the North Central region, as there is a tendency to lax the long high vowels, thus [i] becomes more like [ɪ] in quality, and [e] like [ɛ]. This region is also distinct from the South in that the diphthongal quality of [a͡ɪ] is maintained. Labov, Ash, and Boberg (1997) divide the Midland into two sections: South and North. The consistently noted feature of the South Midland is the fronting of [o͡ʊ] resulting in an [ʌ]-like quality. For example, [to͡ʊd] may sound in the direction of [tʌd]. Exceptions are Louisville, Kentucky, and Savannah, Georgia. According to this criterion, Philadelphia is a member of the South Midland, while Pittsburgh and St. Louis are considered North Midland.

THE WEST. The diversity of dialects decline steadily as one moves westward, resulting in a diffusion of Northern, Midland, and Southern characteristics. While there are exceptions, characteristics of the West are aligned with those of the Midland. The most prominent feature of Western phonology is the merger of [ɑ] and [ɔ]; however, as noted previously, this is not unique to the West. The second feature that emerges is the fronting of the vowel [u]. Although these two characteristics are also noted in the South Midland, there appears to be a much higher frequency of occurrence in the West.

Regional dialects are related to geographical regions within the United States. As noted, these regional boundaries have shifted over the years. Certain phonological changes have occurred and continue to occur, demonstrating the dynamic nature of language. Other important variables of dialect have also been recognized in the study of American English: Two of these are the social and ethnic dimensions of dialect. This next section will examine these two aspects as they relate to phonological variations within the United States.

FOCUS 4: *Which four regional areas were defined?*

Social and Ethnic Dialects

Although the social dimension of dialect has been recognized for decades within the study of language variation, it was typically assigned a secondary role in large-scale surveys. However, over the past years, due to the interest and possible impact of socially based differences in language, these issues have become a primary rather than a secondary focus in many dialect studies (Wolfram & Schilling-Estes, 2006). Social dialectology, or the study of **social dialects**, that is, dialects correlated to social differences, is now a recognized specialization within dialectology.

Research that correlates linguistic behavior with social stratification must be grounded in valid social classifications. Although social status may be subjectively evaluated, the challenge for the researcher is to reduce these subjective, rather abstract notions to objective, measurable units that can be correlated to linguistic variation. Typical variables include occupation, level of education, income, and type of residential dwelling, which are then associated with ranked levels within each category. The overall ranking obtained from combining scores for the different variables is the socioeconomic status, or SES.

In recent years, these socioeconomic scales have been scrutinized and criticized. These scales seem to overwhelming reflect the values of white male mainstream speakers of middle and higher classes and ignore important variables such as the status of the female in the household, for example (Kiesling, 1998). An alternative solution has been relying on community members to make judgments about status differences. However, this type of assignment also has its problems. Different pictures of social class may emerge from representatives of different segments of the community. The lower class may, for example, perceive the entire social class structure very differently from the upper class.

There are other social variables that intersect with social class, including region, age, and gender, to mention a few. One important correlate of linguistic difference relates to the so-called linguistic marketplace (Sankoff & Laberge, 1978). In this evaluation, the person's economic activity, broadly defined, is associated with language variation. For example, people in certain occupations tend to use more standard varieties of a language than members of the same social class who hold other occupations. Thus, teachers or salespeople, who deal on a continual basis with the public's expectations of "standardness," typically use more standard forms than individuals of the same social class in other occupations. On the other hand, working-class males may use more vernacular variations as a means of projecting economic power. These individuals have occupations associated with physical toughness and manliness and hence, it is hypothesized, more vernacular language features (Kiesling, 1998).

The social significance of language forms also changes over time. For example, the historical study of the English language supports the fact that the use of "ain't" and double negatives was once socially insignificant but now has become a stigmatized form (Labov, 1996). The social significance of certain pronunciation patterns also varies over time, shifts sometimes taking place from one generation to the next. Within a period of fifty years, the use of postvocalic "r" in New York City has moved from having little social significance to a well-defined pattern of social stratification in younger speakers (Labov, 1996). The presence of postvocalic "r" ([kɑ͡ɚt] in "cart") is more highly valued than its absence ([kɑt] for "cart"). Also the lack of postvocalic "r" was at one time considered very prestigious in the South, following the model of British English. This has, however, changed over the decades and is now considered a social delineation for either rural speakers or older speakers; urban upper-class speakers tend to pronounce the postvocalic "r."

Another factor that plays an important role in changing patterns of language is ethnicity. Ethnicity relates to those groups of individuals that share a common language, customs, or traditions. The impact of ethnicity on language change will be discussed in the next section.

FOCUS 5: *Why is it difficult to define social dialects?*

Ethnicity

Often *race*, *culture*, and *ethnicity* are used interchangeably within professional literature and informal conversations. However, there are distinctions between each of these terms. **Race** is a biological label that is defined in terms of observable physical features (such as skin color, hair type and color, and head shape and size) and biological characteristics (such as genetic composition). **Culture** may be defined as a way of life developed by a group of individuals to meet psychosocial needs. It consists of values, norms, beliefs, attitudes, behavioral styles, and tradition. **Ethnicity** refers to commonalities such as religion, nationality, and region. While race is a biological distinction, it can take on ethnic meaning if members of a biological group have evolved specific ways of living as a subculture (Battle, 1993).

There are several different kinds of relationships that may exist between ethnicity and language variation. For ethnic groups that maintain a language other then English, there is the potential of language transfer. **Transfer** indicates the incorporation of language features into a nonnative language, based on the occurrence of similar features in the native language. In some Hispanic communities in the Southwest, the use of "no" as a generalized tag question (You go to the movies a lot, no?) may be attributable to the transfer from Spanish. Other phonological features that are attributable to Spanish transfer include the merger of /ʃ/ and /tʃ/ ("shoe" sounds like "chew"), the devoicing of /z/ to /s/ ("lazy" becomes [le͡ɪsi]) and the merger of /i/ and /ɪ/ ("pit" as "peat" or "rip" as "reap").

While some of the linguistic characteristics found among ethnic groups may be directly attributable to transfer from another language, others may be possibly related to certain strategies as the individual acquires English as a second language. In addition, some of the ethnically correlated variation may not be traceable to previous language background at all. Some of the variation may simply be related to assimilation with respect to regional and social dialects. For example, native Italian, Jewish, and Irish speakers in Boston are all at somewhat different stages in respect to specific vowel changes that are typical of that region.

One of the most publicized ethnic dialects is African American English, or African American Vernacular English. A survey of published research in American English shows that more than five times as many publications are devoted to it than to any other group of American English dialects (Schneider, 1996). The next section will examine some of the general and phonological characteristics of this dialect.

African American Vernacular English

African American Vernacular English is the best known and most controversial dialect of American English. Even the name of this dialect has undergone considerable change and debate. More recently the labels Black English, Vernacular Black English, Afro-American English, Ebonics, African American Vernacular English, and African American Language have been used.

In discussing African American Vernacular English, it seems to still be important to start with a disclaimer about language and race. There is no foundation that there is a racial (biological characteristics such as physical features or genetic composition) for the language differences shown by some Americans of African descent. There are many documented instances of individuals of African descent who are raised in European American communities (Standard English communities) who talk no differently than their peers. Conversely, Americans who learn their language and interact primarily with speakers of African American Vernacular English will adopt these features (Wolfram & Schilling-Estes, 2006). (The author recalls a research project at a Florida school-based prekindergarten school consisting of 40 percent white European Americans in which all of the children spoke "African American Vernacular English" due to their neighborhood environments.) There is a continuing need to confront and set straight the controversy about language and race. In the following discussion, it should be understood that dialect issues are related to ethnic, social, and environmental issues rather than genetically determined language differences.

Although African American Vernacular English shares many commonalities with Standard American English and Southern English, there are certain characteristics that distinguish this dialect. These differences affect the phonological, morphological, syntactical, and semantic systems. In this section only the phonological variations will be addressed.

As noted previously, not all African Americans use African American Vernacular English, and among those who do, the degree of use differs significantly. There are several variables that influence the use of African American Vernacular English: age, gender, and socioeconomic status being the most noted. Relative to age, there is evidence that the use of this dialect decreases as the individual becomes older. Elementary school children use a type of dialect that varies the most from the mainstream language, while dialect features that appear prominently in adolescence level off in adulthood (Washington, 1998).

Gender differences in the use of African American Vernacular English have also been reported. As noted previously, males often exhibit increased use of vernacular, nonstandard forms relative to females. This increase in use within the male population possibly represents differential socialization along gender lines; more positive values of masculinity are associated

Although this dialect is now popularly referred to as Ebonics, most professionals prefer *not* to use this label. The term "Ebonics" tends to evoke strong emotional reactions and, according to Wolfram and Schilling-Estes (2006), has "unfortunately given license to racist parodies of various types in recent years" (p. 211). Most professionals prefer to use more neutral labels such as African American Vernacular English or African American English.

with more frequent use of vernacular forms, while women, particularly middle-class women, use standard forms more frequently (Labov, Yaeger, & Steiner, 1972).

Differences in the use of African American Vernacular English according to socioeconomic status are also apparent. Lower- and working-class African Americans reportedly use this dialect more frequently than middle- or upper-middle-class African Americans. This distinction may also reflect differences in educational background. Terrell and Terrell (1993) suggest that there is a continuum of dialect use from those who do not use the dialect at all to those who use it in almost all communicative contexts. This continuum is significantly influenced by social status variables. In addition, African Americans from middle- and upper-middle-class backgrounds appear to be more adept at **code switching**, changing back and forth between two or more languages or dialects—in this case, African American Vernacular English and Standard American English—than lower- and working-class counterparts.

There appear to be three major issues related to a discussion of African American Vernacular English: (1) how specific features, in this case phonological features compare to other dialects of the United States; (2) the historical roots and development of this dialect; and (3) the nature of language change that is presently taking place in African American Vernacular English.

If a comparison is made between the documented phonological features of African American Vernacular English and other dialects within the United States, four types of phonological distinctions can be noted. First, there are those features that could occur in all dialects of American English but are either more frequent or occur in a wider range of communicative contexts in African American Vernacular English. In Table 6.1, the first four

Table 6.1 Frequently Cited Features of African American Vernacular English

Features that appear in most dialects of American English and appear to be more prevalent in African American Vernacular English

Feature	Example
1. Final consonant cluster reduction (loss of second consonant)	first girl → firs' girl; cold → col; hand → han
2. Unstressed syllable deletion (initial and medial syllables)	about → 'bout; government → gov'ment
3. Deletion of reduplicated syllable	Mississippi → miss'ippi;
4. Vowelization of postvocalic [l] (replacement of a consonant by a vowel)	table → [teɪbə]; pool → [puə]

Features that appear in vernacular dialects of American English but not in standard dialects

5. Loss of "r" after consonants (after [θ] and in unstressed syllables)	throw → [θoʊ], professor → [pəfɛsɚ]
6. Labialization of interdental fricatives	bath → [bæf]; teeth → [tif]
7. Syllable-initial fricatives replaced by stops (especially with voiced fricatives)	those → [doʊz]; these → [diz]
8. Voiceless interdental fricatives replaced by stops (especially when close to nasals)	tenth → [tɛnt]; with → [wɪt]

(continued)

Features that appeared in old-fashioned Southern dialects

9. Metathesis (exchanging of sounds) of final /s/ + stop	ask → [æks]; grasp → [græps]
10. Loss of r-coloring of stressed central vowel [ɝ]	bird → [bɜd]; word → [wɜd]
11. Loss of r-coloring of centering diphthongs with [ɚ]	fear → [fiə]; farm → [faəm]
12. Loss of r-coloring of unstressed central vowel [ɚ]	father → [faðə]; never → [nɛvə]

Features that are recently evolving in Southern and African American Vernacular dialects

13. Reduction of diphthong [aɪ] to [a] before voiced obstruents and in the final-syllable position	tied → [tad]; lie → [la]
14. Centering of offglide in [ɔɪ] to [ɔə]	oil → [ɔəl]; boil → [bɔəl]
15. Merger of [ɛ] and [ɪ] before nasals	pen → [pɪn]; when [wɪn]
16. Merger of tense and lax vowels before [l] ([i] → [ɪ]; [e] → [ɛ])	bale and bell → [bɛl]; feel and fill → [fɪl]
17. Fricatives become stops before nasals	isn't → [ɪdn̩]; wasn't → [wʌdn̩]

Features that are apparently unique to African American Vernacular English

18. Stressing of initial syllables, shifting the stress from the second syllable	police → ['poʊ.lis]; Detroit → ['di.trɔət]
19. Deletion of final nasal consonant but nasalization of vowel preceding this deletion (noted by ˜ above the vowel)	man → [mæ̃]; thumb → [θʌ̃]
20. Final-consonant deletion (especially affects nasals) with lengthening of the vowel (noted by : after the vowel)	mean → [mi:]; fine → [fa:]
21. Final-stop devoicing (without shortening of preceding vowel)	bad → [bæ:t]; dog → [da:k]
22. Coarticulated glottal stop with devoiced final stop	bad → [bæ:tʔ]; dog → [dɔkʔ]
23. Loss of [j] after specific consonants (loss of palatalization in specific contexts)	computer → [kamputə]; Houston [hustn̩]
24. Substitution of [k] for [t] in [str] clusters	street → [skrit]; stream → [skrim]

Sources: Stockman (1996); Wolfram (1994).

items belong to this category. Second, some phonological variations occur in not only African American Vernacular English but in other nonstandard vernacular dialects as well, however, not in formal or informal standard dialects. Items 5 through 8 in Table 6.1 represent these features. Third, there are phonological features that represent those noted in the phonology of the South. Some of these features (items 9–12 on Table 6.1) are old-fashioned features of Southern phonology and are rapidly disappearing from present-day speech. Others (items 13–17) do not appear or only rarely appear in earlier records of African American Vernacular or Southern dialect but have emerged during the last quarter of the nineteenth century and are expanding rapidly in both the speech of African American Vernacular English and Southern dialect. The last set of features (items 18 through 24 in Table 6.1) seem to be unique to African American Vernacular English.

Beginning Case Study

JULIE, THE KINDERGARTEN TEACHER

Julie realized that many of the vowel differences that she heard were a part of the features of both Southern and African American Vernacular English. For example, while she said "eye" [aɪ̂], the children in her classroom said something like "ah" [ɑ]. And while you could definitely tell the difference between "pen" and "pin" in Julie's speech, this was not always the case with the children. Often both words sounded like "pin." This might prove to be a complication when teaching the children to write and read these two words. It was also interesting to find out that the end consonants in words could be deleted in African American Vernacular English. The fact that the vowel preceding the deleted nasal usually had a nasal quality demonstrated that the children understood that a nasal consonant was part of the word. This would be helpful when teaching them reading. Also she understood that the th-sounds could be replaced by "f" and "d" in African American Vernacular English ("fum" for "thumb" and "dese" for "these"), so that these should not be considered speech sound problems. And the occasional loss of "r" on words such as "mother" and "father" could also be a dialect feature. Julie felt that she was beginning to understand some of the dialect differences that she might have to work with as a teacher with a Western dialect immersed in a different region and culture.

FOCUS 6: *What is African American Vernacular English? What features are unique to this dialect?*

The second issue that is important when examining African American Vernacular English is the origin and development of this dialect. While it is not within the scope of this text to examine historical aspects in detail, they are most certainly a portion of the heritage of the United States, and some basic information is warranted.

There are two major hypotheses concerning the origin of this dialect: the Creolist Hypothesis and the Anglicist Hypothesis. The Creolist Hypothesis states that African American Vernacular English developed from a creole language. A **creole** is a pidgin language that has become the mother tongue of a community (Crystal, 1987). A **pidgin** language is a system of communication that has grown up among people who do not share a common language but who want to talk to each other. Pidgins have a limited vocabulary, a reduced grammatical structure, and a much narrower range of function when compared to other languages. Pidgins and creoles are two stages in a single process of linguistic development. First, within a community an increasing number of people begin to use a pidgin as their principal means of communication. As a consequence, their children hear the pidgin more than any other language, and gradually it takes on the status of a mother language. Within a generation or two it has become consolidated, the structure more expanded, and thus, a vernacular language in its own right. The Creolist Hypothesis maintains that the creole upon which African American Vernacular English is based was fairly widespread in the South before the Civil War. Vestiges of this creole are still found today in Gullah, more popularly called "Geechee," which is spoken by a small number of African Americans in the Sea Islands off the coast of South Carolina and Georgia. This hypothesis states that this particular creole was common among the descendants of Africans on Southern plantations but was not spoken to any extent by the whites (Wolfram & Schilling-Estes; 2006).

The second hypothesis, the Anglicist Hypothesis, maintains that the roots of African American Vernacular English can be traced to the same source as Anglo American dialects—the dialects of English spoken in the British Isles. Thus, the hypothesis is that the language contact situation was roughly comparable to that of other groups of immigrants. Under this scenario, slaves brought with them to North America a number of different African languages. Over the course of generations, only a few minor traces of these ancestral languages remained as African Americans learned the regional and social varieties of surrounding white speakers. According to the Anglicists, creoles did not play a significant role in the history of the vernacular dialect. Creoles such as Gullah are considered to be anomalies based on a special set of social and physical circumstances unique to the isolated Sea Islands. Although the Creolist Hypothesis was clearly favored up until the 1980s, data have emerged in the form of written records of ex-slaves, interviews, and a limited set of audio recordings that seem to support the Anglicist Hypothesis (Bailey, Maynor, & Cukor-Avila; 1991). If these data are analyzed, it does seem that earlier African American Vernacular English was not nearly as distinct from postcolonial Anglo American English varieties as would have been predicted from the Creolist Hypothesis.

The last issue related to African American Vernacular English examines the direction of change of this dialect: Is the direction of change one of divergence or convergence? Although it might be assumed that this dialect is converging with other dialects of American English, research conducted by Labov (1985) supports the premise that African American Vernacular English is actually diverging from surrounding vernaculars. Although the examples given are grammar related, there is also evidence that the vowel shifts, such as the unique vowel system noted in Philadelphia or the Northern Cities vowel shift, are not spreading to African American Vernacular speakers. Also, the Southern vowel shift seems to be predominantly found among Anglo Americans within that region and not African American speakers of this dialect.

To summarize, this section has first defined social and ethnic dialects. Examples have been provided that attempt to delineate these two areas while at the same time pointing out the difficulties inherent in objectively quantifying their stratification. The most prominent example of an ethnic dialect is African American Vernacular English. The second part of this section examined the phonological characteristics that are found in this dialect. Very often, these features overlap with other vernacular dialects and with those noted in the South. However, there are certain distinct sound patterns that seem to be found only in African American Vernacular English. These features and examples were provided. The last portion briefly discussed the historical roots and development of African American Vernacular English and the nature of language change that is presently taking place within this particular dialect.

The next portion of this chapter will explore the phonological variations that occur when American English is the second language. These are

A new dialect is emerging based on rap lyrics. Due to the popularity of this music, young teenagers of every social and ethnic background are adopting the words, pronunciation, and melodic patterning of rap. This is officially labeled *rap dialect* (Mallinson, 2004).

the characteristics that we perceive as being a foreign accent when listening to speakers whose native language is Japanese or Spanish, for example. Many of these features are a direct result of the sound systems of the native language and can be predicted; others are influenced by regional and social contacts. As the population within the United States increasingly becomes a melting pot of languages, information relevant to foreign dialects will become important when working with both children in the public schools and adults in the workplace.

Phonological Variations: Foreign Dialects

The number of immigrants coming to the United States has increased, averaging close to a million per year since 1990 (*Yearbook of Immigration Statistics*, 2003). These individuals come from a wide array of countries and backgrounds. They bring to the United States a wealth of different languages. One way to examine the types and numbers of non-English language backgrounds is through the statistics provided by the Office of English Language Acquisition in the data they have collected for **limited English proficient students** within the United States.

According to their latest statistics (OELA, 2002), there were more than 460 languages spoken by limited English proficient students nationwide. The data submitted indicate that Spanish is the native language of the great majority of limited English proficient students (79.2%), followed by Vietnamese (2%), Hmong (1.6%), Cantonese (1%), and Korean (1%). All other language groups represented less than 1% of the limited English proficient student population. Languages with more than 10,000 speakers included Arabic, Armenian, Chuukese, French, Haitian Creole, Hindi, Japanese, Khmer, Lao, Mandarin, Marshallese, Navajo, Polish, Portuguese, Punjabi, Russian, Serbo-Croatian, Tagalog, and Urdu.

These national figures, however, mask substantial regional variations in linguistic diversity. For example, in eight states Spanish was not the

Reflect on This: Clinical Application

WHAT IS A "LIMITED ENGLISH PROFICIENT" STUDENT?

The term "limited English proficient" is used for any individual between the ages of 3 and 21 who is enrolled or preparing to enroll in an elementary or secondary school who was not born in the United States or whose native language is a language other than English. Also individuals who are Native Americans or Alaska Natives and come from an environment where a language other than English has had a significant impact on the individual are included in this definition. Difficulties in speaking, writing, or understanding the English language compromise the individual's ability to successfully achieve in classrooms where the language of instruction is English or to participate fully in society (P.L. 107-110, The No Child Left Behind Act of 2001). Title III funds are provided to ensure that limited English proficient students, including immigrant children and youth, develop English proficiency and meet the same academic content and academic achievement standards that other children are expected to meet.

dominant language among limited English proficient students: Blackfoot was the top language in Montana, French in Maine, Hmong in Minnesota, Ilocano in Hawaii, Lakota in South Dakota, "Native American" in North Dakota, Serbo-Croatian in Vermont, and Yup'ik in Alaska. Table 6.2 contains the three top languages spoken by limited English proficient students by state (2001–2002 statistics).

With this large variety of languages, this text will examine the phonological systems of only the top five languages represented in this survey and Arabic. Therefore, the following section will contrast the vowel, consonant, and suprasegmental systems of Spanish, Vietnamese, Hmong, Cantonese, Korean, and Arabic to the phonological system of American English. This contrast is provided as a way to possibly predict which sounds or features might be difficult for individuals learning English as a second language. Although other factors play a role in second language acquisition, such as the length of time in the United States and the age at which the individual came to the United States, it still appears that a primary cause of difficulty is the interaction or transfer between the native language and American English (Yeni-Komshian, Flege, & Liu, 2000).

FOCUS 7: *What are limited English proficient students?*

Spanish American English

There are many dialects and language variations of Spanish that all fall under this one rather large categorization. Immigrants within the United States who speak Spanish seem to fall basically into five major origins: those from (1) Mexico, (2) Central and South America, (3) Puerto Rico, (4) Cuba, and (5) other countries that were not specifically identified in the 2000 census (U.S. Census Bureau, 2000). Figure 6.7 gives an estimate of the distribution of Spanish-speaking individuals within the United States according to this census.

This discussion will first examine some basic qualities of the vowel and consonant system of Mexican Spanish and then attempt to note those differences that might occur in the various dialects of Spanish such as Puerto Rican Spanish or Nicaraguan Spanish.

There are five vowels in Spanish: /i/, /e/, /u/, /o/, and /a/. There are no central vowels in Spanish, neither those without r-coloring nor those with r-coloring. In addition, all Spanish vowels are long and tense. Thus, for the Spanish student of English, the contrasts between "beat" and "bit," "pool" and "pull," "boat" and "bought," and "cat," "cot," and "cut" are difficult. In addition, the [e] and [o] vowels are monophthongs in Spanish. So while easily recognizable, they will sound somewhat different. There is some comparability between the diphthongs of Spanish and English: /aɪ/, /aʊ/, and /ɔɪ/. However, the gliding action between onglide and offglide is quicker and reaches a higher, more distinct articulatory position (Gonzáles, 1988).

The consonants of Spanish show many similarities. The voiced and voiceless stop-plosives are present in Spanish; however, the /t/ and /d/ are articulated as dentals as opposed to the alveolar production of the American English /t/ and /d/. For the Spanish productions, the tip of the tongue is against the edges of the inner surfaces of the upper front teeth. The

Table 6.2 Top Three Languages Spoken by Limited English Proficient Students (LEPS) by State

States	# LEPS	First Language	%	Second Language	%	Third Language	%
USA	4,552,403	Spanish	79.00%	Vietnamese	2.00%	Hmong	1.60%
Alabama	7,434	Spanish	74.7%	Vietnamese	5.80%	Korean	1.90%
Alaska	19,896	Yup'ik	38.6%	Inupiak	11.20%	Spanish	10.00%
Arizona	198,477	Spanish	85.0%	Navajo	7.80%	Apache	1.30%
Arkansas	10,600	Spanish	87.%	Lao	2.40%	Vietnamese	2.20%
California	1,511,299	Spanish	83.40%	Vietnamese	2.50%	Hmong	1.80%
Colorado	71,199	Spanish	81.80%	Vietnamese	2.60%	Asian	unspecified
Connecticut	21,492	Spanish	67.60%	Portuguese	5.30%	Polish	2.80%
Delaware	2,371	Spanish	72.30%	Haitian Creole	7.6%	Korean	3.3%
DC	5,435	Spanish	76.40%	Vietnamese	3.90%	Amharic	2.50%
Florida	249,821	Spanish	75.80%	Haitian Creole	12.4%	Portuguese	2.2%
Georgia	64,849	Spanish	70.10%	Vietnamese	4.40%	African	unspecified
Hawaii	11,687	Ilocano	31.80%	Samoan	12.40%	Marshalles	9.10%
Idaho	19,298	Spanish	78.80%	Native American (unsp)	5.60%		
Illinois	140,540	Spanish	77.60%	Polish	4.40%	Arabic	1.70%
Indiana	20,467	Spanish	64.40%	Penn.Dutch	3.7%	Japanese	1.5%
Iowa	11,402	Spanish	62.30%	Serbo-Croatian	11.60%	Vietnamese	6.70%
Kansas	19,075	Spanish	81.30%	Vietnamese	4.40%	Lao	1.60%
Kentucky	5,119	Spanish	47.30%	Serbo-Croatian	13.00%	Vietnamese	6.40%
Louisiana	6,346	Spanish	48.50%	Vietnamese	25.10%	Arabic	4.40%
Maine	2,737	French	16.80%	Spanish	12.90%	Passamaquoddy	10.70%
Maryland	12,183	Spanish	53.00%	Korean	6.00%	Haitian Creole	3.4%
Massachusetts	24,165	Spanish	69.40%	Portuguese	10.00%	Khmer	5.10%
Michigan	36,463	Spanish	44.80%	Arabic	22.50%	Chaldean	5.00%
Minnesota	46,601	Hmong	34.10%	Spanish	28.30%	Somali	6.60%
Mississippi	63,116	Spanish	60.40%	Vietnamese	18.80%	Choctaw	7.10%
Missouri	2,954	Spanish	44.20%	Serbo-Croatian	19.20%	Vietnamese	6.60%
Montana	11,525	Blackfoot	25.20%	Crow	15.60%	Dakota	10.60%
Nebraska	7,575	Spanish	76.80%	Vietnamese	6.10%	Nuer	3.30%
Nevada	10,301	Spanish	91.50%	Tagalog	1.90%	Chinese	unspecified
N. Hampshire	38,902	Spanish	38.70%	Serbo-Croatian	10.50%	Portuguese	3.80%
New Jersey	3,321	Spanish	67.3%	Portuguese	3.8%	Korean	3.3%
New Mexico	52,701	Spanish	78.8%	Navajo	14.6%	Vietnamese	.5%
New York	58,308	Spanish	62.2%	Cantonese	5.2%	Russian	3.0%
North Carolina	165,238	Spanish	77.6%	Hmong	5.6%	Vietnamese	2.2%
North Dakota	52,482	Native American	85.9%	Serbo-Croatian	4.5%	Spanish	2.2%
Ohio	7,.190	Spanish	39.20%	Arabic	8.20%	Somali	8.00%
Oklahoma	19,814	Spanish	51.70%	Cherokee	20.20%	Choctaw	4.20%
Oregon	43,410	Spanish	72.50%	Russian	8.40%	Vietnamese	3.60%
Pennsylvania	44,126	Spanish	52.90%	Vietnamese	5.00%	Khmer	3.60%
Rhode Island	31,277	Spanish	69.80%	Portuguese	6.70%	Kabuverdianu	4.9%
South Carolina	10,164	Spanish	77.30%	Russian	2.80%	Vietnamese	2.4%
South Dakota	6,900	Lakota	57.40%	Spanish	8.80%	German	8.6&
Tennessee	5,848	Spanish	61.20%	Vietnamese	4.80%	Arabic	4.20%
Texas	12,350	Spanish	93.40%	Vietnamese	1.90%	Cantonese	0.70%
Utah	558,773	Spanish	65.30%	Navajo	6.70%	Vietnamese	2.50%
Vermont	41,057	Croatian	26.70%	Vietnamese	16.70%	Spanish	12.30%
Virginia	998	Spanish	60.40%	Korean	5.20%	Vietnamese	4.80%
Washington	35,298	Spanish	60.90%	Russian	7.50%	Vietnamese	6.40%
West Virginia	57,409	Spanish	26.30%	Arabic	8.60%	Khmer	8.5%
Wisconsin	1,139	Spanish	47.80%	Hmong	40.10%	Lao	1.10%
Wyoming	29,037	Spanish	90.40%	Vietnamese	6.00%	Russian	3.60%

Source: Adapted from statistics in the Survey of the States' Limited English Proficient Students and Available Educational Programs and Services 2000–2001 Summary Report, by the Office of English Language Acquisition, 2002, Washington, DC: National Clearinghouse for English Language Acquisition and Language Instruction Educational Programs: Washington D.C.

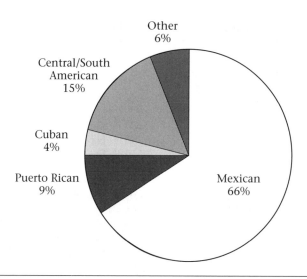

Figure 6.7 Distribution of Spanish-Speaking Individuals Within the United States

production is transcribed as [t̪] and [d̪]. Other shared consonants include /j, w, f, m, l, s, tʃ, and n/, while /θ/ may occur in some dialects but not in others. The consonants /v, z, h, ð, ʃ, dʒ, ʒ, ŋ/ are present in English but not in Spanish, although both /ŋ/ and /ð/ are allophones of other phonemes. In addition, the "r" is pronounced differently in Spanish. Spanish distinguishes two "r" phonemes: /ɾ/ and an alveolar trill. The /ɾ/ has been introduced in Chapter 5 and is a flap, tap, or one-tap trill, which in American English can be an allophonic variation of /t/ or /d/ when these sounds are produced between two vowels. For example, in casual conversation the word "ladder" or "better" can be pronounced [læɾɚ] or [bɛɾɚ]. The second "r" of Spanish is an alveolar trill (which according to the IPA is transcribed [r] but to eliminate confusion will be symbolized here as /r̄/) in which the apex of the tongue flutters rapidly against the alveolar ridge with either two or three vibrations. Therefore, the transference of the Spanish "r" to English will end up with a qualitatively somewhat different-sounding "r." Figures 6.8 and 6.9 demonstrate the vowel and consonant sounds of Hispanic Spanish according to González (1988).

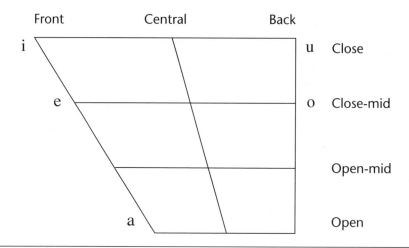

Figure 6.8 Vowels of Spanish

	Bilabial	Labio-dental	Dental	Alveolar	Post-alveolar	Palatal	Velar	Labio-velar
Stop	p b			t d¹			k g	
Fricative		f		s			x	
Affricate					tʃ			
Nasal	m			n		ɲ²		
Lateral				l				
Flap				ɾ				
Trill				r̄				
Glide						j		w

¹These sounds are often pronounced with the tongue behind the incisors, thus are dentalized productions.

²This is a nasal sound that is made by pressing the middle of the tongue firmly against the palate while the apex is tucked down behind the lower teeth.

Figure 6.9 Consonants of Spanish

Reflect on This: Clinical Application

These differences lead to the following problems, which are noted in Penfield and Ornstein-Galacia (1985) and Perez (1994).

1. Variable production of [tʃ] and [ʃ], thus [tʃoʊ] for "show" and [ʃɛk] for "check."
2. Devoicing of /z/ in all environments, especially in word-final position.
3. Devoicing of /v/ in word-final position, thus [hæf] for "have."
4. Realization of [v] as [β] (a voiced bilabial fricative) or [b] especially between two vowels, thus [aβan] for "oven." Note that the central vowels might be replaced by the Spanish [a] vowel.
5. Realization of [θ] and [ð] as [t] and [d], thus [tɪŋk] for "think" and [deɪ] for "they."
6. Realization of [j] for [dʒ] in word-initial position, thus [jas] for "just."
7. Devoicing of [dʒ] between two vowels and in word-final positions, thus [tineɪtʃɚ] for "teenager" and [læŋwɪtʃ] for "language."
8. Realization of [a] for [ʌ] in stressed syllables, thus [drag] for "drug."
9. Tensing of /ɛ/ to /e/, especially preceding nasals, thus [frend] for "friend."
10. Inconsistent realizations of [i]–[ɪ], [e]–[ɛ], [ɛ] and [æ], and [u]–[ʊ]. Thus, "speak" may be pronounced [spɪk].
11. Velarization of /h/ to the Spanish velar fricative /x/, thus [xi] for "he."
12. Reduction of consonant clusters in word-final position, thus "war" for "ward" or "star" for "start."
13. Deletion of intervocalic flaps and occasionally other consonants, thus [lɪl] for "little" and [læɚ] for "ladder." Syllables may be reduced as well.
14. Trilling of the "r" that may result in [ɾ or r̄] for "r," thus, [əɾaʊnd] or [ər̄aʊnd] for "around."
15. Intrusive [h], thus for "and it" the Spanish speaker could say [hændhɪt].
16. Unstressed syllable deletion, such as [spleɪn] for "explain."

(continued)

17. Shift of major stress on noun compounds from the first word to the second word, thus mini'skirt instead of 'mini-skirt.
18. Shift of major stress on verb particles from the second word to the first word, thus 'show up instead of show 'up.
19. Shift of stress on specific words, such as 'ac cept for ac 'cept.
20. Differences in sentence intonation patterns. Penfield and Ornstein-Galacia (1985) note five different patterns. These are summarized in Table 6.3.

Cuban American English

The Cuban Americans are considered the oldest population of Hispanic immigrants in the United States. Most of the Cuban Americans today live in New York, New Jersey, California, and Florida. Cuban Spanish is categorized as a variety of Caribbean Spanish that includes the three Antillean islands as well as the coastal areas of Mexico, Panama, Columbia, and Venezuala (Otheguy, Garcia, & Roca, 2000).

Table 6.3 Differences in Sentence Intonational Patterns: Spanish-Influenced English

Rising glides at any point in an intonational contour to highlight or emphasize specific words, e.g., "hair":

| I | have | to | cut | my | h a i r | now |

Rising glides are maintained even at the end of a neutral, declarative sentence, e.g., "awake":

| I | want | to | be | a | w a k e |

Initial sentence contours begin above the normal pitch of voice, e.g., "All":

| All | | sports | I | like. |

Declarative, neutral statements terminated with a one-pitch contrast:

| Give | her | to | mom |

Rise-fall glides in sentence-final contours, e.g., "good":

| That | | sounds | g o o d |

Source: Adapted from *Chicano English: An Ethnic Dialect*, by J. Penfield and J. Ornstein-Galacia, 1985, Philadelphia: John Benjamin.

Reflect on This: Clinical Application

According to Hidalgo (1987), the main phonological features of Cuban American Spanish are as follows:

1. In word-final position, /s/ is deleted in Cuban Spanish. This could lead to deletion of the final /s/ if a transfer is made between Spanish and English.
2. The consonants /l/ and /r̄/ are frequently interchanged before consonants and in word-final position. Inconsistent realizations of /l/ and /r/ could result in American English.
3. Deletion of intervocalic and word-final /d/ production could lead to a similar deletion pattern in American English.
4. The Spanish /r̄/ may be pronounced like /h/ or as a uvular approximate. This could impact the quality of the r-productions in American English.
5. The labio-dental /v/ is used as a variant of /b/, particularly in words spelled with "v."

Puerto Rican American English

Before the invasion of Puerto Rico by the United States in 1898, this island had belonged to Spain for approximately 400 years (Zentella, 2000). Since that time, Puerto Rico has experienced intense Americanization. New York presently has the largest population of Puerto Ricans, although there are a considerable number of Puerto Ricans living in Massachusetts, Florida, and Pennsylvania (Zentella, 2000). The use of Spanish and English varies according to the situation; however, the issue of generation will also play an important role. For example, parents who grew up in Puerto Rico speaking Spanish and move to the United States will have a tendency to use Spanish at home with their children, whereas their children will speak both English and Spanish.

Reflect on This: Clinical Application

The following phonological distinctions were noted by Zentella (2000).

1. The use of /s/ for /z/ and /tʃ/, especially before /i/ and /eɪ/, can result in pronunciation differences such as [sip] for "cheap" or [sen] for "chain."
2. Similarities noted in numbers 2, 4, and 5 on the Penfield and Ornstein-Galacia (1985) and Perez (1994) list: devoicing of /z/ in all environments, especially in word-final position; realization of /v/ as /β/ (a voiced bilabial fricative) or /b/, especially between two vowels, thus [aβan] for "oven"; and realization of /θ/ and /ð/ as /t/ and /d/, thus [tɪŋk] for "think" and [deɪ] for "they."
3. The consonants /l/ and /r̄/ are frequently interchanged before consonants and in word-final position. Inconsistent realizations of /l/ and /r/ could result in American English.
4. The Spanish /r̄/ may be pronounced as a uvular approximant in the middle of words and word-initially. This could impact the quality of the r-productions in American English.

Reflect on This: Clinical Application

Some of the phonological features of Nicaraguan American Spanish include the following:

1. Weak production of the intervocalic /j/. In words such as "yoyo" or "oh yes," the /j/ may be perceived as possibly a sound deletion.
2. Velarization of word-final [n], which could result in an inconsistent distinction between /n/ and /ŋ/ at the end of words, thus "sun" could be produced as "sung."
3. The Spanish /r̄/ may be pronounced as a velar approximate in the middle of words and word-initially. This could impact the quality of the r-productions in American English.

Nicaraguan American English

Most of the immigration of Nicaraguans to the United States took place during the Somoza regime in the middle of the 1970s with the uprising of the Sandinista group (Lipski, 2000). Nicaraguans are primarily concentrated in New York City, Los Angeles, New Orleans, and Miami. Within the Nicaraguan population, there is a group of individuals who speak one of two indigenous languages from this area: Miskito or Caribbean Creole English. This last group of Nicaraguans, due to their English-language skills, was able to integrate almost immediately into the job market of the United States (Lipski, 2000). The Spanish of the Nicaraguans shares many similarities with the other noted groups of Spanish speakers within the United States.

Vietnamese American English

With the end of the Vietnam War in 1975 and the subsequent rule of Vietnam by a Communist government, an influx of immigrants came from Indochina to the United States in search of political asylum. Vietnamese is part of the Viet-Muong grouping of the Mon-Khmer branch of the Austroasiatic language family. This family also includes Khmer, which is spoken in Cambodia, the Munda languages spoken in northeastern India, and others in southern China. Vietnamese is a tone language. Thus differences in tones do signify meaning. There are three dialects of Vietnamese that are mutually intelligible: North Vietnamese (Hanoi dialect), Central Vietnamese (Hué dialect), and Southern Vietnamese (Saigon dialect). The tones in each of these dialects vary slightly, but the Hué dialect is more markedly different than the others. Figure 6.10 demonstrates the vowels of Vietnamese according to Cheng (1994) and Ruhlen (1976).

A few unfamiliar vowels include /ɐ/, /ɯ/, and /ɤ/. As can be seen from the vowel quadrilateral, /ɐ/ is a low-central vowel, and /ɯ/ is a high-back vowel similar to /u/ but without lip rounding. The /ɤ/ is mid-back vowel, similar to /o/ but again without lip rounding. The lax vowels /ɪ/ and /ɛ/ are not present in Vietnamese, and for words containing these vowels, the tense /i/ and /e/ vowels may be substituted in American English. Figure 6.11 is a chart of the consonants of Vietnamese.

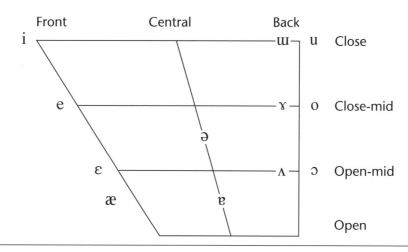

Figure 6.10 Vowels of Vietnamese

	Bilabial	Labio-dental	Dental	Alveolar	Post-alveolar	Palatal	Velar	Labio-velar	Glottal
Stop	p b		t d t' t[1]			c[2]	k g		
Fricative		f v[3]		s z[3]	ʃ[3] ʒ[3]		x ɣ		h
Affricate					tʃ				
Nasal	m			n		ɲ	ŋ		
Lateral				l					
Flap									
Trill				r[3]					
Glide						j[3]		w	

[1][t] as well as [t'] (a voiceless dental/alveolar ejective) and [ʈ] (a retroflex variation of [t] exist in Vietnamese (Cheng, 1994).

[2]This sound is a voiceless palatal plosive with the articulatory closure between [t] and [k].

[3]Sound may be present in certain dialects but not others.

Figure 6.11 Consonants of Vietnamese

Concept Exercise EJECTIVES

Ejectives are produced by closing the glottis and compressing the air in the mouth between the glottis and the consonant closure farther forward in the vocal tract (International Phonetic Association, 1999). Therefore, there is a build-up of air pressure behind the point of contact and an explosive glottalized release. Try making an ejective by first starting out with a glottal stop (the vocal folds are held tightly together). Do you feel how you close off the glottis? Now take a deep breath, close off the glottis again, and put your tongue in the articulatory position for [t] without releasing your breath. After a second, release the [t], still keeping the glottis closed. You should be able to hear a faint popping sound. That is the ejective [t'].

Hmong American English

Many people think that the Hmong came to the United States to enjoy the economic benefits, but in fact, most are here to escape the death and horror of a genocidal war against them. The long campaign of the Laotian and Vietnamese governments to destroy the Hmong is vengeance for Hmong support of the United States in the Vietnam War. The Hmong people in the United States are largely concentrated in Wisconsin, Minnesota, and California. Several million Hmong people remain in China, Thailand, and Laos, speaking a variety of Hmong dialects. The Hmong language group is a monosyllabic, tonal language (seven to twelve tones, depending on the dialect). There appear to be two basic dialects of Hmong: Mong Leng and Hmong Der. These two dialects are mutually intelligible. The following consonant and vowel inventories are based on the Mong Leng dialect and are offered by Mortensen (2004). The phonology of Hmong Der can be found in Ratliff (1992). Figure 6.12 depicts the vowels of this dialect of Hmong.

The /ɨ/ vowel is a rounded centralized vowel with a high tongue position. The tongue position is moved horizontally so that the maximum ele-

Reflect on This: Clinical Application

Based on the absence of certain consonants and the discussion by Cheng (1994), the following possible pronunciation difficulties may arise in the Vietnamese speaker of American English.

1. The affricates /tʃ/ and /dʒ/ do not exist in Vietnamese and may produce difficulties.
2. There is a limited number of final consonants in Vietnamese. The consonants /p, k, m, ŋ/ and a /ŋm/ consonant combination are the only final consonants that are used by all three dialects of Vietnamese. Depending on the dialect, there is variable use of /t/, /c/ (a palatal stop), /n/, and /ɲ/ as final consonants. Therefore, the Vietnamese speaker may have problems realizing the other consonants in the word-final position.
3. There are no word-initial consonant combinations in Vietnamese. The Vietnamese speaker may either reduce the combination to a singleton production or insert a schwa sound between the blend. Thus, the word "stew" might become [sətu].
4. Depending on the dialect, an "r" sound might not be present. In addition, there are no central vowels with r-coloring. This sound, especially its prevalence in American English, might be problematic for Vietnamese speakers of American English.
5. Depending on the dialect, other sounds may not be present in the inventory of Vietnamese and, thus, may need to be learned. These include /v, z, ʃ, θ, ð, ʒ/, and /j/. There will be a tendency to substitute the voiceless counterparts /f/ and /s/, which do exist in Vietnamese, for the voiced consonants. In addition, the voiceless and voiced velar fricatives /x, ɣ/ may be substituted for other fricative sounds.

vation of the tongue is mediopalatal rather than prepalatal as it is with /i/. Also, /æ/ and /a/ are variants of one /a/-type vowel; they can be used interchangeably. Three nasalized vowels exist in this dialect: /ĩ/, /ũ/, and /ã/. Figure 6.13 demonstrates the consonants of Mong Leng Hmong.

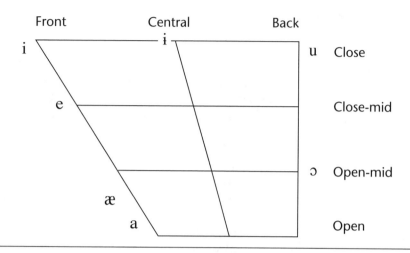

Figure 6.12 Vowels of Mong Leng Hmong

	Bilabial	Bilabial with Lateral Release	Labio-dental	Dental	Alveolar	Retroflex	Palatal	Velar	Uvular	Glottal
Stop	p pʰ[1]	pˡ pˡ2			t d tʰ dʰ	ʈ ʈʰ	c cʰ[1]	k kʰ	q qʰ	ʔ
Pre-Nasalized Stop	ᵐb[3] ᵐbʰ	ᵐbˡ ᵐbɬ			ⁿd ⁿdʰ	ⁿɖ ⁿɖʰ	ᶮɟ ᶮɟʰ	ᵑg ᵑgʰ	ᴺɢ ᴺɢʰ	
Fricative			f v		s[4]	ʂ[4] ʐ	ç ʝ[5]			h
Affricate										
Pre-Nasalized Affricate					ⁿdz ⁿdzʰ	ⁿɖʐ̩ ɖʐ̩ʰ				
Nasal	m	mˡ mɬ			n		ɲ	ŋ		
Lateral					l ɬ					
Glide							j			

[1]The elevated /ʰ/ indicates that these sounds have an aspirated sound that has phonemic value.

[2]The /ɬ/ symbol indicates that the lateral release is similar to the lateralized /s/ that was introduced on page 137.

[3]The nasal symbols located to the left of the symbol indicate the corresponding nasal that is involved in the nasalized stop. Thus, bilateral stops have bilateral nasals, /m/, while the uvular stop has an accompanying uvular nasal.

[4]There is an aspirated /s/ that may be produced by some speakers.

[5]This sound is a voiceless palatal fricative that is similar (but with a narrower opening between the active and passive articulators) to a voiceless /j/.

Figure 6.13 Consonants of Mong Leng Hmong

Reflect on This: Clinical Application

Based on the absence of certain consonants, the following possible pronunciation difficulties may arise in the Hmong speaker of American English.

1. Voiced stop-plosives that do not demonstrate prenasalization do not exist in Hmong. There is the possibility of substituting the prenasalized voiced stops for these sounds.
2. The voiced fricative /z/ does not exist in Hmong. Again, the Hmong speaker of American English may substitute the voiceless fricative /s/ in words containing /z/.
3. The consonant /w/ is not within the inventory of Hmong. This may need to be learned.
4. An "r" sound is not present in Hmong. In addition, there are no central vowels with r-coloring. This sound, especially its prevalence in American English, might be problematic for Hmong speakers of American English.
5. The affricates in Hmong are prenasalized. There could be a tendency to substitute the prenasalized affricates for /tʃ/ and /dʒ/. In addition, /ʃ/ and /ʒ/ do not exist in Hmong.
6. The Hmong language has many stop-plosives with a lateral release such as /pˡ/ and /pⁱ/. These might be substituted for /pl/, for example.
7. There are no word-final consonants in Hmong. This could be difficult for the Hmong speaker to realize.
8. Most words are monosyllabic in Hmong. This could pose difficulties when trying to pronounce multisyllabic words and manipulating word stress.

Cantonese American English

The majority of Chinese Americans are from the Canton Province in Southern China. They generally settled in California but gradually dispersed to larger cities such as New York City, Chicago, etc. Today approximately 40 percent of the Chinese Americans reside in the state of California. The two metropolitan areas that have the largest population of Chinese Americans are San Francisco and Los Angeles. In the San Francisco Bay area alone, there are approximately 400,000 Chinese Americans.

As one of the Chinese languages, Cantonese belongs to the Sino Tibetan language family, which also includes Tibetan and Lolo Burmese and Karen (both spoken in Burma). The major languages within Chinese are Mandarin, Wu, Min, Yue (Cantonese), and Hakka (Li & Thompson, 1987). Given all the dialects that exist within Cantonese, the language is sometimes referred to as a group of Cantonese dialects, and not just Cantonese. Oral communication is virtually impossible among speakers of some Cantonese dialects. For instance, there is as much of a difference between the dialects of Taishan and Nanning as there is between Italian and French. According to its linguistic characteristics and geographical distribution, Cantonese can be divided into four dialects: Yuehai (including

Zhongshan, Chungshan, and Tungkuan), as represented by the dialect of Guangzhou City; Siyi (Seiyap), as represented by the Taishan city (Toishan and Hoishan) dialect; Gaoyang, as represented by the Yangjiang city dialect; and Guinan, as represented by the Nanning city dialect, which is widely used in Guangxi Province. If not otherwise specified, the term *Cantonese* often refers to the Guangzhou dialect, which is also spoken in Hong Kong and Macao. Figure 6.14 demonstrates the vowels of a Hong Kong dialect of Cantonese (Lee, 1999).

The /y/ vowel is a front vowel, similar to /i/ but with lip rounding. The vowel /ə/ is a central vowel with lip rounding, while /œ/ is a vowel similar to /ɛ/ but with lip rounding. There are long and short variants of many of the vowels and many diphthongs in Cantonese; officially, Cantonese counts fifty-two vowels (Cheng, 1994). Figure 6.15 shows the consonants of Hong Kong Cantonese.

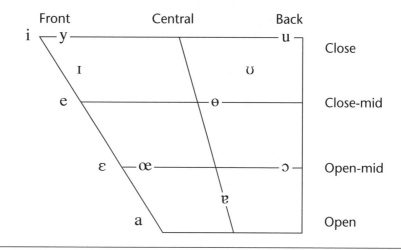

Figure 6.14 Vowels of Hong Kong Cantonese

	Bilabial	Labio-dental	Dental	Alveolar	Post-alveolar	Palatal	Velar	Labio-velar	Glottal
Stop	p pʰ1		t tʰ				k kʰ	kʷ2	
Fricative		f		s					h
Affricate					ts dz tʰs dʰz				
Nasal	m			n			ŋ		
Lateral				l					
Glide						j		w	

[1]The raised /ʰ/ indicates that these sounds have an aspirated and a nonaspirated variation that is phonemic and, therefore, distinguishes meaning between words.

[2]The /kʷ/ is a coarticulated consonant, as the /k/ and /w/ are articulated together.

Figure 6.15 Consonants of Hong Kong Cantenese

Reflect on This: Clinical Application

The following learning difficulties for Cantonese speakers of American English are outlined by Chan and Li (2000).

1. There are no voiced syllable-final plosives in Cantonese; therefore, learners of English tend to substitute /p, t, k/ for /b, d, g/ in the word-final position. In addition, there is a tendency to not release the voiceless plosives in Cantonese, which is transferred to American English. Thus, "rope" and "robe" or "mate" and "maid" are practically indistinguishable. Cantonese learners of English also have a tendency to devoice plosives in syllable-initiating position.
2. Due to the absence of voiced /v/ and /z/, Cantonese speakers of English tend to substitute their voiceless counterparts, /f/ and /s/.
3. As /ʃ/ and /ʒ/ do not exist in Cantonese, /s/ will often be used as a substitute for these sounds.
4. Cantonese does not have "th" sounds, and the Cantonese speaker of English will often substitute /t/ or /f/ for /θ/ ([tɪn] for "thin") and /d/ or /f/ for /ð/ ([deɪ] for "they").
5. The affricates /tʃ/ and /dʒ/ do not exist, and Cantonese speakers of English will often substitute /ts/ and /dz/ for /tʃ/ and /dʒ/.
6. Cantonese speakers of English often have trouble distinguishing /l/, /n/, and /r/. When the /r/ is in a word-initial position, they tend to substitute an l-like sound for /r/. Other speakers may substitute /w/ for /r/. In syllable-initial position, /n/ may be substituted by /l/, while in final position the /l/ may be deleted or a /u/ sound is used, rendering "wheel" as [wiu].
7. Long and short vowels are problematic for Cantonese speakers of American English. Thus word pairs with /i/–/ɪ/ and /u/–/ʊ/ may be difficult.
8. When /i/ or /ɪ/ occur at the beginning of a word, there is a tendency to add a /j/ sound, thus "east" and "yeast" sound the same. This is a transfer from Cantonese, as the vowel /i/ in syllable-initial position is preceded by /j/.
9. Cantonese contains no consonant clusters, and speakers will have a tendency to delete these clusters in words or insert a schwa vowel between the consonant sounds of the cluster.

Korean American English

In 1903, the first Korean immigrants to the United States arrived in Honolulu, Hawaii. Today, a little over one million Korean Americans live throughout the United States, representing one of the largest Asian American populations in the country. The largest concentration of Korean Americans is found in the five-county area of Los Angeles, which includes Los Angeles, Orange, San Bernardino, Riverside, and Ventura counties. About one-quarter of all the Korean Americans living in the United States reside in this region. The next largest area of concentration is the New York region, including New York City, northern New Jersey, and the Connecticut/

Long Island area. This area constitutes about 16 percent of the entire Korean American population in the United States.

The Korean language belongs to the Altaic language group but contains many words of Chinese origin (Ball & Rahilly, 1999). There are nineteen consonants and eight vowels, which occur distinctively long or short. These vowels are depicted in Figure 6.16 from Lee (1999).

As can be seen from Figure 6.16, some of the long vowels change their tongue position relative to the short vowels: For example, /a:/ is a more back placement, while /ʌ:/ is a higher and more central placement.

Figure 6.17 is a consonant inventory of Korean (Ladefoged & Maddieson, 1996; Lee, 1999).

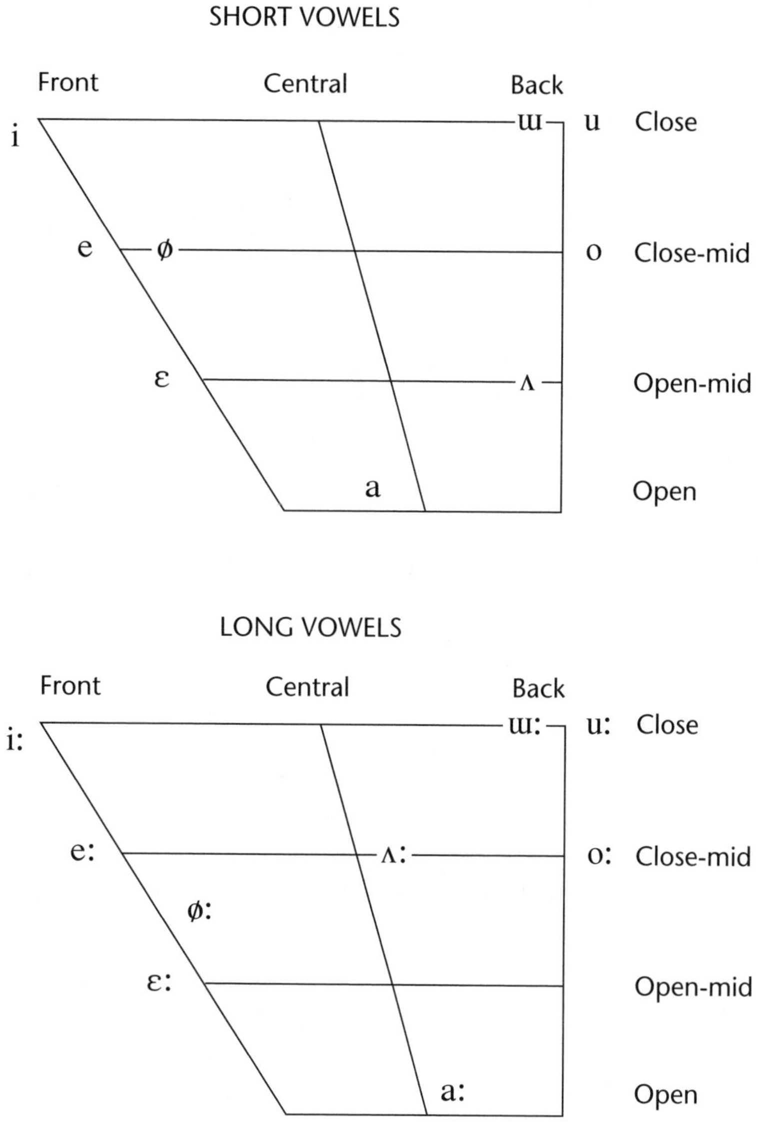

SHORT VOWELS

LONG VOWELS

Figure 6.16   Vowels of Korean

	Bilabial	Labio-dental	Dental	Alveolar	Post-alveolar	Palatal	Velar	Labio-velar	Glottal
Stop	p pʰ¹		t d¹ tʰ				k kʰ		
Fricative				s z					h
Affricate					tʃ dʒ tʰʃ dʰʒ²				
Nasal	m			n			ŋ		
Lateral				l				w	
Glide									

¹Syllable-initially, these sounds are voiceless unaspirated or slightly aspirated, while intervocalically they are voiced.

²Lee (1999) describes this affricate as containing postalveolar stops ([c] and [ɟ]), while Ladefoged and Maddieson (1996) use the symbols that are noted above.

Figure 6.17 Consonants of Korean

Reflect on This: Clinical Application

The following areas are considered problematic for Korean speakers of American English (Cho, 2004):

1. Korean differs considerably from English in the phonetic realization of word-final stops. Word-final Korean stops are always unreleased, i.e., produced without audible aspiration, whereas English stops are either released or unreleased. This, together with the differences in voicing and aspiration initiating a syllable and intervocalically, can lead to confusion of /p/–/b/, /t/–/d/, and /k/–/g/ pairs of words, such as "cap" and "cab."

2. Several English consonant sounds do not exist in the Korean speech sound system. These include the fricatives /f/, /v/, /θ/, and /ð/. These sounds are produced as [p], [b], [t], and [d] respectively, and the /p/ and /f/ and /b/ and /v/ sounds in particular are very often confused.

3. Korean speakers make no distinction between /r/ and /l/. The equivalent Korean consonant is alveolar and is somewhere between the two. This, together with the fact that there are no central vowels with r-coloring, leads to problems with r-sounds and the stereotyped /r/ and /l/ mix up.

4. There are differences in the structure of syllables between Korean and English. In Korean, consonants are not released unless they are followed by a vowel in the same syllable, and word-final consonants are never released. This causes the insertion of a vowel at the end of every English word that ends with a consonant. For example, "Mark" becomes [maku] and "college" becomes [kaləsdʒi]. This is a strong characteristic of the speech of beginning learners of English in Korea.

5. The Korean syllable form usually follows a CVC pattern, with a single consonant in the initial-word position followed by a vowel. In English two to three consecutive consonants can occur at the beginning of a word, such as "treat" or "street." In these cases, Korean students follow the Korean syllabic

pattern and insert an extra vowel between the consonants. Thus, "plight" could be pronounced "polite."

6. Korean is a syllable-timed language, and Korean learners of English may have difficulties with the patterns of stressed and unstressed syllables in English words. One of the tasks for Korean students is to gain familiarity with American English stress and rhythm.

7. Korean has a very different syntactic structure from English. Because of that and the syllable-timed language factor, Korean learners of English may pronounce each word in a sentence with equal emphasis. They have difficulty producing and perceiving weak forms in English.

Arabic American English

In terms of speakers, Arabic is the largest living member of the Semitic language family (206 million speakers). Classified as Central Semitic, it is closely related to Hebrew and Aramaic. The Semitic languages are a family of languages spoken by more than 300 million people across much of the Middle East, North Africa, and the Horn of Africa. Modern Standard Arabic has its historical basis in Classical Arabic that is the only surviving member of the Old North Arabian dialect group, which has documented inscriptions since the sixth century. Classical Arabic has been a literary language and a liturgical language of Islam since the seventh century. There are many issues when proposing a phonological system of Standard Arabic. The following vowel and consonant categorizations are based on Huthaily (2003), Newman (2002), and Thelwall and Sa'Adeddin (1999).

There are three vowels in Arabic—/i/, /u/, and /a/—that appear in long and short variations. The tongue position for the short forms is somewhat lower for /i/ and /u/, resembling /ɪ/ and /ʊ/ respectively, while the short /a/ vowel qualitatively approaches /æ/. Arabic also has two diphthongs, /a͡ʊ/ and /e͡ɪ/. Figure 6.18 demonstrates the vowels of Arabic.

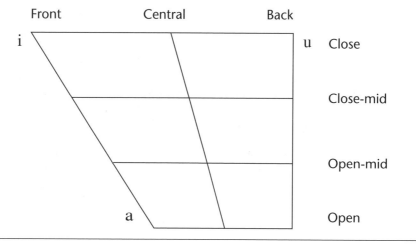

Figure 6.18 Vowels of Arabic

Some of the consonants of Arabic are unique to those previously presented. The /t/ and /d/ are dental productions. In addition, /t/ and /d/ have pharyngealized productions that have phonemic value. Pharyngealization involves a secondary approximation of the back and root of the tongue into the pharyngeal area. These pharyngealized consonants are categorized as emphatic consonants. There is some discussion as to whether these sounds are pharyngeal or epiglottal in their production. Ladefoged and Maddieson (1996) maintain, based on more recent possibilities to directly observe the laryngeal area, that there is epiglottal activity. However, they are noted as pharyngealized consonants in Figure 6.19. As noted in Figure 6.19, several other consonants have pharyngealized forms as well.

	Bilabial	Labio-dental	Dental	Alveolar	Post-alveolar	Palatal	Velar	Uvular	Pharyngeal	Glottal
Stop	b		t[1] d tˁ[2] dˁ				k	q		ʔ ʔˁ
Fricative		f	θ ð ðˁ	s z sˁ	ʃ	x ɣ			ħ	h
Affricate					dʒ					
Nasal	m		n[1]							
Trill				r̄[3]						
Lateral				l lˁ[4]						
Glide						j	w			

[1]According to Thelwall and Akram Sa'Adeddin (1999), for example, these sounds are dentalized productions.

[2]The /ˁ/ symbol indicates a pharyngealized production.

[3]Although Thelwall and Sa'Adeddin (1999) describe the /r/ as an alveolar trill, Watson (2002) describes it as a dental tap or postvelar fricative depending on the dialect.

[4]The pharyngealized /l/ is noted in Classical Arabic only in the word /alˁlˁah/.

Figure 6.19 Consonants of Arabic

Reflect on This: Clinical Application

The following possible pronunciation difficulties may arise in the Arabic speaker of American English (Altaha, 1995; Kharma & Hajjaj, 1989; Power, 2003; Val Barros, 2003; Watson, 2002).

1. In Arabic there is typically a one-to-one correspondence between sounds and letters, and letters stand directly for their sounds. Therefore, if given written words to pronounce, the Arabic student will often be confused by the lack of sound-letter correspondence in English. The influence of the

written form can lead to several different pronunciation difficulties, both with vowels and consonants for the Arabic student.

2. The central vowels with and without r-coloring do not exist in Arabic. Therefore, the /a/ - /æ/ variation (typically /æ/) or /u/ are substituted for /ʌ/. The Arabic r-sound will probably replace the central vowels with r-coloring, which might lead to some differences in the quality of these r-sounds.

3. The distinctions between specific vowels, especially open, lax, short vowels such as /ɪ/, /ɛ/, and /ʊ/ will be problematic for the Arabic speaker. According to Power (2003), the /ɪ/ vowel becomes lengthened and lowered to /e/, whereas /ɛ/ may be produced as /i/ or /æ/.

4. The following consonant distinctions seem to be problematic for Arabic speakers learning American English: /p/ - /b/, /f/ - /v/, /tʃ/ - /dʒ/ - /ʃ/. This is due to the absence of these oppositions in Arabic. For example, /p/, /v/, and /tʃ/ do not exist in Arabic.

5. Other consonants exist in Arabic, but they have different phonetic realizations and, thus, present problems in pronunciation. Although /n/ and /ŋ/ exist in Arabic, they are both allophones of the same phoneme /n/. In English, on the other hand, they are distinct phonemes. In addition, /ŋ/ never occurs at the end of a word in Arabic, thus, Arabic speakers have a tendency to add /k/ to the end of words that end in /ŋ/. This results in pronunciations such as [baɪɪŋk] for "buying" or [sɪŋk] for "sing." The phonotactics of /l/ are quite different in Arabic, and these speakers have a tendency to use the light /l/ in all word positions. In Arabic the "d" is always unreleased and voiceless in word-final position. Words such as "bad," "rod," and "mad" will often be pronounced "bat," "rot," and "mat." Although the phoneme /r/ exists in Arabic, it is pronounced as a trill. The American English approximant is unfamiliar to Arabic speakers, and they will have a strong tendency to produce this sound the way they know it in Arabic. While this may not cause misinterpretation, it will strongly contribute to the foreign accent. Speakers from Egypt will also evidence difficulties with /dʒ/ and /ð/. In modern spoken varieties of Egyptian Arabic, /dʒ/ is replaced by /ʒ/, and /h/ by /ð/ (Val Barros, 2002).

6. Arabic has far fewer consonant clusters both in the word-initial and word-final positions, and three-segment consonant clusters do not exist in Arabic. In contrast to English, which has 78 three-segment clusters and 14 four-segment clusters occurring at the end of words, Arabic has none. Clusters are often pronounced with a short vowel inserted to aid in pronunciation. Other clusters contain sounds that are not in the Arabic consonant inventory or have different pronunciations; for example, /sp/, /gr/, /spl/, and /str/. These clusters will be problematic for the Arabic learner of English. Again, a short vowel may be inserted between segments.

7. In Arabic, word stress is regular and predictable. Arabic speakers often have problems grasping the unpredictable nature of English word stress and the concept that stress can alter meaning, as in convict' (verb) versus con' vict (noun). Thus, word stress may be a problem for Arabic speakers learning English.

To summarize, this last section examined the vowel and consonant inventories of Spanish (including Hispanic, Cuban, Puerto Rican, and Nicaraguan Spanish), Vietnamese, Hmong, Cantonese, Korean, and Arabic. Based on the noted features, and incorporating the suprasegmental features of these languages, clinical implications were noted for speakers of each of these languages as they are acquiring American English skills.

Case Study

Sam was the new kid in town. He had just moved to a small town in New Mexico and was trying to make friends. Some of the children were finding that they had a hard time understanding Sam's speech. Later that day, Sam's teacher talked to Sam and referred him to the speech-language clinician at the school with a note that Sam had r-problems. The clinician listened to Sam's speech. She noticed that the characteristic r-coloring of central vowels, which was typical for that New Mexico area, was not being realized by Sam. Thus, "bird" sounded like [bɜd] and "father" like [fɑðə]. However, his [r] in "rabbit" or "ring" sounded fine. But there was something definitely different about Sam's speech. The speech clinician started to talk to Sam about how he was dealing with his move and where he had moved from. Sam slowly explained that he had moved from Maine and that his speech was just fine there. The speech clinician explained to Sam that his speech was indeed fine. The differences that everyone was noticing were regional dialect differences. The lack of r-coloring on rhotic vowels was characteristic of the regional dialect of the Eastern New England area, which includes Maine.

Summary

FOCUS 1: *What is the difference between Standard English and vernacular dialects?*

There appear to be two sets of representations of Standard English, a formal and an informal version. Formal Standard English, which is applied primarily to written language and the most formal spoken language situations, tends to be based on the written language and is exemplified in guides of usage or grammar texts. When there is a question as to whether a form is considered Standard English, then these grammar texts are consulted. Informal Standard English takes into account the assessment of the members of the American-English-speaking community as they judge the "standardness" of other speakers. This notion exists on a continuum ranging from standard to nonstandard speakers of American English. It relies far more heavily on grammatical structure than pronunciation patterns. In other words, listeners will accept a range of regional variations in pronunciation but will not accept the use of socially stigmatized grammatical structures. For example, a rather pronounced Boston or New York regional dialect is accepted, but structures such as "double negatives" would not be considered Standard English. On the other hand, vernacular dialects refer to those varieties of spoken American English that are considered outside the continuum of Informal Standard English. Vernacular dialects are signaled by the presence of certain structures. Therefore, a set of nonstandard English structures mark them as being vernacular. For example, the presence of double negation, lack of subject–verb agreement, and using variations from standard verb forms would be features that would label the speaker as utilizing a vernacular dialect. Although there may be a core of features that exemplify a particular vernacular dialect, not all speakers display the entire set of structures described. Therefore, differing patterns of usage exist among speakers of one particular vernacular dialect.

FOCUS 2: *What are the main types of dialects?*

One can describe a dialect according to its hypothesized causative agent. In this way, two main categories are formed: (1) those dialects corresponding to various geographical locations, which are considered regional dialects, and (2) those that are in general related to socioeconomic status and/or ethnic background, labeled social or ethnic dialects. In addition, dialects are classified according to their linguistic features. This would include the phonological, morphosyntactical, semantic, and pragmatic differences that are distinctive when the speakers representing that dialect are compared to those speaking informal Standard English.

FOCUS 3: *What are the three variables that seem to have an overall effect on the regional dialects? Explain these three variables.*

(1) Chain shifts, (2) the merging of specific vowels, and (3) the variations of r-productions.

1. Chain shifts are systematic changes in vowel systems in which the vowels shift in respect to their articulatory features. They demonstrate the tendency of sound systems to maintain specific phonemic distinctions. That means that surrounding vowels also change so there is a rotation of the *entire* vowel system. Thus, as one vowel changes its production features, other vowels shift to accommodate this change. This maintains articulatory distance between the vowels. If the entire system did not change, but only the articulatory features of one or two vowels, then the productions of certain vowels might become so close that we could perceive them as one and the same vowel. The Northern Cities and the Southern vowel shifts were provided as examples of chain shifts within the United States.
2. Mergers neutralize features, and phonemic distinctions are lost. Thus, two sounds, in this case two vowels, tend to become more like each other. The phonemic boundary between the two becomes indistinct, and one vowel may emerge as the prevalent pronunciation. There are basically two types of mergers: (1) unconditioned mergers, which affect the phonemes wherever they appear, and (2) conditioned mergers, which occur in a specific phonemic environment. The only unconditioned merger in the vowel system of General American English is the collapse of the distinction between /ɑ/ or /a/ and /ɔ/. The conditioned

merger within the United States was noted as being the /ɪ/–/ɛ/ merger before /m/ and /n/.

3. Variations of r-production refer to the centering rhotic diphthongs, such as /ɑɚ/ in "car" and /ɛɚ/ in "bear," and the central vowels with r-coloring, such as /ɝ/ in "bird." Several production possibilities may occur with these r-sounds. First, the r-coloring is completely absent. For example, "bird" would be pronounced [bɜd] and "car" as [kɑə]. The second possibility is that the characteristic r-quality has been weakened, often attributed to less retroflexion of the tongue. Finally, this r-sound may be totally preserved, which is the case in many regions of the United States.

FOCUS 4: *Which four regional areas were defined?*

The four regional areas were (1) the North, (2) the South, (3) the West, and (4) the Midland. The first three demonstrate a relatively uniform development of the sound shifts of American English, each moving in somewhat different directions. The fourth region, the Midland, has considerably more diversity, and most of the individual cities have developed dialect patterns of their own.

The North is divided into the North Central region, the Inland North, Eastern New England, New York City, and Western New England. For the short vowels, these areas all evidence the Northern Cities vowel shift. For the long vowels, which include the diphthongs, the North Central and the Inland North regions maintain a long-high position, which is typical of the vowel quadrilateral that has been presented in this text. The r-coloring of postvocalic r-productions, such as in "farm" ([fɑɚm]) is also maintained in these areas.

On the other hand, the Eastern New England area demonstrates r-lessness. In addition, /ɑ/ and /ɔ/ are merged into an intermediate vowel, typically /ɑ/ or, more frequently, /a/.

New York City appears to have a unique dialect that is not reproduced farther west and, therefore, cannot fit neatly into any larger regional groupings. The long vowels maintain a high position that is similar to that noted for the North Central and Inland North areas. There is consistent r-lessness of postvocalic "r," except for the central vowel with r-coloring /ɝ/ and when a final "r" is followed by a vowel in the next word, as in "the car is here." In addition, the /æ/ vowel splits into a lax and tense form, and the production differences between /ɑ/ and /ɔ/ are maximal, the /ɔ/ vowel being raised to a mid-high position.

The South demonstrates the Southern shift, which was noted in detail earlier. However, a small area of the Southeast is distinct from the rest of the South, including the two cities of Charleston and Savannah. In these cities, there is a low level of monophthongization and, subsequently, the Southern shift. Another characteristic of the Southern region is the /ɑ/–/ɔ/ distinction. With the exception of the margins of the South—west Texas, Kentucky, Virginia, and the city of Charleston—this distinction is marked not by a change in the vowel quality but by a back upglide for /ɔ/.

Speakers in the Midland area do not seem to participate in either the Northern Cities shift or the Southern shift. They are distinct from the North Central region, as there is a tendency to lax the long-high vowels, thus /i/ becomes more like /ɪ/ in quality and /e/ like /ɛ/. This region is also distinct from the South as the diphthongal quality of /aɪ/ is maintained.

The diversity of dialects declines steadily as one moves westward, resulting in a diffusion of Northern, Midland, and Southern characteristics. While there are exceptions, characteristics of the West are aligned with those of the Midland. The most prominent feature of Western phonology is the merger of /ɑ/ and /ɔ/; however, as noted previously, this is not unique to the West. The second feature that emerges is the fronting of the vowel /u/, as in "two" or "do," for example. Although these two characteristics are also noted in the South Midland, there appears to be a much higher frequency of occurrence in the West.

FOCUS 5: *Why is it difficult to define social dialects?*

Although social status may be subjectively evaluated, the challenge for the researcher is to reduce these subjective, rather abstract notions to objective, measurable units that can be correlated with linguistic variation. Typical variables include occupation, level of education, income, and type of residential dwelling, which are then associated with ranked levels within each category. The overall ranking obtained from combining scores for the different variables is the socioeconomic status, or SES.

In recent years, these socioeconomic scales have been criticized. These scales seem to overwhelming reflect the values of white male mainstream speakers of middle and higher classes and ignore important variables, such as the status of the female in the household, for example. An alternative solution has been relying on community members to make judgments about status differences. However, this type of assignment also has its problems. Members of the lower class may, for example, perceive the entire social class structure very differently from those in the upper class.

There are other social variables that intersect with social class, including region, age, and gender, to mention a few. In addition, the social significance of language forms also changes over time. For example, the historical study of the English language supports the fact that the use of "ain't" and double negatives was once socially insignificant but now has become a stigmatized form.

FOCUS 6: *What is African American Vernacular English? What features are unique to this dialect?*

African American Vernacular English, or what has been called Black English or African American English, is a systematic, rule-governed dialect that is spoken by many but not all African American people within the United States. Although it shares many commonalities with Standard American English and Southern English, there are certain differences that distinguish this dialect. These differences affect the phonological, morphological, syntactical, and semantic systems.

Although many different features were noted in Table 6.1, features unique to this dialect include (1) stressing of initial syllables, shifting the stress from the second syllable, (2) deletion of final nasal consonant but nasalization of preceding vowel, (3) final-consonant deletion (especially affects nasals), (4) final-stop devoicing (without shortening of preceding vowel), (5) coarticulated glottal stop with devoiced final stop, (6) loss of [j] after specific consonants (loss of palatalization in specific contexts such as "comp<u>u</u>ter"), and (7) substitution of /k/ for /t/ in /str/ clusters.

FOCUS 7: *What are limited English proficient students?*

The term *limited English proficient* is used for any individual between the ages of 3 and 21 who is enrolled or preparing to enroll in an elementary or secondary school and who was not born in the United States or whose native language is a language other than English. Also individuals who are Native American or Alaska Native and come from an environment where a language other than English has had a significant impact on the individual are included in this definition. The difficulties in speaking, writing, or understanding the English language compromise the individual's ability to successfully achieve in classrooms where the language of instruction is English or to participate fully in society (P.L. 107-110, The No Child Left Behind Act of 2001). Title III funds are provided to ensure that limited English proficient students, including immigrant children and youth, develop English proficiency and meet the same academic content and academic achievement standards that other children are expected to meet.

Further Readings

Labov, W. (2001). *Principles of linguistic change, Volume 2: Social factors.* Oxford, UK: Blackwell.

Ladefoged, P., & Maddieson, I. (1996). *The sounds of the world's languages.* Oxford, UK: Blackwell.

Smitherman, G. (1994). *Black talk: Words and phrases from the hood to the amen corner.* Boston: Houghton Mifflin.

Wolfram, W., & Schilling-Estes, N. (2006). *American English: Dialects and variations* (2nd ed.). Malden, MA: Blackwell.

Key Concepts

chain shifts p. 156
code switching p. 169
consonant cluster variations p. 154
creole p. 171
culture p. 167
dialect p. 150
ethnic dialects p. 154
ethnicity p. 167
formal Standard English p. 152
informal Standard English p. 152
limited English proficient
   students p. 173

mergers p. 159
phonotactic processes p. 154
pidgin p. 171
prosodic variability p. 155
race p. 167
regional dialects p. 154
social dialects pp. 154, 166
substitution processes p. 154
transfer p. 167
vernacular dialects p. 152

Think Critically

1. Make a list of words that could be articulated with the /ɔ/–/ɑ-a/ distinction, such as "caught" and "cod." Also make a list of minimal pair words that contain /ɪ/ and /ɛ/ preceded by the nasals /m/ and /n/, such as "pin" and "pen." First, see if you produce these distinctions, and then ask several of your friends to say these words and note whether they produce these distinctions. Try to find friends that might come from a different regional area of the United States and see if they make these distinctions.

2. What words or pronunciations are you familiar with from "rap dialect"? Make a list of these.

3. Based on the state that you are in, what are the three non-English languages that are spoken (see Table 6.2)? Go onto the Web and see if you can find three interesting things about the culture or the language of individuals speaking these languages.

4. What does it mean that aspiration (such as [p] and [pʰ] in Cantonese, for example) has phonemic value? Which other consonants on the foreign language charts (Spanish, Cantonese, Hmong, Vietnamese, Korean, Arabic) also demonstrate features that have phonemic value in that language but not in American English?

5. Examine the features on Table 6.1, Frequently Cited Features of African American Vernacular English. The first four features are those that appear in most dialects of American English. Go through each of the four and see if you ever use those features. List some examples if you do use any of the four listed features.

Test Yourself

1. Dialects that are related to the particular geographic area are called
   a. regional dialects.
   b. social dialects.
   c. ethnic dialects.
   d. all of the above.

2. African American English is an example of which of the following dialects?
   a. regional dialect
   b. social dialect
   c. ethnic dialect
   d. all of the above

3. If someone says [pɪksbɚg] for "Pittsburgh," this is an example of which type of phonological variation?
   a. substitution process
   b. consonant-cluster variation
   c. prosodic variability
   d. a and b

4. The Northern Cities vowel shift and the Southern vowel shift are

a. very comparable: Similar vowel chain shifts are happening in both.

b. examples of mergers.

c. moving the vowels in the vowel chains in opposite directions, thus, the two dialects are becoming more dissimilar.

d. chain shifts of vowels that took place in the 1800s.

5. Monophthongization of [aɪ] is characteristic of

a. the New York City area.

b. the New England area.

c. most of the South.

d. the Midland area.

6. When referring to social dialects, the linguistic marketplace was noted as a social variable. This refers to

a. the difference in speech patterns relative to low and high socio-economic levels.

b. the value placed upon using vernacular dialects.

c. the fact that certain occupations (economic activities) tend to use more standard varieties of a language than other members of the same social class with different occupations.

d. all of the above.

7. A pidgin language is a

a. form of informal Standard English.

b. language that was spoken in the British Isles during the last century and has influenced American English.

c. language spoken in northwestern Pennsylvania.

d. system of communication that has grown up among people who do not share a common language, but who want to talk to one another.

8. Which one of the following groups of Spanish-speaking individuals is the largest in the United States?

a. Mexican

b. Puerto Rican

c. Cuban

d. Central and South American

9. Several of the foreign languages that were summarized were tone languages. A tone language is a language in which

a. all words end with a rising pitch.

b. the meaning of a syllable (morpheme) changes with the systematic use of specific pitch variations.

c. all words have only one syllable.

d. words do not have final consonants.

10. Which one of the following languages has the same vowel system as American English?

a. Hmong

b. Korean

c. Spanish

d. none of the languages

Answers: 1. a   2. c   3. d   4. c   5. c   6. c   7. d   8. a   9. b   10. d

For additional information, go to www.phonologicaldisorders.com

CHAPTER 7

Speech in Context and Diacritics

Chapter Highlights

- What is coarticulation?
- What is assimilation? What are the different types of assimilation?
- What are pitch, tone, intonation, and speech melody?
- What is stress? Which variables are associated with stress?
- What is tempo? What is rhythm?
- What are diacritics? What type of features can they add to a particular speech sound?

Chapter Application: Case Study

Jeri had just started her new job working in a private practice. There were several speech-language clinicians who were working in the same facilities; however, Jeri had been hired to work fairly exclusively with preschool children who had phonological disorders. She had really liked working with these children when she was in graduate school and hoped to get some real experience in this private practice. She was scheduled to assess three children this morning between the ages of 4 and 6 years old. The first child, Andrew, who was 4 years old, was fairly straightforward. He produced /t/ for /k/ and /d/ for /g/ in all word positions. He also had difficulties with later-developing sounds such as /θ/ and /ð/. Jeri decided she would leave the th-sounds for later. The second child, Nicole, was 6 years old and had trouble with /s/ and /ʃ/ productions. Jeri listened carefully and tried to see how Nicole was producing her /s/. She decided that the tongue placement was too far forward: The /s/ almost sounded like a th-sound, but not really. The /ʃ/ was clearly produced without the typical lip rounding. Jeri would need to go back to her notes and find out how to transcribe these sounds: a too-far-forward tongue placement on /s/ and lack of lip rounding on /ʃ/. She knew it had to do with diacritics that she had learned that were added to the phonetic symbol. And then child number three appeared. Justin was 4 years old and really unintelligible. He seemed to have /d/, /m/, /n/, and /b/ sounds; especially /d/ was used as a substitution for many other sounds. Jeri noted also lots of consonant and vowel distortions that she was going to have difficulty transcribing. Also, the melody of his speech sounded unusual. She was not clear how to document this or what notation system to use. Justin was going to be a challenge.

Up to this point, the production characteristics of consonants and vowels have been treated as isolated units. However, in connected speech the production features of vowels and consonants are constantly being modified due to the impact of several variables. Two of these factors that will be discussed in this chapter are coarticulation and suprasegmental (prosodic) features. **Coarticulation** refers to the changes in the production features of consonants and vowels as they are influenced by surrounding sounds. **Suprasegmental features**, or **prosodic features**, typically include those modifications that occur that are related to intonation, stress, and timing. These features will be defined and examples given in the following section. Both coarticulatory and suprasegmental aspects of speech production will be important variables as we examine consonants and vowels in words and utterances. Therefore, the first goal of this chapter is to define, explain, and give examples of coarticulation and suprasegmental features as they impact the articulation of vowels and consonants in words and conversational speech.

The second portion of this chapter will introduce the diacritics that can be used to document modifications in vowel and consonant production. **Diacritics** are small, letter-shaped symbols or marks that can be added to a vowel or consonant symbol to modify or refine its phonetic value. These diacritics are very important as we attempt to transcribe the speech of children and adults with speech difficulties. Diacritics associated with consonant, vowel, and suprasegmental productions will be introduced and clinical examples provided. The accompanying DVD gives audio and video examples of the various diacritics.

Sounds in Context: Coarticulation and Assimilation

Speech is not a series of discrete segments but rather consists of overlapping motor movements. These constantly changing articulatory patterns can result in several types of modifications to the sounds in context and are influenced by the neighboring sounds and, therefore, by the phonetic context in which the sound occurs. These modifications are grouped together under the term *coarticulation*. **Coarticulation**, in a broad manner, refers to the fact that a phonological segment is not realized identically in all environments, but often apparently varies to become more like an adjacent or nearby segment (Kühnert & Nolan, 2000). The influences of coarticulation often extend well beyond the boundaries of a particular segment and appear to be the influence of both spatial and temporal linking of articulatory gestures.

Although the term *coarticulation* dates from the 1930s (Menzerath & De Lacerda, 1933), the fact that speech sounds influence each other and vary, often substantially, according to the adjacent phonetic context has been known for much longer. It is in part based on the fact that the stream of speech cannot be divided into separate segments corresponding to "sounds," which has been documented since the 1800s (e.g., Paul, 1898; Rousselot, 1897–1901; Sievers, 1876). However, speech-language clinicians often do not recognize this phenomenon nor account for the fact that coarticulation can and does have an impact on a child's speech production. These changes are often quite normal variations and should not be

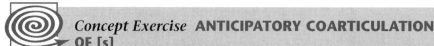

labeled as error patterns. In addition, coarticulation should be considered when establishing the phonetic context for treatment. In other words, the phonetic context should be evaluated when selecting words and phrases for newly acquired sounds.

To exemplify, one type of coarticulation is called *spreading*. Spreading refers to the expansion of an articulatory feature beyond its segmental unit. One type of spreading that has been extensively researched is the lip rounding associated with the /u/ vowel. This lip rounding, labeled as anticipatory coarticulation, is initiated as many as four to six segments before the actual target vowel, regardless of syllable or word boundaries (Benguerel & Cowan, 1974; Sussman & Westbury, 1981). Assume that we are working with a child with an s-problem. If you say [s] in isolation, you will note that typically there is lip spreading. (This is actually one of the articulatory features of /s/ that we often use when attempting to establish an /s/ that sounds within normal limits. We will often ask the child to "smile" when attempting the sound.) Now assume that our client is barely able to say [s], and we have the first attempts at an [s] articulation that sounds "correct." If we attempt this sound in the context of /u/ in words such as "soup" or "Sue," the phenomenon of coarticulatory spreading would necessitate that the [s] will be produced with lip rounding. For the child's unstable production, this could lead to articulatory difficulties.

It should also be kept in mind that, in general, children demonstrate more variable phonetic patterns than adults (e.g., Kent & Forner, 1980; Sharkey & Folkins, 1985). This has led to the hypothesis that children's productions might be characterized by more, rather than less, coarticulation (Nittrouer, Studdert-Kennedy, & McGowan, 1989; Nittrouer & Whalen, 1989). This view, which is consistent with the gestural approach of Browman and Goldstein (1986), assumes that children rely to a larger extent on syllable-based speech production units and only gradually narrow their extent of articulatory organization. Thus, the coarticulatory overlap of gestures would be more prominent at early ages. Coarticulation is an important aspect of speech production. The next section will look at the result of coarticulation, which is referred to as assimilation.

FOCUS 1: *What is coarticulation?*

Assimilation is the adaptive articulatory change that results in neighboring sound segments becoming similar in their production. Assimilatory changes may affect any or all of the sound's phonetic properties. Thus, the active and passive articulators, manner, and/or voicing characteristics of a consonant may change due to assimilation. Assimilation appears to be the result of motor simplification processes; these changes promote economy of effort, facility of movement, and take less time. Therefore, assimilation processes are natural consequences of normal speech production. Although certain types of assimilation are characteristic of children's speech, they occur continually in the speech of adults as well.

There are different types and degrees of assimilation. Due to the fact that neighboring speech sounds become more alike, these processes have also been referred to as **harmony processes**.

1. Assimilation, or harmony processes, can affect those sounds that are directly adjacent to one another or are separated by one or more sounds within a word or utterance. When one segment affects a sound that directly precedes or follows it, this is referred to as **contact** or **contiguous assimilation**. The influence of the rounded, high-back vowel [u] resulting in lip rounding of [s] during the production of "Sue" (as opposed to the normally occurring lip spreading of [s]) is an example of contact, or contiguous, assimilation. If at least one other segment separates the sounds in question, especially when the sounds are in two different syllables, this is labeled **remote** or **noncontiguous assimilation**. With very small children, one can hear the pronunciation of [gag] for "dog" or [gʌk] for "duck." These are examples of remote or noncontiguous assimilation. In these cases, the active and passive articulators for [g] and [k] (postdorsal-velar) have assimilated the coronal-alveolar placement of [d]. Although they are not in two different syllables, the vowel is separating the two consonants.

Some common examples of contact and remote assimilation are as follows:

"news" [nuẕ] versus "newspaper" [nus̱peɪpɚ]

Although the word "news" has a voiced [z] at the end, in the context of "newspaper" this [z] becomes devoiced resulting in [s]. This is a contact assimilation that results from the influence of the voiceless [p] that follows the normally voiced fricative.

"phone" [foʊn̲] versus "phonebooth" [foʊm̲buθ]

The [n] at the end of "phone" is assimilated typically to an [m] in "phonebooth." This is due to the following bilabial stop-plosive [b], which has a tendency to change the coronal-alveolar [n] to a bilabial nasal [m].

The following example is often heard in the speech of young children:

"yellow" [j̠ɛl̲oʊ] → [l̲ɛl̲oʊ]

This is a remote assimilation of the active and passive articulators as well as the manner of articulation, which is influenced by the [l] in the second syllable; the mediodorsal-mediopalatal central approximant [j] becomes an apico-alveolar lateral approximant.

2. Assimilation, or harmony, processes can also be labeled according to the direction of the influence. If the influence is moving forward, i.e., a sound segment modifies a following sound, this is termed **progressive** or **perseverative assimilation**. If the influence is moving backward, i.e., a sound segment modifies a preceding sound, this is termed **regressive** or

Reflect on This: Clinical Application

The following assimilation processes were noted in the results of a child's articulation test:

Contact Assimilation

    "jumping" [dʒʌmpɪn] → [dʒʌmbɪn]

A contact assimilation of voicing: The voiced [m] (and probably the influence of the voiced vowel) impacted the normally voiceless [p].

    "skunk" [skʌŋk] → [stʌŋk]

A contact assimilation of the active and passive articulators: The placement of [s] (apico-alveolar) influenced the usual postdorsal-velar production of [k], changing it to a coronal-alveolar [t].

Remote Assimilation

    "telephone" [tɛləfoʊn] → [tɛdəfoʊn]

A remote assimilation of the active articulator and the manner of articulation: under the influence of [t], the apico-alveolar lateral approximant was changed to [d], a coronal-alveolar stop-plosive.

---

anticipatory assimilation. The previous example with "yellow" is an example of regressive (or anticipatory) assimilation.

The following examples can often be heard:

    "cabin" [kæbən] → [kæbm̩]

This is a progressive assimilation in which the bilabial [b] influences the final nasal, which is typically a coronal-alveolar placement. It now becomes a bilabial nasal, thus [m].

    "intact" [ɪntækt] but "incubate" [ɪŋkjubeɪt]

This is a regressive assimilation in which the [k], a postdorsal-velar consonant, influences the normally coronal-alveolar nasal. This nasal becomes more like the [k], thus assimilating to a postdorsal-velar nasal.

    "fish sandwich" [fɪʃ sænwɪtʃ] → [fɪs sænwɪtʃ]

This is a regressive assimilation in which the "s" of "sandwich" influences the preceding [ʃ]. The result is that the [ʃ] is assimilated to an [s].

    "pumpkin" [pʌmkɪn] → [pʌŋkɪn]

This is an example of a regressive assimilation of the active and passive articulators: Under the influence of the postdorsal-velar stop-plosive [k], the bilabial nasal [m] is changed to a postdorsal-velar nasal [ŋ].

3. Assimilation or harmony processes can also be labeled according to the degree of assimilation. If the number of features affected is such that the altered segment is perceived to be a different speech sound altogether, i.e., a different phoneme, this is considered **phonemic assimilation** (Ball & Rahilly, 1999). Phonemic assimilation can be partial or total. **Partial assimilation** is encountered when the changed segment is closer but not identical to the sound that was the source of the change. Examples of partial assimilation include the previously noted "pumpkin" ([pʌmkɪn] → [pʌŋkɪn]) or "phonebooth" ([foʊnbuθ] → [foʊmbuθ]). **Total assimilation** is the label given when the changed segment and the source of the change become identical. Total assimilation would include "panty hose" ([pænti

Reflect on This: Clinical Application

The following assimilation processes were noted in the results of a child's articulation test:

Progressive Assimilation

"ice cream" [aɪskrim] → [aɪstrim]

Progressive assimilation of the active and passive articulators: Under the influence of the apico-alveolar fricative [s], the [k] is assimilated from a postdorsal-velar to a coronal-alveolar stop-plosive.

"television" [tɛləvɪʒən] → [tɛdəvɪʒən]

Progressive assimilation of the active and passive articulators: The coronal-alveolar stop-plosive [t] impacts the [l], changing it from an apico-alveolar lateral approximant to a coronal-alveolar stop-plosive.

Regressive Assimilation

"ice cream cone" [aɪskrimkoʊn] → [aɪskrinkoʊn]

Regressive assimilation of the active and passive articulators: The coronal-alveolar nasal [n] influences the [m], assimilating it from a bilabial to a coronal-alveolar nasal.

The following assimilation was noted in a child with speech sound difficulties. Note that [b] can be produced; it is present at the end of the word "bathtub."

"bathtub" [bæθtəb] → [θæθtəb]

Regressive assimilation of all production features: Influenced by the following voiceless apico-dental fricative [θ], the voiced bilabial stop-plosive is totally changed to [θ].

hoʊz] → [pæni hoʊz]) and "yellow" ([jɛloʊ] → [lɛloʊ]). If the number of features affected is such that the altered segment is perceived to be an allophonic variation of the speech sound, i.e., it does not change the phoneme value, this is considered an **allophonic similitude**. The lip rounding noted on [s] in the word "Sue" or the nasalization that is typically noted on vowels in the environment of nasal consonants, such as in the word "man" [mæ̃n], would be examples of allophonic similitude. A further type of assimilation is termed *coalescence*. **Coalescence** occurs when two neighboring speech sounds are merged and form a new and different segment. An example of coalescence was noted on the word "sandwich" ([sænwɪtʃ]) when a child responded with [sæmɪtʃ]. Here the nasal qualities of [n] and the bilabial influence of [w] combine to form a new sound, [m], a bilabial nasal.

In addition to assimilation processes, speech sounds in context are influenced by suprasegmental or prosodic features. These features, which include pitch, loudness, and tempo, extend over more than one segment. The following discussion is an introduction to the suprasegmental aspects of speech.

FOCUS 2: *What is assimilation? What are the different types of assimilation?*

The Suprasegmentals

The prefix *supra-* indicates "beyond the limits of," "outside of." Therefore, *suprasegmental* indicates those aspects of speech production that are outside of the segmental units. Suprasegmental aspects of speech transcend the actual consonants and vowels of an utterance extending throughout the entire utterance. *Prosody* refers to modulations of voice, from the Greek verb indicating "to sing with" or "accompanying"

Sound segments, which are combined to produce syllables, words, and sentences, relate to *what* we say. At the same time that we articulate these sound segments, our pronunciation varies in other respects as well. For example, we vary the pitch of our voice, we use different loudness levels, or we may speed up or draw out a word or sound. Consider the sentence, "You bought that." This could be said as a statement, with a falling tone at the end of the word, such as [ju bɑt ðæt ↘], or it could be said as a question, [ju bɑt ðæt ↗]. In the first case, the pitch decreased at the end of the sentence; in the second case it increased. Imagine now that you want to say the same thing, but you are indicating that whatever was bought was totally unbelievable. You might make "that" louder or you might even lengthen the vowel somewhat. By varying our pitch, loudness, and duration, the meaning that we want to convey is changed. Prosodic, or suprasegmental, features relate to *how* we say something to convey meaning.

Suprasegmental features occur across segments and include pitch, loudness, and durational variations. Pitch, the first suprasegmental parameter, is often used synonymously with the terms *melody, tone,* or even *intonation*. To keep these terms somewhat differentiated, the following definitions are suggested. **Pitch** will be used to refer to the perceptual correlate of frequency. The physiological mechanism associated with frequency is the number of cycles per second the vocal folds vibrate, known as the fundamental frequency (these terms were covered in Chapter 2). Thus, how we perceive the changes in fundamental frequency of the vocal folds is pitch.

Tone refers to the changes in fundamental frequency, perceived as pitch, when they function linguistically at the word (morpheme) level. The best examples are the so-called tone languages. In these languages, systematic fundamental frequency changes; thus, pitch changes have phonemic value. Thus, pitch changes create words with different meanings. In well over half of the languages of the world, it is possible to change the meaning of a word simply by changing the pitch level at which it is spoken. An example of this is the sound segment /si/ in Cantonese. By varying primarily the tone of the word, six different meanings emerge. Figure 7.1 shows pitch tracks of the six productions of /si/. The numbers on the left, represented in Hz, demonstrate the fluctuations in fundamental frequency. It should be kept in mind that these Hz figures are relative. The word /si/ was spoken by a woman; typically, a male's voice would produce overall lower fundamental frequencies.

The third term, **intonation**, refers to the feature of pitch when it functions linguistically at the sentence level. Therefore, the difference between a statement "I saw him" and a question "I saw him?" relates to intonation. Intonation also carries nonlinguistic meaning: the use of features (such as tempo) at the sentence level to reflect the attitudes of the speaker and the relative urgency of the message. There is an interaction between the linguistic and the attitudinal aspects of intonation; they cannot be clearly separated. This is exemplified by the inability to find a correlation between grammatical and lexical sentence types and intonation contours. For example, in several studies no special question-intonation contour could be clearly established (Hadding-Koch, 1961; Uldall, 1960). The elevated question type, such as "Is she there?" looked the same as certain "reactions" by speakers. Thus, although linguistic and attitudinal intonation should be clearly separated, this is not often an objectively easy task.

To simplify matters, there seem to be a few common intonation contours (MacKay, 1987).

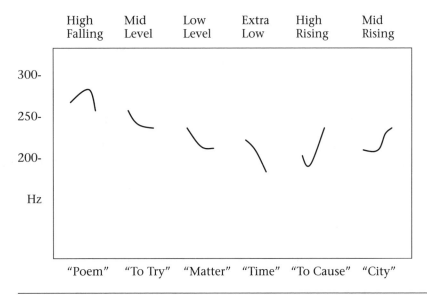

Figure 7.1 Approximate Pitch Levels Showing the Tones of the Cantonese Syllable /si/

Source: Adapted from Ladefoged (2005).

Statements: The intonation is usually relatively level with a slight rise and fall in intonation at the end of the sentence.

Examples:

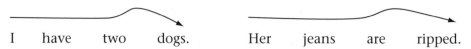

Questions: The pitch level is generally higher throughout the utterance with a short drop then rise at the end of the question.

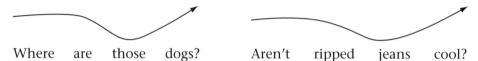

Exclamations: This type of sentence has a pattern similar to that of the statement, but there is a sharper fall in pitch at the end.

Often, short sentences will look like longer, compressed sentences of similar syntactic type. In addition, each breath group of a sentence, each place that you would pause in a sentence, may have its own intonation pattern. The following is question intonation followed by two short statement intonation patterns.

Short sentence:

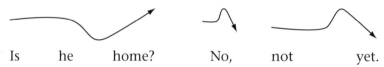

The following sentence demonstrates three breath groups (each breath group is within parentheses with their own intonation pattern):

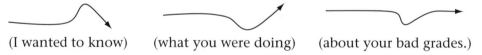

Also if a list of items is presented, then each individual item is marked with a specific intonation pattern, and the end of the list is also marked.

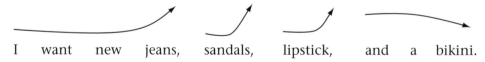

These are just basic intonation patterns. Obviously, other intonation patterns exist, and these same sentences could be stated with various other intonation contours depending on the context. These are just offered as an introduction.

The last term, melody or, better, **speech melody,** is a general term used to reference pitch fluctuations relative to their linguistic function. According to Abercrombie (1967), melody at the sentence level is referred to as *intonation*, at the word (morpheme) level, *tone*. If one uses this definition, then speech melody is a broader term encompassing both intonation and tone. Languages can also be classified according to the two speech melody parameters: intonation languages and tone languages. In the case of intonation languages, the function of the speech melody patterns is a part of the structure of sentences. In tone languages, the function of the speech melody patterns is a portion of the structure of the morphemes. American English is an intonation language; Chinese is a tone language.

FOCUS 3: *What are pitch, tone, intonation, and speech melody?*

A second parameter of the suprasegmentals is stress. **Stress** refers to the degree of force of an utterance or the prominence produced by means of respiratory effort (Lehiste, 1977). Syllables can be stressed. For example, if we examine the word "<u>con</u>tract" versus "con<u>tract</u>," we find that the placement of the stress (first syllable as opposed to the second syllable) changes the meaning of the word. Stress can also be on a word in a sentence. Consider the sentence "I drove her home." If stress is put on "I," then it could indicate that I—as opposed to someone else—drove her home. By changing the stress to "home," "I drove her <u>home</u>" becomes a question of where you drove her—home as opposed to somewhere else.

As can be seen from the above examples, there are at least two different types of stress: word stress and sentence stress, which is typically called phrasal stress (MacKay, 1987). *Word stress* refers to the prominence of a certain syllable in a word. Although we differentiate three levels of stress in multisyllabic words, typically only two are marked: primary and secondary stress. The phonetic symbols used for primary and secondary stress are covered in the section on diacritics. However, some examples of word stress and phrasal stress would be helpful.

Most words in American English are stressed on the first syllable, such as "<u>ho</u>-li-day," "<u>win</u>-ter," "<u>loo</u>-king." However, there are many different words that have stress on the second syllable, such as "a-<u>way</u>," "for-<u>get</u>," and "un-<u>wrap</u>." There are also words in which the stress can be on other syllables, such as "re-cre-<u>a</u>-tion" or "pa-tho-<u>lo</u>-gi-cal." Noun and verb pairs can be contrasted in American English using stress. The noun "<u>rec</u>-ord" versus the verb "re-<u>cord</u>" and "<u>sub</u>-ject" versus "sub-<u>ject</u>" are two examples of this type of stress.

Prominence is also given within the grammatical phrase in American English to show grammatical and semantic relations among the words in the phrase. This is termed *phrasal stress*. For example, in an adjective-noun combination, the noun usually takes primary stress:

It's a black <u>bird</u>.
It's my dog's <u>house</u>.

However, if it is a compound noun, then the first element of the compound may take primary stress:

It's a <u>black</u>bird.
Hunter is in his <u>dog</u>house.

Just as word stress can distinguish between two word meanings, phrasal stress creates distinctions between such phrases as "<u>hot</u> dog" (I ate a <u>hot</u> dog) and "hot <u>dog</u>" (Hunter was in the sun; he's a hot <u>dog</u>) or "hearing-impaired <u>teacher</u>" (She taught child with hearing losses; she was a hearing impaired teacher) and "<u>hearing impaired</u> teacher" (She had a hearing loss and was a teacher; she was a <u>hearing impaired</u> teacher.)

Stress can also function at the sentence level. In American English, content words are given more prominence than function words. Content words are those containing the most information and consist of nouns, verbs, adjectives, and adverbs. Low-semantic-content words include prepositions and articles. Look at the following sentences:

He caught a cold.
His grades were really bad.

The words with emphasis include "He" and "cold" in the first sentence. The word "caught," though, has more emphasis than "a." Words that are emphasized in the second sentence include "grades," "really," and "bad." However, sentence emphasis also depends on the context. One could imagine a context in which "were" in the second sentence could have primary emphasis. "His grades <u>were</u> really bad," indicating that now they are not.

Sentence emphasis can also function contrastively in what has been termed new information versus old information. Those words that give the listener new information, as opposed to the old, "setting the stage" information, are in this case stressed.

I lost the <u>dog</u>.
<u>Which</u> dog?
The big one, <u>Hunter</u>.
Where did you see him <u>last</u>?
He <u>was</u> in the <u>backyard</u>.

Unlike intonation, which can be traced directly back to the changing fundamental frequency of the vibrating vocal folds, stress is an elusive factor. There is no single mechanism that can be attributed to stress. If it is defined from the speaker's viewpoint, then stress is attributed to greater effort; more effort is exerted in the production of a stressed syllable than

Reflect on This: Clinical Application

Clients with dysarthrias may have difficulty with word stress and sentence emphasis. The following transcription exemplifies such a possible displacement of stress.

"umbrella"   Speaker with dysarthria: [ʌm brɛ lə]
"He <u>needed</u> his um<u>bre</u>lla"   Speaker with dysarthria: [hi nidəd hɪz ʌm brɛ lə]

an unstressed one. However, if stress is defined from a listener's viewpoint, then it is claimed that stressed syllables are louder than unstressed ones. However, already decades ago (Black, 1949; Fairbanks, House, & Stevens, 1950; Lehiste & Peterson, 1959; Liberman, Cooper, Harris, & MacNeilage, 1963) it was found that perception of stress is very subjective. If loudness, measured in amplitude of the signal, is objectively manipulated, there is not a direct correlation between loudness levels and the perception of stress. Listeners also tend to perceive those vowels that are produced with greater articulatory effort, such as [i] and [u], as being louder, even though objectively they were not. Although stress seems to be related to greater articulatory effort, the objective measurements of stress demonstrate that, typically, increased loudness, a higher fundamental frequency, and a longer duration are noted in stressed versus unstressed syllables.

Beginning Case Study

JERI, THE SPEECH-LANGUAGE CLINICIAN

Jeri had noted that Justin's speech melody was somehow different. As she listened more to his speech, she noticed that word stress and sentence emphasis were different. He seemed often to use equal stress on multisyllabic words, and sentence emphasis was often on the first word of the sentence, regardless of the content.

Here are some examples that Jeri had noted:

<u>Where</u> is that red car? (as opposed to the green one that he had)

<u>I</u> want that one. (in a choice between this one and that one)

<u>Do</u> you have it? (asking about a special toy)

<u>Can</u> I have the blue one? (referring to the blue crayon he needed it to finish his picture)

Jeri thought that the sentence emphasis should be on different words. Which words would you think that Justin should have emphasized in the four sentences?

FOCUS 4: *What is stress? Which variables are associated with stress?*

The third suprasegmental is duration. Every speech sound has a certain time interval. The relative speed of an utterance is referenced by tempo. **Tempo** is the speed of speaking. It is possible to speed up or slow down the rate at which syllables, words, and sentences are produced to convey several different meanings and emotions. A faster tempo may indicate urgency, a slower one contemplation. A rapid, clipped single syllable may convey irritation; a slowly drawled syllable, more personal reflection. Consider the two sentences:

"Are you leaving?" asked Janet. "Yes," snapped Larry.

"Are you leaving?" asked Janet. "Yeeeeeesss," replied Larry thoughtfully stroking his chin.

Pitch, loudness and tempo together enter into a language's expression of rhythm. **Rhythm** refers to the manner in which stressed and unstressed syllables succeed each other, i.e., how syllables are distributed across time. Each language has its own rhythmical pattern, which is one of the most fundamental things about it. Languages fall basically into two types of rhythmical patterns: stress-timed, or isochronous, rhythm and syllable-timed rhythm. In a stressed-timed language, each breath group has more or less the same duration. Typically, breath groups contain about five syllables, although it is possible to have a breath group of only one syllable. On page 208, breath groups for a sentence were placed in parentheses. Breath groups are those places in a sentence where normal pauses occur. That means that the unstressed syllables will be spoken rather quickly to compensate for the stressed syllable, which is longer in duration. If the breath group has an unusually high number of syllables, the whole group of syllables will be speeded up, the stressed syllable still taking relatively more time. In a stress-timed language, usually, but not always, the stressed syllable in the breath group contains new information. Therefore, by altering the duration of a specific syllable, the meaning can change. When a stressed-time language is spoken faster, vowels are shortened, reduced (to schwa /ə/ typically), or deleted so that more syllables can be inserted between the two stressed syllables. English is considered to be a classical example of a stressed-time language.

On the other hand, in syllable-timed languages each syllable is thought to take up roughly the same amount of time. That means that each breath group varies in duration. However, if a breath group has an unusually high number of syllables, each syllable will be spoken more quickly to fit within a single breath. The term *machine-gun rhythm* has been used figuratively to describe this pattern with each underlying unit being of the same duration as the bullet noise of a machine-gun. French is considered to be a syllable-timed language.

FOCUS 5: *What is tempo? What is rhythm?*

To summarize, suprasegmental, or prosodic, features extend over several sound segments. At least three parameters can be observed: pitch, loudness, and duration. These three factors function linguistically as intonation, stress, and tempo. The combined effect of intonation, stress, and tempo is referred to as the rhythm of a particular utterance or language.

The next section will examine the diacritics; those markers that are added to the phonetic symbol to give it added meaning. There are diacritics that are used specifically for vowels, those for consonants, and a set of symbols that categorize the suprasegmentals. These diacritics will often be used when transcribing disordered speech.

Diacritics

Phonetic transcription systems were originally designed to transfer standard speech events into readable signs. For example, sounds and words of a particular foreign language could be transcribed using the International

Phonetic Alphabet. If you knew this system, you would actually have a good idea of how to pronounce those words even though you might not know the foreign language at all. For this purpose, phonemic or broad transcription of a language using the given consonant and vowel symbols of the IPA would probably be adequate. However, speech-language pathologists are often transcribing aberrant patterns of speech. For this special purpose, the given vowels and consonants might not be enough to describe the production detail. Additional symbols may be frequently required to denote the special production features demonstrated by individuals with speech disorders. These additional symbols are termed *diacritics*. As noted previously, diacritics are marks added to transcription symbols in order to give them a particular phonetic value. Figure 7.2 is an excerpt from the International Phonetic Alphabet chart showing the diacritics.

For example, in the box of Figure 7.2, the first two are *voiceless*, indicated by a small circle, and *voiced*, indicated by a symbol looking like a rather open "v." These diacritics, which are typically placed below the symbol in question, would be used if a normally voiced sound was produced partially voiceless, [z̥], for example, or if a sound that is typically voiceless demonstrated a partial voiced quality, exemplified by [s̬]. In each of these examples, the diacritic adds a special production feature to the symbol. The basic concept is an important one; diacritics are supplemental markers that can be added to the sound symbol to document an atypical production feature.

While the diacritics noted on the IPA chart functioned fairly effectively in their attempt to portray disordered speech, at the 1989 convention of the International Phonetic Association, a committee of individuals was established to draw up recommendations for the transcription of disordered

DIACRITICS Diacritics may be placed above a symbol with a descender, e.g. ŋ̊

̥	Voiceless	n̥ d̥	̤	Breathy voiced	b̤ a̤	̪	Dental	t̪ d̪
̬	Voiced	s̬ t̬	̰	Creaky voiced	b̰ a̰	̺	Apical	t̺ d̺
ʰ	Aspirated	tʰ dʰ	̼	Linguolabial	t̼ d̼	̻	Laminal	t̻ d̻
̹	More rounded	ɔ̹	ʷ	Labialized	tʷ dʷ	̃	Nasalized	ẽ
̜	Less rounded	ɔ̜	ʲ	Palatalized	tʲ dʲ	ⁿ	Nasal release	dⁿ
̟	Advanced	u̟	ˠ	Velarized	tˠ dˠ	ˡ	Lateral release	dˡ
̠	Retracted	e̠	ˤ	Pharyngealized	tˤ dˤ	̚	No audible release	d̚
̈	Centralized	ë	̴	Velarized or pharyngealized	ɫ			
̽	Mid-centralized	e̽	̝	Raised	e̝	(ɹ̝ = voiced alveolar fricative)		
̩	Syllabic	n̩	̞	Lowered	e̞	(β̞ = voiced bilabial approximant)		
̯	Non-syllabic	e̯	̘	Advanced Tongue Root	e̘			
˞	Rhoticity	ɚ a˞	̙	Retracted Tongue Root	e̙			

Figure 7.2 Diacritics

Source: *International Phonetic Alphabet* (2005). Copyright © 2005 by the International Phonetic Association.

ExtIPA SYMBOLS FOR DISORDERED SPEECH
(Revised 1997)

CONSONANTS (other than those on the IPA Chart)

	bilabial	labiodental	dentolabial	labioalv.	linguolabial	interdental	bidental	alveolar	velar	velophar.
Plosive		p̪ b̪	p͆ b͆	p̺ b̺	t̼ d̼	t̪ d̪	▓			▓
Nasal			m̪	m̺	n̼	n̪	▓			
Trill					r̼	r̪	▓		▓	
Fricative: central			f̪ v̪	f̺ v̺	θ̼ ð̼	θ̪ ð̪	h̪ h̪			fŋ
Fricative: lateral+ central	▓	▓	▓	▓			▓	ʪ ʫ	▓	▓
Fricative: nareal	m̃						▓	ñ̥	ŋ̃	
Percussive	ʬ						ʭ			
Approximant: lateral	▓	▓	▓	▓	l̼	l̪	▓			

Figure 7.3 Extensions to the IPA (ExtIPA) for Disordered Speech

Source: From the *International Clinical Phonetics and Linguistic Association*, 1997. Copyright 1997 by the ICPLA. Reproduced with permission.

speech. Their report, published in 1990 (Duckworth, Allen, Hardcastle, & Ball) contained a list of symbols that were termed "Extensions to the IPA" or, in its common abbreviated form, "ExtIPA." These symbols were adopted by the International Clinical Phonetics and Linguistics Association and published in the 1994 publication of the *Journal of the International Phonetic Association*. The ExtIPA has also been revised, the newest revision dating to 1997. Figure 7.3 is a partial list of the ExtIPA symbols.

There are numerous diacritics in use today. Most of them are part of the IPA notation system. Others will have to be modified to meet our clinical needs. Still others might have to be invented to represent a special articulatory situation. The following is a list of diacritics that are often utilized. Unless otherwise noted, these diacritics are those proposed by the latest modification of the International Phonetic Alphabet (IPA, 2005).

Diacritics Used with Consonants

CHANGES IN THE ACTIVE OR PASSIVE ARTICULATORS FOR CONSONANTS. These symbols describe deviations from normal tongue placement for consonants.

Reflect On This: Clinical Application

THE ExtIPA AND MULTIPLE INTERDENTALITY

Multiple interdentality is a label dating back to at least the 1930s (Froeschels, 1931). It is used to describe an immature speech habit in which children produce [t], [d], [l], and [n] with their tongue tip too far forward. In other words, the tongue tip is between their teeth, making it an interdental production. Looking at the ExtIPA chart, we see that there is a way to transcribe these sounds. They would be transcribed in the following manner:

[t̪], [d̪], [l̪], [n̪]

Children with multiple interdentality often have difficulty with [s] and [z], as well. These sounds are also produced interdentally and end up sounding like th-sounds, [θ] and [ð].

---

1. Dentalization. Dentalization refers to an articulatory variation in which the tongue approaches the upper incisors. It is marked by [̪] placed under the IPA symbol. For example, the symbol /s/ represents an apico-alveolar voiceless fricative. A dentalized realization results when the tip of the tongue does not approximate the alveolar ridge but approaches the upper incisors instead. A dentalized realization is transcribed as

[s̪] = dentalized [s]

Dentalized s-sounds, [s̪] and [z̪], frequently occur in the speech of children (Van Riper, 1978; Weiss, Gordon, & Lillywhite, 1987).

Transcription Example:

house $\quad$ h a͡ʊ s̪

sun $\quad$ s̪ ʌ n

scissors $\quad$ s̪ ɪ z̪ ɚ z̪

2. Palatalization. Another modification of consonant articulation is *palatalization.* Only sounds for which the palate is not the passive articulator can be palatalized. Therefore, palatalization can occur with sounds that have the passive articulator anterior or posterior to the hard palate region. If the passive articulator is the alveolar ridge or the upper incisors, the term *palatalization* would be used if the anterior portions of the tongue approach anterior parts of the palate, i.e., when the active and passive articulators are positioned somewhat posteriorly. For velar consonants, palatalization indicates the movement of the active and passive articulators in the direction of the palate, to a more anterior articulation. Palatalization causes a typical change in the quality of the sound(s) in question. The diacritical mark for palatalization is an elevated [ʲ], which is placed behind the symbol in question. The term *palatalization* is also used to indicate a secondary articulation that is often heard as a [j]-type glide following the consonant concerned (Ball & Rahilly, 1999). Secondary articulations are usually predictable coarticulatory effects related to neighboring sound segments.

> [sʲ] = palatalized [s], the tongue placement is farther back than is normally the case
>
> [lʲ] = palatalization of [l], which can occur before [ju] in words such as "evaluate"

Transcription Example:

sushi _____ sʲuʃi _____

zipper _____ zʲɪpɚ _____

evaluate _ ɪvælʲueɪt _____

3. Velarization. Velarization refers to the posterior movement of the tongue placement (in the direction of the velum) for palatal sounds. The auditory impression of this change in the articulators can be exemplified by the so-called "dark" /l/, which in General American English is usually heard in word-final positions (also as a syllabic), preceding a consonant, and following back vowels (Bronstein, 1960; Carrell & Tiffany, 1960). The velarization in these cases is often so prominent that even main phonetic characteristics of [l], the articulation of the tongue tip against the alveolar ridge, are sometimes no longer present. In such a case, the velarization actually replaces the typical apico-alveolar l-articulation. The velarized production is an allophonic variation of /l/. Velarized [l]-productions are transcribed [ɫ]. However, other sounds may become velarized as well. According to the IPA, the symbol for velarization is an elevated [ˠ] placed after the symbol in question.

> [kuɫ] = velarized [l]
>
> [tˠub] = velarized [t]

Transcription Example:
Typically, velarized [l] is not transcribed in contexts in which it normally occurs. However, the following examples demonstrate how it could be transcribed.

calm _ kaɫm _____

loop _ ɫup _____

4. Lateralization. /l/ is the only lateral in General American English; only nonlateral speech sounds can be lateralized. If during any consonant production other than /l/, air is released laterally, we speak of *lateralization*. Occasionally, [s] is produced as a lateralized consonant by children with speech difficulties.

A lateral [s]-production can also be caused by coarticulatory conditions. For example, when [l] immediately follows [s], the lateral release of the l-sound may trigger a lateralized [s]. Lateralization is considered a pri-

Reflect on This: Clinical Application

LATERAL s-ARTICULATION IN CHILDREN

Articulations of [s] and [z] require a highly accurate placement of frontal parts of the tongue (apical or predorsal) *approximating* the alveolar ridge. This precarious position must be maintained throughout the entire sound duration, a motorically difficult task, especially for young children. To make things easier, children sometimes establish direct contact between the active and passive articulators. Under these circumstances, the airstream can, of course, not escape centrally any longer. In an attempt to maintain the fricative effect of [s], the child now releases the air laterally into the cheeks. The result is a conspicuous [s] variation, a lateral lisp.

mary articulation; thus, for a lateral [s] production, a completely different symbol is used.

[ɬ] = **lateralized voiceless [s]**
[ɮ] = **lateralized voiced [z]**

Transcription Examples:

Santa ɬæntə

soap ɬoʊp

zoo ɮu

Reflect on This: Clinical Application

THREE VARIATIONS OF [s] MISARTICULATIONS

As previously noted, there are at least three ways in which /s/ can be misarticulated. If the tongue is placed more anteriorly, a dentalized [s] occurs: [s̪]. If the tongue is more posteriorly located than is normally the case, a palatalized [s] may result, thus [sʲ]. Lateralized [s] and [z], [ɬ] and [ɮ], result when the tongue tip comes into direct contact with the alveolar ridge and the lateral edges of the tongue are lowered. This allows for lateral air escape, which may occur on one side, unilaterally, or on both sides, bilaterally.

Differentiating between dentalized, palatalized, and lateralized [s]-productions may seem difficult at first. However, there are clear perceptual qualities that distinguish the three forms of [s] actualizations. Dentalized [s]-sounds, [s̪], have a "dull" quality; they lack the sharp high-frequency characteristic of norm [s] productions. On the other hand, lateralized [s] sounds, [ɬ] and [ɮ], have a distinct noise component to them that is typically as disagreeable as it is conspicuous. Palatalized [s] variations, [sʲ], approach [ʃ] perceptually due to the somewhat posterior placement of the articulators.

VOICE SYMBOLS

1. Devoicing of voiced consonants. Under normal circumstances, vowels and more than half of our consonants are voiced. If these sounds become devoiced in a speech sample, it needs to be marked. In cases of *total* devoicing, the IPA symbol for the voiceless counterpart of the voiced sound, its unvoiced cognate, is usually indicated.

[k̂eɪt] for "gate"
[tɑg] for "dog"

2. Partial devoicing. Often, however, the sound in question is only partially devoiced. The diacritic for *partial devoicing* is a small circle placed under the sound symbol.

[d̥ɑg] for "dog"

If that placement interferes with the clarity of the basic symbol, it is acceptable to put the circle above the sound symbol.

[g̊eɪt] instead of [g̥eɪt]

It should be noted that, in normal conversational speech, voiced final consonants are often partially or totally devoiced. Therefore, such pronunciations as [dɪʃəs] for [dɪʃəz] (dishes) or [sto͡uf] for [sto͡uv] (stove) would be considered normal pronunciations. Although these articulations should be marked, they are not typically considered misarticulations.

3. Voicing of voiceless consonants. Voiceless consonants may become partially or totally voiced. If voiceless consonants become totally voiced, the segment is transcribed with the respective symbol.

[zu] "Sue" = total voicing of the normally voiceless fricative

---

Reflect on This: Clinical Application

The following transcriptions are from Daniel, age 4;7.

stove	[sto͡uv]	→	[sto͡uf]	total devoicing
slide	[sla͡ɪd]	→	[sla͡ɪd̥]	partial devoicing
flag	[flæg]	→	[flæg̊]	partial devoicing
nose	[no͡uz]	→	[no͡us]	total devoicing

The general devoicing tendency in final positions suggests that realizations like these should probably not be considered aberrant productions. However, one should check other productions by Daniel to be certain that his devoicing does not occur excessively or in other word positions.

---

4. Partial voicing. If voiceless consonants become *partially* voiced, the diacritical mark is a lowercase "v" under the respective sound symbol.

[s̬u] "Sue" = partial voicing of the normally voiceless fricative

Transcription Example:

fan f̬æn

think θ̬ɪŋk

5. Aspiration and nonaspiration of stop-plosives. Stop-plosives (as well as other consonants) are often described according to two parameters: fortis and lenis. As noted in Chapter 5, *fortis* refers to more articulatory effort, whereas lenis refers to comparatively less. Most voiceless sounds are realized as fortis consonants, while voiced sounds are usually articulated as lenis productions. (One can note the increased articulatory effort on the level of air pressure by contrasting [t] and [d] with your hand in front of your mouth.) The sudden release of the articulatory effort in fortis stop-plosives leads typically to aspiration. This aspiration is noted by using a small, elevated "h" following the voiceless stop-plosive sound.

tune   [tʰun]

Stop-plosives, which are normally aspirated, are not marked unless the aspiration is excessive.

Voiceless stop-plosives that are typically aspirated may be produced without this fortis aspiration. In this case, the diacritic for unaspirated stops could be added, [⁼].

pie   [p⁼aɪ]

This example indicates that a normally aspirated [p] has occurred without aspiration.

Transcription Examples:

touch tʰʌtʃ

pen pʰɛn

kite kʰaɪt

◎ *Concept Exercise* ASPIRATION

With your hand in front of your mouth, say [p] and note the puff of air that accompanies the production. Try the same thing with [b], and you will find that there is not nearly as much air pressure generated. In this case, [p] has considerably more air pressure, i.e., [p] is aspirated when compared to [b]. Now try the word "two" versus "stew." You should be able to feel the difference between the aspiration of [t] in the word-initial position as opposed to the lack of aspiration when [t] is preceded by [s].

6. Unreleased stop-plosives. Stop-plosives can be modified in yet another manner. Unreleased consonants result when the articulatory closure is maintained, and not released as usual. While voiceless unreleased stops are more obvious because of their loss of aspiration, voiced stops can be unreleased as well. Unreleased stops typically occur at the end of an utterance or in word-final positions. To indicate an *unreleased* articulation, the diacritical mark [̚] is added after the stop-plosive.

The pop is hot.

[ðə pɑp ɪz hɑt̚]

Transcription Examples:

hot ___hat̚___

tap ___tæp̚___

7. Syllabic consonants. Unstressed syllables can become reduced syllables in which the vowel nucleus disappears, and the following consonant becomes a syllabic; it becomes the peak of that syllable. That is especially the case in unstressed final syllables when a nasal or the lateral [l] follow the preceding vowel. The proper diacritic mark for such an occurrence is a straight line directly *under* the syllabic consonant:

lesson = [lɛsən] → [lɛsn̩]

Reflect on This: Clinical Application

Unreleased consonants should be noted *during* the simultaneous transcription of a client's speech. Just listening to and transcribing from tape recordings can be misleading; when taped, unreleased consonants can sound similar to consonant omissions. Confusing this unreleased production with a final-consonant deletion could lead to an inaccurate diagnosis. During live transcriptions, we can hear and at least partially see the actual articulation. This provides a much better basis for our judgment: unreleased consonant production or consonant deletion.

The articulatory position of the syllabic relative to the final consonant of the preceding syllable is important. Some authors (e.g., Edwards, 2003) state that there needs to be a homorganic relationship between the final consonant of the preceding syllable and the syllabic. Thus, the active articulator must be the same (or approximately the same) for both consonants. In order for a syllabic to occur, the consonants /p/ and /b/ must precede /m/, while /t/, /d/, /s/, and /z/ must precede /n/, and /k/ and /g/ must precede /ŋ/ (Edwards, 2003). Other authors (e.g., Small, 2005) state that, although the preceding consonant is not homorganic (the same active articulator), "many individuals still use the syllabic in transcription because the vowel between the consonants is almost nonexistent" (Small, 2005, p. 125). This can be confusing for students beginning transcription and working with diactrics. *Please check with your instructor as to how she or he would like you to use the syllabic diacritics.* The author finds it easier for students to simply apply the rule that the preceding consonant and the syllabic consonant must be homorganic. Consider also the following examples:

"dog and cat"	[dɑg ænd kæt] → [dɑgŋ kæt]
"cut and bruised"	[kʌt ænd bruzd] → [kʌt n̩ bruzd]
"up and away"	[ʌp ænd əweɪ͡] → [ʌp m̩ əweɪ͡]

Again, the consonant preceding the syllabic determines the reduction of the word "and" in each case.

However, there are exceptions to this rule. Edwards (2003) notes that /t/ preceding the syllabic /l/ will typically cause the /t/ to be pronounced as [ɾ], while /t/ before the syllabic /n/ will result in [ʔ], the glottal stop. Examples include the following:

| "cattle" | [kætəl] → [kæɾl̩] |
| "button" | [bʌtən] → [bʌʔn̩] |

Transcription Examples:

redden rɛdn̩

bottle bɑtl̩

8. Labialization/non-labialization of consonants. Consonants, with the exception of /ʃ/ and /w/, are typically produced without lip rounding. If a normally unrounded consonant is produced with lip rounding, this is referred to as labializing the sound in question. When /ʃ/ or /w/ are produced without lip rounding, this is a nonlabialized production. According to the International Phonetic Alphabet diacritic chart (2005), the diacritic for *labialized* consonants is an elevated "w" placed after the symbol. The diacritic for nonlabialized consonants is an arrow placed under the symbol in question (ExtIPA, 1997). Labialized consonants can be the result of assimilation processes, as in the following example:

soup [sʷup] = labialized [s]

The labialized /s/ is the result of a regressive assimilation due to the lip rounding of the following /u/. Labialization of normally unrounded

Reflect on This: Clinical Application

In spontaneous speech, adults often reduce the unstressed final syllable, as in the following example:

He was batting them hard.
[hi wʌz bæʔn̩ m̩ hɑ͡ɚd]

In spontaneous speech, and often during an articulation test, children will also demonstrate the use of syllabics.

kitten	[kɪʔn̩]
losing	[luzn̩]
golden	[go͡ʊldn̩]

While such syllabics obviously need to be noted and transcribed, they are considered norm realizations.

consonants due to assimilation is noted, however, not considered a speech sound problem. On the other hand, /ʃ/ is usually produced with at least some degree of lip rounding. The following example indicates /ʃ/ without lip rounding:

ship [ʃɪp] = nonlabialized [ʃ]

Unrounded [ʃ] realizations can also be due to assimilation; however, there are children who unround [ʃ] in all contexts. This should be noted and is considered an aberrant production.

Transcription Example:

shade ___ʃe͡ɪd___
sandwich ___sʷæ͡nwɪtʃ___

Beginning Case Study

JERI, THE SPEECH-LANGUAGE CLINICIAN

Nicole, one of the children on Jeri's caseload, had an s-production in which her tongue was too far forward. This is a dentalized production and would be transcribed as [s̪] and [z̪]. In addition, this child produces the /ʃ/ without the characteristic lip rounding. The transcription for this is [ʃ] with an arrow placed under it, thus [ʃ].

9. Derhotacization. Derhotacization is the loss of r-coloring for the consonant /r/ and the central vowels with r-coloring, /ɜ/ and /ə/, respectively. Derhotacized central vowels are transcribed as [ɜ] and [ə]. The consonant /r/ as in "run" can also lose its r-coloring. Children often substitute [w] for this sound; however, that is not considered derhotacization.

Transcription Examples:

mother ___mʌɜ̩ə___

bird ___bɜd___

shirt ___ʃɜt___

Diacritics Used with Vowels

1. Rounding/unrounding of vowels. There are vowels that are normally rounded and others that are normally unrounded: /u/, rounded, versus /i/, unrounded, for example. The rounding or unrounding of the lips is an important feature of vowel realizations. However, for several reasons some clients might delete or inappropriately add these characteristics. This results in a distortion of the respective sound quality. The International Phonetic Alphabet offers two symbols to indicate rounding and unrounding of vowels. The signs are placed directly *under* the vowel symbol in question and consist of a small c-type notation that when open to the right indicates unrounding (or less rounding than is considered norm). When this "c" is inverted, creating an opening to the left, it denotes rounding (or more rounding than is normally the case).

> **[u̜] = [u] with less rounding than is usual**
> **[ɔ̹] = [ɔ] with more rounding than is usual**

Transcription Examples:

tune ___tu̜n___

tin ___tɪ̹n___

2. Changes in tongue placement for vowels. Deviations in tongue positioning affect vowel as well as consonant articulations. Two main factors that determine vowel quality pertain to the location of the raised portion of the tongue (front and back dimensions) and the extent to which the tongue is raised in the direction of the hard or soft palate (high and low dimensions).

RAISED/LOWERED TONGUE POSITION. The IPA system offers a set of diacritics that signal the direction of tongue heights on the *vertical* plane leading to deviations from norm vowel productions. There are tongue symbols for *too raised* or *too lowered*, a "hump" location for the norm production of the vowel in question. The diacritic [˔] under the vowel symbol marks a lower elevation, while the diacritic [˕] under the vowel marks a higher elevation of the tongue than is normally the case for the vowel production.

For example,

[sɪ̞t]

would indicate that the high-front elevation of the tongue for standard [ɪ] articulation has not been reached in this realization, i.e., the tongue articulation was lower than normal, resulting in a perceptible off-quality for [ɪ]. If we try to describe our auditory impression of this sound, we would say that it shifted in the direction of (but did not reach) the sound quality of [e].

Similarly, the transcription

[bɪ̝t]

would indicate a higher-than-normal elevation of the tongue for [ɪ], resulting in a quality that approaches [i] characteristics.

ADVANCED/RETRACTED TONGUE POSITION. There are also diacritics signaling variations in tongue placement on the *horizontal* plane that result in qualitative changes. They indicate a tongue "hump" location that is *too far forward* or *too far back* for a norm production of the vowel in question. The diacritic for vowels produced with a tongue elevation more advanced than usual is [+]. More retracted protrusions are marked by the diacritic [–] under the vowel symbol: [ɔ̠], for example.

Transcription Examples:

hot ___hɑ̟t___
beet ___bi̠t___

Beginning Case Study

JERI, THE SPEECH-LANGUAGE CLINICIAN

Jeri noted that Justin had some vowel distortions. She listened very carefully, and these were the distortions that she thought she was hearing:

Word	Typical Production	Justin's Production
tree	[tri]	[di̞]
spoon	[spun]	[pṵn]
cup	[kʌp]	[tʊp]
shovel	[ʃʌvəl]	[dʊbə]
duck	[dʌk]	[dʊt]
lamp	[læmp]	[wæ̝m]
bath	[bæθ]	[bæ̝t]
frog	[frɑg]	[dɑ̝d]

Justin has a tendency to lower high vowels such as [i] and to raise low vowels such as [æ] and [ɑ]. He also retracts the tongue on the central vowels to the point that [ʌ] often sounds like [ʊ].

Reflect on This: Clinical Application

Changes in the position of the tongue for vowel realizations are often perceptually difficult to target. Although transcribers are aware that the vowel quality is "off," they might not be sure in which direction. If the tongue hump has been lowered or raised, the vowel quality will sound somehow similar to the neighboring vowel on the vertical plane of the vowel quadrilateral. Thus, a lowered [ɛ] will have a certain [æ] quality, or a raised [ʊ] will approach [u]. The best reference source in these cases is the vowel quadrilateral. However, this is not as simple if the tongue movements pertain to the horizontal plane, i.e., to a tongue position that is too far forward or retracted. One point of reference is that front vowels that demonstrate a retracted tongue position and back vowels that demonstrate a more advanced tongue position sound somewhat "centralized"; their distinct quality appears reduced. Therefore, although the vowel can still be identified as the respective front or back vowel, it approaches a [ʌ]-type quality. See Figure 7.4.

NASALITY SYMBOLS. During the production of most General American English speech sounds, the velum is elevated to block the expiratory air from escaping through the nasal cavity. There is only one exception to this rule: the nasals. In reality, the conditions are not always so clear-cut. If a nasal follows a vowel, for example, nasality often seeps into the vowel segment; the preceding vowel becomes nasalized. As long as the nasality does not overstep the boundary line of natural assimilatory processes, this nasality remains unmarked. Speakers and listeners perceive these variations as normal. However, if the nasality is perceived as being excessive, *hypernasal*, we need to place the tilde (which may have been introduced in

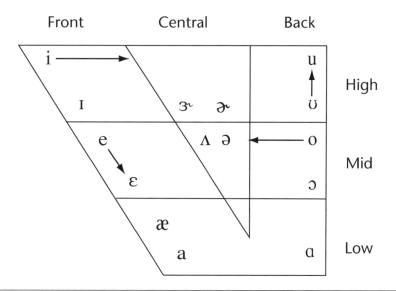

Figure 7.4 Raising and Lowering Vowels, Forward and Retracted Position of Vowels

French and Spanish language classes) over the respective sound(s). As speech-language specialists, we encounter hypernasality prominently in the speech of clients with dysarthria and cleft palates.

knock [nãk] = nasalized [a]

In addition, the nasal consonants /m/, /n/, and /ŋ/ can be articulated without the characteristic nasality resulting in denasalized productions. This could occur, for example, if a child has a cold or swollen adenoids or tonsils. In this case, the tilde that is used for nasality is implemented, but with two lines through it. Thus, m̃ would be a denasalized [m] production.

Transcription Examples:

tune ___tuñ̃___

song ___sã̂ŋ___

run ___rã̃n___

FOCUS 6: *What are diacritics? What types of features can they add to a particular speech sound?*

Diacritics for the Suprasegmentals: Stress, Juncture, and Duration

STRESS MARKERS.   Every multisyllabic word has its own *stress pattern* that might or might not be realized in a regular manner by our clients. The main purpose for all stress realizations is to emphasize certain syllables over others, thus creating a hierarchy of prominence among them. Although three levels of stress can be noted, typically only two levels are marked: primary and secondary stress.

1. Primary stress.   The order of prominence is actualized by differences in loudness, pitch, and duration, the loudness differences being the most striking of the three. Generally, two different loudness levels are observed. The loudest syllable is said to have the *primary stress*. It is marked by a superscript, short, straight line in front of the respective syllable.

lovely	[ˈlʌvli]
rotation	[roʊˈteɪʃən]
communication	[kəmjunəˈkeɪʃən]

2. Secondary stress.   The next loudest syllable bears the *secondary* stress. It is indicated by a *sub*script short straight line in front of the syllable in question.

supermarket	[ˈsupɚˌmɑɚˌkət]
linguistic	[lɪŋˈgwɪstɪk]
articulation	[ɑɚˌtɪkjuˈleɪʃən]

Reflect on This: Clinical Application

One of the characteristics of African American dialect is the total regressive assimilation of postvocalic nasals (e.g., Haynes & Moran, 1989; Wolfram, 1986). The assimilation process is *regressive* in that the nasal following the vowel changes the characteristic of the preceding vowel into a nasalized vowel. It is considered a *total* assimilation process because the postvocalic nasal consonant is totally replaced. The following examples demonstrate this process:

pen	[pɛn]	→	[pɛ̃n]	→	[pɛ̃]
thumb	[θʌm]	→	[θʌ̃m]	→	[θʌ̃]

The following examples were noted on an articulation test from a child, age 4;3, speaking African American Vernacular English:

broom	[brum]	→	[brũ]
telephone	[tɛləfon]	→	[tɛləfõ]
sandwich	[sænwɪtʃ]	→	[sæ̃wɪtʃ]
spoon	[spun]	→	[spũ]

Since these variations are dialectal in nature, they would not be considered aberrant pronunciations. In African American Vernacular English, they represent a rule-governed pronunciation possibility.

Some people find it difficult to distinguish between the loudness differences that characterize stress. For them, it might be of help to know that in General American English different loudness levels characterizing stress go usually (but not always) hand in hand with changes in pitch. Thus, the stressed syllable is higher in pitch. To pay attention to pitch differences first, then, might aid in discriminating between differing levels of loudness in stressing. It is also helpful to know that many (but again not all) words in General American English have their primary (or secondary) stress emphasis on the first syllable. A third possibility for those with difficulty in distinguishing stress differences is to systematically vary the loudness in each of the syllables of the word in question: [ˈjɛ lou̯] versus [jɛ ˈlou̯], for example. Typically, one version of that particular word will sound clearly more acceptable than the other. By a process of elimination, then, one can often ascertain the appropriate stressing pattern.

Transcription Examples:

away ___ əˈweɪ̯ ___

phonetics ___ fəˈnɛˌtəks ___

JUNCTURE SYMBOLS. During continuous speech, all sounds seem to connect rather seamlessly. Occasionally, however, short gaps separating words or sounds are necessary to avoid misunderstanding. Consider the realizations of the following sentences:

It's a nice treat.

It's an ice treat.

In cases like this, the placement of the gaps, or open junctures, becomes a distinguishing element between the two different sentences and their meanings. In phonetic transcription, open junctures can be marked with the diacritic sign "+" between the two elements in which a gap or pause occurs. The sample sentences would be transcribed accordingly.

It's a nice treat.   [ɪts ə + na͡ɪs trit]

It's an ice treat.   [ɪts ən + a͡ɪs trit]

A closed juncture, without a pause or gap, is considered to be normal and is, therefore, unmarked.

A terminal juncture marks the end of an utterance. These have been addressed in the section on suprasegmentals, pages 206–209.

Transcription Examples:

ice cream ___a͡ɪs + skrim___

I scream ___a͡ɪ + skrim___

DURATION SYMBOLS.   Sounds take up different amounts of time in continuous speech. Fricatives, for example, are normally longer than stops, while vowels are shorter before voiceless (fortis) consonants than before their voiced (lenis) counterparts.

Consider these minimal pairs:

beat   bead
pick   pig

We are so used to these measurable differences in sound duration that we register differences in usual lengths automatically as "too short" or "too long." If that is our perceptual impression, we have to indicate it by means of diacritical markers. Normal, i.e., inconspicuous, sound duration remains unmarked.

1. Lengthening.   Longer-than-normal duration is signaled by either one or two dots following the sound symbol in question. The more dots the longer the sound.

[fit]   standard vowel length
[fi·t]   slightly longer than normal vowel duration
[fi:t]   clearly longer than normal vowel duration

2. Shortening.   Shorter-than-normal speech sound productions also occur. As mentioned above, different *degrees* of shortening are, as a rule, not indicated. The diacritic mark for any shortened sounds is [˘] placed above the respective sound symbol.

Shortening of sounds can lead to cutting off a portion of their phonetic properties. Young children with unstable /s/ sounds sometimes shorten the (normally fairly long) segments to something that might sound like the release portion of [t]. If onset and holding portions of [t] are also identifiable, the obvious transcription would be [t]. However, if that is not the case, i.e., if we indeed had an /s/-impression, we would transcribe this as [š].

Transcription Examples:

sit ___ š̆ɪt ___

and ___ æeːnd ___

SYLLABLE BOUNDARIES. Syllable boundaries are indicated by a period placed between the syllables.

| articulation | [ɑɚ̯.tɪk.ju. ˈleɪ̯.ʃən] |
| communication | [kə.mjun.ə˞ ˈkeɪ̯.ʃən] |

As you looked through the words, did you possibly think that you would have put the syllable boundaries differently? For example, the syllable boundaries for "communication" might be [kə.mju.nə. ˈkeɪ̯.ʃən]? There are no set rules for syllable boundaries, so it is important that we listen carefully to the individual that we are transcribing. Both children and adults with phonological disorders could establish syllable boundaries in an atypical manner.

Transcription Examples:

contact ___ kan.tækt ___

combine ___ kɔm.baɪn ___

wonder ___ wʌn.dɚ ___

Case Study

By using diacritics, a far more accurate diagnosis can be established. The following broad and narrow transcription of Brad, age 7;3, emphasizes this point.

Brad, Age 7;3: Broad transcription

Word	Transcription	Word	Transcription
shop	[ʃɑp]	shoe	[ʃuː]
see	[ʃiː]	seat	[ʃiːt]
ship	[ʃɪp]	wash	[wɑʃ]
sip	[ʃɪp]	yes	[jɛʃ]
rush	[rʌʃ]	kiss	[kɪʃ]
cushion	[kʊʃən]	messy	[mɛʃi]

Based on the broad transcription, this child demonstrates a collapse of phonemic function, as both [s] and [ʃ] are produced as one phoneme [ʃ]. The clinician noted, however, that the productions sounded somewhat different. The [ʃ] did not always sound the same. She carefully listened again and utilized diacritics for a transcription of the same words. The following transcription resulted:

Word	Transcription	Word	Transcription
shop	[ʃɑp]	shoe	[ʃuː]
see	[sʲiː]	seat	[sʲiːt]
ship	[ʃɪp]	wash	[wɑʃ]
sip	[sʲɪp]	yes	[jɛsʲ]
rush	[rʌʃ]	kiss	[kɪsʲ]
cushion	[kʊʃən]	messy	[mɛsʲi]

This transcription has been modified from the examples given by Ball and Kent (1997, p. 2).

It appears clear that Brad does actually make articulatory distinctions between [s] and [ʃ]. He uses a palatalized [s] ([sʲ] for /s/), distinguishing it from the accurate production of [ʃ]. Therefore, Brad does not demonstrate a collapse of the contrast between [s] and [ʃ]. This would be an important detail for this child's diagnosis.

Summary

FOCUS 1: *What is coarticulation?*

Coarticulation refers to the fact that a phonological segment is not realized identically in all environments but often apparently varies to become more like an adjacent or nearby segment. The influences of coarticulation often extend well beyond the boundaries of a particular segment and appear to be the influence of both spatial and temporal linking of articulatory gestures.

It has also been hypothesized that children's productions might be characterized by more, rather than less, coarticulation. This view assumes that children rely to a larger extent on syllable-based speech production units and only gradually narrow their extent of articulatory organization. Thus, the coarticulatory overlap of gestures would be more prominent at early ages.

FOCUS 2: *What is assimilation? What are the different types of assimilation?*

Assimilation is the adaptive articulatory change that results when neighboring sound segments become similar in their production. Assimilatory changes may affect any or all of the sound's phonetic properties. Thus, the active and passive articulators, manner, and/or voicing characteristics of a consonant may change due to assimilation. Assimilation appears to be the result of motor simplification processes; these changes promote economy of effort, facility of movement, and take less time. Therefore, assimilation processes are natural consequences of normal speech production. Although certain types of assimilation are characteristic of children's speech, they occur continually in the speech of adults as well.

There are different types and degrees of assimilation.

1. Assimilation, or harmony, processes can affect those sounds that are directly adjacent to one another. This is known as contact (or contiguous) assimilation. If at least one other segment separates the sounds in question, especially when the sounds are in two different syllables, this is labeled remote (or noncontiguous) assimilation.
2. Assimilation processes can also be labeled according to the direction of the influence. If the influence is moving forward, i.e., a sound segment modifies a following sound, this is termed progressive (or perseverative) assimilation. If the influence is moving backward, i.e., a sound segment modifies a preceding sound, this is termed regressive (or anticipatory) assimilation.
3. Assimilation processes can also be labeled according to the degree of assimilation. If the number of features affected is such that the altered segment is perceived to be a different speech sound altogether, i.e., a different phoneme, this is considered phonemic assimilation. Phonemic assimilation can be partial or total. Partial assimilation is encountered when the changed segment is closer to but not identical to the sound that was the source of the change. *Total assimilation* is the label given when the changed segment and the source of the change become identical.
4. If the number of features affected is such that the altered segment is perceived to be an allophonic variation of the speech sound, i.e., it does not change the phoneme value, this is considered an allophonic similitude.
5. Coalescence occurs when two neighboring speech sounds are merged and form a new and different segment.

 FOCUS 3: *What are pitch, tone, intonation, and speech melody?*

Pitch will be used to refer to the perceptual correlate of frequency. The physiological mechanism associated with frequency is the number of cycles per second the vocal folds vibrate, known as the fundamental frequency. Thus, how we perceive the changes in fundamental frequency of the vocal folds is pitch.

Tone refers to the changes in fundamental frequency, perceived as pitch, when they function linguistically at the word (morpheme) level. The best examples are the so-called tone languages. In these languages, systematic fundamental frequency changes and thus, pitch changes have phonemic value.

Intonation refers to the feature of pitch when it functions linguistically at the sentence level. Therefore, the difference between the statement "I saw him" and the question "I saw him?" relates to intonation. Intonation also carries nonlinguistic meaning: the use of features (such as tempo) at the sentence level to reflect the attitudes of the speaker and the relative urgency of the message.

Speech melody is a broader term, encompassing both intonation and tone. Languages can also be classified according to the two speech melody parameters: intonation languages and tone languages. In the case of intonation languages, the function of the speech melody pattern is a part of the structure of sentences. In tone languages, the function of the speech melody pattern is a portion of the structure of the morphemes. American English is an intonation language; Chinese is a tone language.

 FOCUS 4: *What is stress? Which variables are associated with stress?*

Stress refers to the degree of force of an utterance or the prominence produced by means of respiratory effort. Syllables can be stressed. For example, if we examine the words "'con tract" versus "con 'tract," we find that the placement of the stress (first syllable as opposed to the second syllable) changes the meaning of the word. Stress can also be on a word in a sentence.

Unlike intonation, which can be traced directly back to the changing fundamental frequency of the vibrating vocal folds, stress is an elusive factor. There is no single mechanism that can be attributed to stress. If it is defined from the speaker's viewpoint, then stress is attributed to greater effort; more effort is exerted in the production of a stressed syllable than an unstressed one. However, if stress is defined from a listener's viewpoint, then it is claimed that stressed syllables are louder than unstressed ones. Although stress seems to be related to greater articulatory effort, the objective measurements of stress demonstrate that, typically, increased loudness, a higher fundamental frequency, and a longer duration are noted in stressed versus unstressed syllables.

 FOCUS 5: *What is tempo? What is rhythm?*

Tempo is the speed of speaking. It is possible to speed up or slow down the rate at which syllables, words, and sentences are produced to convey several different meanings and emotions. A faster tempo may indicate urgency, a slower one contemplation. A rapid, clipped single syllable may convey irritation; a slowly drawled syllable, more personal reflection.

Pitch, loudness, and tempo together enter into a language's expression of rhythm. *Rhythm* refers to the manner in which stressed and unstressed syllables succeed each other. Each language has its own rhythmical pattern, which is one of the most fundamental things about it. There are two types of rhythmical patterns in languages: stress-timed, or isochronous, rhythm and syllable-timed rhythm. English is considered to have a stress-timed rhythm, while French has a syllable-timed rhythm.

 FOCUS 6: *What are diacritics? What types of features can they add to a particular speech sound?*

Additional symbols may be frequently required to denote the special production features demonstrated by individuals with articulation or phonological disorders. These additional symbols are termed *diacritics*. Diacritics are marks added to transcription symbols in order to give them a particular phonetic value.

There are many different diacritics that can be used with consonants. A few of the more useful ones for speech-language clinicians include diacritics that can be used to note changes in the articulatory position of the active or passive articulators, voicing, aspiration or lack of aspiration, unreleased stop-plosives, syllabics, and lip rounding (or lack of lip rounding). Diacritics used with vowels include rounding and unrounding of the vowel in question or changes in tongue placement. There are also diacritics that mark stress, duration, juncture, and syllable boundaries.

Further Readings

Ball, M., Rahilly, J., & Tench, P. (1996). *The phonetic transcription of disordered speech.* London: John Wiley & Sons.

Fox, A. (2002). *Prosodic features and prosodic structure: The phonology of suprasegmentals.* Oxford, UK: Oxford University Press.

Lehiste, I. (1970). *Suprasegmentals.* Cambridge: Massachusetts Institute of Technology.

Key Concepts

allophonic similitude p. 206
anticipatory assimilation p. 204
assimilation p. 202
coalescence p. 206
coarticulation p. 201
contact assimilation p. 203
contiguous assimilation p. 203
diacritics p. 201
harmony process p. 203
intonation p. 207
noncontiguous assimilation p. 203
partial assimilation p. 205
perseverative assimiliation p. 203

phonemic assimilation p. 205
pitch p. 206
progressive assimilation p. 203
prosodic features p. 201
regressive assimilation p. 203
remote assimilation p. 203
rhythm p. 212
speech melody p. 208
stress p. 209
suprasegmental features p. 201
tempo p. 211
tone p. 207
total assimilation p. 205

Think Critically

1. The following transcription is from Matthew, age 4;6. Discuss what the diacritics/transcriptions indicate for each of the sounds. Which productions would be considered norm articulation, possibly resulting from assimilation processes, and which would be considered misarticulations?

This morning I snuck up on my cat.

[ðɪʤ mõə̃nən âɪ s̪nʌk ʌp ɑn mâɪ kæt]

I like my cat, Tigger.
He's a big fur ball.

[ʔâɪ lâɪk mâɪː k̚æt tɪɣə]
[hisʲ ə bɪg fɝ b̥ɑl]

He's brown and on his tummy   [hiz braʊn ænd ɑn hɪz tʌmĭ
he has white all over him.   hi hæʂ waɪt ɑl ovə hɪm]

2. Explain the following assimilation processes. Are they contact–remote or progressive–regressive?

"bet you" [bɛt ju] → [bɛtʃu]
"Pontiac" [pɑntiæk] → [pɑniæk]

A child says,

"window" [wɪndoʊ] → [wɪnoʊ]
"kite" [kaɪt] → [taɪt]

but can say "key" or "comb" accurately.

3. Explain the differences in [s]-production that are noted by the use of the following diacritics:

[s̰]

[sʲ]

[ɬ]

4. Give an example of two sentences with different intonation patterns. Mark the pattern using the examples from page 208.

5. Give an example of three words with stress on the first syllable and three words with stress on the second syllable. Mark these with the appropriate diacritics.

Test Yourself

1. The change in the production features of consonants and vowels as they are influenced by surrounding sounds is referred to as
   a. speech melody.
   b. coarticulation.
   c. timing.
   d. prosodic features.

2. Intonation, stress, and timing are a portion of the concept of
   a. suprasegmentals.
   b. coalescence.
   c. diacritics.
   d. assimilation.

3. When one sound assimilates a sound that is directly adjacent to it, this is what type of assimilation?
   a. remote
   b. contact
   c. partial
   d. noncontiguous

4. Assimilation processes are also called
   a. suprasegmentals.
   b. diacritics.
   c. speech melody.
   d. harmony processes.

5. The diacritic in the second syllable of "bottle" [bɑtl̩] indicates that
   a. the [l] is a dark l-sound.
   b. the [l] is a lateral production.
   c. [l] is a syllabic.
   d. a sound has been omitted.

6. If a child says [pliz̥], this indicates that
   a. [z] has been partially devoiced.
   b. there is lip rounding on the [z].
   c. the [z] has been lateralized.
   d. the [z] has too much voicing.

7. If the [e] is transcribed [e̞], this would indicate that
   a. the vowel has been raised, sounding more like a [ɪ].
   b. the vowel has been devoiced.
   c. the vowel has been neutralized, approximating [ʌ].
   d. the vowel has been lowered, sounding more like an [ɛ].

8. If a child says [wi:l], this would indicate that
   a. the child is having problems with the [l] production.
   b. the child lengthened the [i] vowel.
   c. the child left out a sound between [i] and [l].
   d. the child had too much aspiration.

9. The manner in which stressed and unstressed syllables succeed each other is known as
   a. tone.
   b. intonation.
   c. stress.
   d. rhythm.

10. Intonation is primarily a product of
    a. changes in vocal fundamental frequency.
    b. changes in sentence timing.
    c. the use of tone in words.
    d. coarticulation.

Answers: 1. b 2. a 3. b 4. d 5. c 6. a 7. d 8. b 9. d 10. a

For additional information, go to www.phonologicaldisorders.com

Phonological Development

PRACTICAL AND THEORETICAL IMPLICATIONS

Chapter Highlights

- What are the prelinguistic stages? What are the features and the approximate ages for each stage?
- Which types of syllable shapes, vowels, and consonants predominate the first-fifty-word stage?
- Why do the age results from the cross-sectional sound mastery studies vary?
- Which sounds appear to be later developing sounds? How does the acquisition of consonant clusters fit into this acquisition process?
- What are distinctive features? How do distinctive features explain the development of the child's phonological system?
- What is natural phonology? What role do phonological processes play in this model?
- What are the basic differences between linear and nonlinear phonologies?

Chapter Application: Case Study

This is Katie's first semester of graduate school in communicative disorders. She is required to sign up for two different types of clinical experiences. One of her assignments is phonology clinic. She has been assigned three children with different types of phonological disorders: Paula, Mikey, and Coulton. All of the children are 4½ years old and seem to have no other problems other than their disordered phonological systems. Paula has problems with /k/ and /g/; she produces [t] and [d] as substitutions. In addition, she produces [w] for /r/ and leaves out the r-coloring on the central vowels /ɝ/ and /ɚ/. She also distorts her s-sounds, producing a dentalized [s]. Mikey leaves off the ends of words and also has difficulty with r- and s-sounds. Coulton uses stop-plosives to replace his fricatives. Therefore, his [f] and [v] productions are [p] and [b], while /s, z, ʃ, ʒ, θ, and ð/ are replaced by [t] and [d]. Katie wonders where to begin. She is aware that these children are still in the developmental process and that some sounds probably do not need to be in their inventory yet. However, the children are in the clinic, so obviously they need work with their phonology. Where should she begin, and which sounds are developmentally appropriate at this age?

T his chapter will discuss the development of speech sound form in children. Although it is clear that this is a gradual process, it is important to know a timeline and approximate acquisition ages for the various sounds of American English. This will be instrumental in our assessment of children with possible articulation and phonological impairments. The diagnosis of articulation and phonological impairments is based in part on the discrepancy between where the child should be in the developmental process and the child's actual level of functioning. In addition, the speech sound developmental sequence is often used as a basis for setting goals in the treatment of articulation and phonological disorders.

The second goal of this chapter is to examine how specific contemporary phonological theories view the speech sound developmental process. These theories attempt to explain how the child slowly changes from a babbling toddler to a child with a fully developed phonemic system. They also provide hypotheses about the error patterns that normally developing children demonstrate as well as those that children with phonological disorders demonstrate. In addition, contemporary theories also provide a basis for assessment procedures and treatment possibilities. First, let's examine the developmental path that children take in the speech sound acquisition process.

Prelinguistic Stages: Before the First Word

Child language development is commonly divided into **prelinguistic behavior**, vocalizations prior to the first true words, and linguistic development, which starts with the appearance of these first words. This division is exemplified by the use of early nonmeaningful versus later meaningful sound productions. Roman Jakobson's *discontinuity hypothesis* (1941/1968) clearly emphasized a sharp separation between these two phases of development. According to his theoretical notion, babbling is a random series of vocalizations in which many different sounds are produced with no apparent order or consistency. Such behavior is seen as clearly separated from the following systematic sound productions evidenced by first words. According to Jakobson, the division between prelinguistic and linguistic phases of sound production is often so complete that the child might actually undergo a period of silence between the end of the babbling period and the first real words. Jakobson's hypothesis was based primarily on observations of many children representing several different languages. However, systematic research has not documented his original findings. This is possibly due to the difference in methodology used or the shift in viewpoint from the infant's being a rather passive to an active learner of speech and language.

For example, research since that time (e.g., Masataka, 2001; Mitchell & Kent, 1990; Oller, 1980; Stark, 1980) has repeatedly found that (1) babbling behavior is not random; rather, the child's productions develop in a systematic manner; (2) the consonant-like sounds that are babbled are restricted to a small set of segments; and (3) the transition between babbling and first words is not abrupt but continuous; late babbling behavior and the first words are very similar in respect to the sounds used and the way they are combined. It also appears that the child's perceptual abilities are rather developed before the first meaningful utterances. For example, some word comprehension is evident at approximately 7 to 9 months of age (Owens, 2008). The ability to associate minimally paired words to different objects has also been documented in very young children (Shvachkin, 1973). Although this ability is a gradual acquisition process, more general contrasts begin at approximately 1 year of age. Findings like these suggest that the child's language system starts to develop prior to the first spoken meaningful words.

It should be kept in mind that it isn't until 6 to 8 months of age that the child's vocal tract approximates its later adult shape, a prerequisite for sound production as we know it (Bosma, 1975). These physiological changes coincide with the beginning of the actual babbling period, which shows refined perception and production skills similar to those later used in the child's first fifty words. It is during the prelinguistic period that the child's phonological development begins. However each child approaches this phase of development somewhat differently. Although specific "stages" are outlined, it should be noted that overlap often does occur between the stages. In addition, the age of acquisition for each stage must be considered as approximations. Some children might approach a stage earlier, others later. In addition, some children seem to stay very briefly in one stage, while others remain longer before moving to the next stage. The following represents an overview of the *prelinguistic stages* of production as described by Stark (1986).

Stage 1: **Reflexive crying and vegetative sounds** (birth to 2 months)

This stage is characterized by a large proportion of reflexive vocalizations. **Reflexive vocalizations** include cries, coughs, grunts, and burps that seem to be automatic responses reflecting the physical state of the infant. **Vegetative sounds** may be divided into grunts and sighs, associated with activity, and clicks and other noises, for example, which are associated with feeding.

Stage 2: **Cooing and laughter** (2 to 4 months)

During this stage, cooing or gooing sounds are produced during comfortable states. Although these sounds are sometimes referred to as vowel-like, they also contain brief periods of consonantal elements that are produced at the back of the mouth. Early comfort sounds have quasi-resonant nuclei, i.e., they are produced as a syllabic nasal consonant or a nasalized vowel (Nakazima, 1962; Oller, 1980). From 12 weeks onward, a decrease in the frequency of occurrence of crying is noted, and primitive vegetative sounds start to disappear in most infants. At 16 weeks, sustained laughter emerges (Gesell & Thompson, 1934).

Stage 3: **Vocal play** (4 to 6 months)

Although there is some overlap between Stages 2 and 3, the distinguishing characteristics of Stage 3 include longer series of segments and the production of prolonged vowel- or consonant-like steady states. It is during this stage that the infant often produces extreme variations in loudness and pitch. Transitions between the segments are much slower than is the case with children or adults. In contrast to Stage 2, Stage 3 vowels demonstrate more variation in tongue height and position (Hsu, Fogel, & Cooper, 2000).

Stage 4: Canonical babbling (6 months and older)

Although canonical babbling usually begins around 6 months of age, most children continue to babble into the time when they say their first words. Stark (1986) divides this stage into two types of babbling behavior: reduplicated and nonreduplicated, or variegated, babbling. **Reduplicated babbling** is marked by similar strings of consonant-vowel productions. There might be slight quality variations in the vowel sounds of these strings of babbles; however, the consonants will stay the same from syllable to syllable. An example of this is [əmama]. **Nonreduplicated** or **variegated babbling** demonstrates variation of both consonants and vowels from syllable to syllable. An example of this is [batə]. Smooth transitions can be noted between vowel and consonant productions.

From the previous description, one might conclude that these babbling stages are sequential in nature, a child first going through reduplicated babbling and then later nonreduplicated babbling. This has indeed been documented by Elbers (1982) and Oller (1980), for example. However, more recent investigators have questioned this developmental pattern. For example, Mitchell and Kent (1990) assessed the phonetic variation of multisyllabic babbling in eight infants at 7, 9, and 11 months of age. Their findings showed that (1) nonreduplicated babbling was present from the point in time the infant began to produce multisyllabic babbling, and did not evolve out of an earlier period of reduplicated babbling, and (2) no significant differences existed in the phonetic variation for the vocalizations when the infants were 7, 9, and 11 months old. In other words, the vocalizations produced by the older children were not more variable in their phonetic composition than those produced by the younger children. These and other findings (Holmgren, Lindblom, Aurelius, Jalling, & Zetterstrom, 1986; Smith, Brown-Sweeney, & Stoel-Gammon, 1989) suggest that both reduplicated and variegated

Reflect on This: Clinical Application

A child age 15 months comes for a speech-language evaluation. The child does not have any words, and true babbling does not seem to be present. Reduplicated and variegated babbling are not noted by the clinician, and the parents reconfirm this. The child does seem to be within the vocal play stage, as you notice that extreme loudness and pitch variations are produced. The child also produces [m] and [n] and some vowel sounds in isolation. Given the information on the stages of development and the approximate ages at which they occur, could you say approximately how far behind this child appears?

forms extend throughout the entire babbling period. At the beginning of this stage, babbling is used in a self-stimulatory manner, it is not used to communicate to adults. Toward the end of this stage (approximately 9 months of age), babbling may be used in ritual imitation games with adults (Kuhl & Meltzoff, 1996; Stark, 1986).

Stage 5: **Jargon stage** (10 months and older)

This babbling stage overlaps with the first meaningful words. The jargon stage is characterized by strings of babbled utterances that are modulated by primarily intonation, rhythm, and pausing (Crystal, 1986). It sounds as if the child is actually attempting sentences, but without actual words. Since many jargon vocalizations are delivered with eye contact, gestures, and intonation patterns that resemble statements or questions, parents are convinced that the child is indeed trying to communicate something to which they often feel compelled to respond (Papaeliou, Minadakis, & Cavouras, 2002; Stoel-Gammon and Menn, 1997).

FOCUS 1: *What are the prelinguistic stages? What are the features and the approximate ages for each stage?*

The following section examines the child's segmental productions toward the end of the canonical babbling stage.

Vowel-like Sounds

One of the earliest series of investigations with a large number of children were those carried out by Irwin and colleagues in the 1940s and 1950s (e.g., Chen & Irwin, 1946; Irwin, 1945, 1946, 1947a, 1947b, 1948, 1951; Irwin & Chen, 1946; Winitz & Irwin, 1958). According to the data on fifty-seven children from 13 to 14 months of age, there was a continued predominance of front and central over high and back vowel-like sounds. Later investigations (Davis & MacNeilage, 1990; Kent & Bauer, 1985) generated similar results.

Consonant-like Sounds

Several authors have investigated the consonant-like sounds that predominate in the late babbling stage (Fisicelli, 1950; Irwin, 1947a; Locke, 1983; Pierce & Hanna, 1974). The most frequent ones were /h/, /d/, /b/, /m/, /t/, /g/, and /w/, followed by /n/, /k/, /j/, /p/, and /s/ (the high frequency of /s/ was noted only in the Irwin, 1947a, study). These twelve most frequently produced consonant-like sounds represented about 95 percent of all the segments transcribed in the three studies (Locke, 1983). These results stand in contrast to earlier statements that babbling consists of a great multitude of random vocalizations. On the contrary, these and other investigations (e.g., Locke, 1990; Vihman, Macken, Miller, Simmons, & Miller, 1985) suggest that only a limited set of phones is babbled.

Syllable Shapes

During the later babbling periods, open syllables are still the most frequent type of syllables. Kent and Bauer (1985) found, for example, that V, CV, VCV, and CVCV structures accounted for approximately 94 percent of all syllables produced. While closed syllables were present, they were found to be very limited in number.

Prosodic Feature Development

The development of prosodic features in infants has gained considerable importance in the last years. Current research begins to document their development and supports the viewpoint of a close interaction between prosodic features, early child-directed speech, and early language development (Hallé, de Boysson-Bardies, & Vihman, 1991; Hane, 2003; Hsu & Fogel, 2001; Masataka, 1993; Robb & Saxman, 1990; Snow & Balog, 2002; Turk, Jusczyk, & Gerken, 1995; Whalen, Levitt, & Wang, 1991). A better understanding of prosodic features and their development may offer us valuable insights into the transition from babbling to the first words and the close interconnection of segmental and prosodic feature acquisition.

Coinciding with the canonical babbling stage, or starting at approximately 6 months of age, the infant utilizes distinct patterns of prosodic behavior. Certain features are now employed consistently, primarily intonation, rhythm, and pausing (Crystal, 1986). Acoustic analysis shows that falling pitch is the most common intonation contour for the first year of life (Kent & Murray, 1982). Prosodic patterns continue to diversify toward the end of the babbling period to such a degree that terms such as *expressive jargon* (Gesell & Thompson, 1934) or *prelinguistic jargon* (Dore, Franklin, Miller, & Ramer, 1976) have been applied to them. These strings of babbles typically end in a manner that is characteristic of adult American English intonation patterns, giving the impression of sentences without words.

The First Fifty Words

Around a child's first birthday, a new developmental era begins, the *linguistic phase.* It starts with the moment when the first meaningful word is produced. This sounds straightforward; however, there are some problems defining the first meaningful word. Must it be understood and produced by the child in all applicable situations and contexts? Must it have an adultlike meaning to the child? What about those utterances that do not resemble our adult representation but are, nevertheless, used as "words" by the child in a consistent manner?

Most define the **first word** as an entity of relatively stable phonetic form that is produced consistently by the child in a particular context. This form must be recognizably related to the adultlike word form of a particular language (Owens, 2008). Thus, if the child says [ba] consistently in the context of being shown a ball, then this form would qualify as a "word."

If, however, the child says [dodo] when being shown the ball, then this would not be accepted as a "word" because it does not approximate the adult form.

Children frequently use "invented words" (Locke, 1983) in a consistent manner, thereby demonstrating that they seem to have meaning for the child. These vocalizations used consistently but without a recognizable adult model have been called **protowords** (Menn, 1978), **phonetically consistent forms** (Dore et al., 1976), **vocables** (Ferguson, 1976), and **quasi-words** (Stoel-Gammon & Cooper, 1984).

The time of the initial productions of words is typically called the *first-fifty-word stage*. This stage encompasses the time from the first meaningful utterance at approximately 1 year of age to the time when the child begins to put two words together at approximately 18 to 24 months. Whether this stage is actually a separate developmental entity might be questioned. The first word might be a plausible starting point, but the strict fifty-word cut-off point is, according to several studies, purely arbitrary (Nelson, 1973). Nevertheless, it appears that the child produces approximately fifty meaningful words before the next generally recognized stage of development begins: the *two-word stage*.

During the first-fifty-word stage, there seems to be a large difference between the production and the perceptual capabilities of the child. For example, at the end of this stage, when children can produce approximately fifty words, they are typically capable of understanding around 200 words (Ingram, 1989a). This fact must have an effect upon the development of semantic meaning as well as on the phonological system. It must be clearly understood that, by analyzing the child's verbal productions during this stage, we are looking at only one aspect of language development. The child's perceptual, motor, and cognitive growth, as well as the influence of the environment, play an indispensable role in this stage of language acquisition.

Segmental Form Development: The First Fifty Words

During the first-fifty-word stage, several authors have noted phonetic variability and a limitation of syllable structures and sound segments (e.g., Ingram, 1989a; Mitchell & Kent, 1990). **Phonetic variability** refers to the rather unstable pronunciations of the child's first fifty words. While this has been well documented, it appears that some productions are more stable than others. To complicate matters, it seems that some children have a tendency to produce more stable articulations from the beginning of this stage. For example, Stoel-Gammon and Cooper (1984) and French (1989) provide data on children whose phonetic realizations were stable from the first real word on.

The second characteristic of this stage is the limitation of syllable structures and segmental productions utilized. From their relatively small repertoire of words, it would seem logical to conclude that children do not produce a large array of syllable structures and sound segments. However, what are the actual limitations during the first fifty words?

First, certain syllable types clearly predominate. These are CV, VC, and CVC syllables. When CVCV syllables are present, they are full or partial syllable reduplications. *Syllable reduplication* refers to the first syllable of a word being reproduced as the second syllable. Thus, productions such as [dada] or [wɑwɑ] are considered reduplications. This, of course, does not mean that other syllable types do not occur. Looking, for example, at the data from Ferguson and Farwell (1975), French (1989), Ingram (1974), Leopold (1947), Menn (1971), Stoel-Gammon and Cooper (1984), and Velten (1943), these syllables are indeed the most frequently occurring. However, the children produced other syllables as well. Menn's Daniel, for instance, produced a CCVC ([njaj]), Leopold's Hildegard a CCVCV ([prɪti]), and Ferguson and Farwell's T, a CVCVVC ([wakuak]). If the individual children are examined to see if patterns emerge, differences can be found. Certain children seem to favor specific types of syllables. For example, some children evidence CVC structures to a moderate degree from the very beginning of this stage. With others, CVC syllables appear only later and do not constitute any major part of the child's phonology until after the fifty-word stage.

Second, what are the speech sound limitations that can be observed during the first-fifty-word stage? More specifically, which vowels and consonants are present, and which ones are not? Two publications that have had a large impact on this question are those presented by Jakobson (1941/1968) and Jakobson and Halle (1956). After studying several diary reports of children from various linguistic backgrounds, they concluded that

the first consonants are labials, most commonly /p/ or /m/;

these first consonants are followed by /t/ and later /k/;

fricatives are present only after the respective homorganic stops have been acquired; and

the first vowel is /a/ or /ɑ/, followed by /u/ and/or /i/.

Over the years, Jakobson's postulated universals have undergone a good deal of scrutiny. Although most of the investigators (e.g., Oller, Wieman, Doyle, & Ross, 1976; Stoel-Gammon & Cooper, 1984; Vihman, Ferguson, & Elbert, 1986) have concentrated on consonant inventories, Ingram (1974) attempted to grapple with the acquisition of vowels. Using the data from four case studies (Ingram, 1974; Leopold, 1947; Menn, 1971; Velten, 1943), Ingram compared the vowels in the first fifty words, noting that most children seemed to follow the acquisitional pattern of [a] preceding [i] and [u].

When early consonants were examined, several investigations have pointed out the wide range of variability among individual subjects (e.g., Ferguson & Farwell, 1975; Stoel-Gammon & Cooper, 1984; Vihman, 1992; Vihman et al., 1986). If one wants to generalize, then the marked use of voiced labial (/m, b/) and coronal-alveolar stops and nasals (/n, d/) has to be underlined. Findings substantiating these generalizations from five different investigations are summarized in Table 8.1, which compares the consonant inventory of twenty-six children from five different research studies.

Thus, voiced labial consonants seem to dominate the first sounds; however, coronal-alveolar and postdorsal-velar sounds are also present. With the exception of affricates, all manners of articulation are represented in these initial consonant productions.

Table 8.1 Consonant Productions Within the First-Fifty-Word Vocabularies

Consonants produced by all children	[b] [m]
Consonants produced by more than half of the children	[p], [t], [d], [k], [g] [n] [w] [h], [ʃ]

Source: Summarized from Ferguson & Farwell (1975), Leonard, Newhoff, & Mesalam (1980), Shibamoto and Olmsted (1978), Stoel-Gammon & Cooper (1984), and Vihman, Ferguson, & Elbert (1986).

The results summarized in Table 8.1 have been documented through cross-sectional research. In other words, several children at various age groups were tested one time, and the results were compared. Longitudinal research follows a child or a group of children over a specific time frame. It has the advantage of observing the acquisition process of individual children. However, longitudinal research is often limited in that only one child or a small group of subjects is evaluated. One notable longitudinal investigation by Stoel-Gammon (1985) investigated a sizable number of children utilizing spontaneous speech. This study gives us a different view of the acquisition process.

Thirty-four children between 15 and 24 months of age participated in this study. The investigation was constructed to look at meaningful speech; therefore, the subjects were grouped according to the age at which they began to actually say at least ten identifiable words within a recording session. This resulted in three groups of children: Group A, children who had ten words at 15 months; Group B, ten words at 18 months; and Group C, ten words at 21 months. The resulting data provide information about early consonant development and can be summarized as follows:

Note the three groups of children in the Stoel-Gammon (1985) study. The time span when children said ten identifiable words ranged from 15 to 21 months. This gives one an indication of the variability among children. While some children had ten identifiable words at 15 months, others had this size of a vocabulary only six months later.

1. A larger inventory of sounds was found in the word-initial than the word-final position.
2. Word-initial inventories contained voiced stops prior to voiceless ones, while the reverse was true for word-final productions.
3. The following phones appeared in at least 50 percent of all the subjects by 24 months of age:

   [h, w, b, t, d, m, n, k, g, f, and s] word-initially

   [p, t, k, n, r, and s] word-finally

4. The "r" nearly always appeared first in a word-final position, thus, as a central vowel with r-coloring or a centering diphthong.
5. If the mean percentage of norm consonant productions was calculated (a percentage based on the total number of consonants produced divided by the number of correct consonants; Shriberg & Kwiatkowski, 1982), 70 percent accuracy was achieved. Since there is obviously a large difference in the inventory produced by 2-year-olds compared to adults, the author states that this accuracy level suggests that children are primarily attempting words that contain sounds within their articulatory abilities.

FOCUS 2: *Which types of syllable shapes, vowels, and consonants predominate the first-fifty-word stage?*

Prosodic Feature Development

As the child moves from the end of the babbling period to first words, the previously noted intonational contours continue. The falling intonation contour still predominates, but both a rise-fall and a simple rising contour have also been observed (Kent & Bauer, 1985).

An important aspect of communication during the first-fifty-word stage is *prosodic variation*. Examples of children's speech during this time have included pitch variations to indicate differences in meaning: for example, a falling pitch on the first syllable, [daꜜda], as daddy entered the room versus [daꜛda], a rising pitch on the first syllable when a noise was heard outside when daddy was expected (Crystal, 1986). Prosodic features are also used to indicate differences in syntactical function. Bruner (1975) labels these prosodic units *place-holders*. A demand or question, for example, is often first signaled by prosody and words added later. For example, a child aged 1;2 first used the phrase "all gone" after dinner by humming the intonation. Approximately a month passed before the child's segmental productions were somewhat accurate (Crystal, 1986). One widely held view is that these prosodic units fulfill a social function. They are seen as a means to signal joint participation in an activity shared by the child and the caregiver.

Intonational changes seem to develop prior to stress. While various pitch contours appear earlier than the first meaningful words, contrastive stress is first evidenced only at the beginning of the two-word stage, or at the age of approximately 1;6. For a more detailed analysis of early intonational development, see Crystal (1986), Snow (1998a, 1998b, 2000) and Snow and Balog (2002).

The Preschool Child

This section gives information on the developing phonology of the child from approximately 18 to 24 months, the end of the first-fifty-word stage, to the beginning of the school years. It is during this time that the largest growth within the phonological system takes place. However, not only is the child's phonological system expanding, large gains are also seen in other language areas. From 18 to 24 months of age, the child's expressive vocabulary has at least tripled, from 50 to 150–300 words (Lipsitt, 1966; Mehrabian, 1970), while the receptive vocabulary has grown from 200 to 1,200 words (Weiss & Lillywhite, 1981). The transition from one-word utterances to two-word sentences, a large linguistic step, is typically occurring at this time. With the production of two-word sentences, the child has entered the period of expressing specific semantic relationships: the beginning of syntactical development.

Around the child's fifth birthday, the expressive vocabulary has expanded to approximately 2,200 words, while about 9,600 words are in the child's receptive vocabulary (Weiss & Lillywhite, 1981). Almost all of the basic grammatical forms of the language, such as questions, negative statements, dependent clauses, and compound sentences, are now present as well. More important, the child knows how to use language to communicate in an effective manner. Five-year-olds talk differently to babies than they do to their friends, for example. They also know how to tell jokes and riddles, and they are quite able to handle the linguistic subtleties of being polite and rude.

A child's phonological development at 18 to 24 months still demonstrates a rather limited inventory of speech sounds and phonotactic possibilities. At this time, speech and language perception seems to precede production; children can now identify single-segment differences between words. By the end of the preschool period, an almost complete phonological system has emerged.

All these changes occur in less than four years. Although this section focuses on phonological development, such a discussion must always be seen within the context of the equally large expansions in morphosyntax, semantics, and pragmatics that occur during this time.

Segmental Development: Cross-Sectional Results

It appears that no discussion on phonological development can be complete without looking at the large sample studies that began in the 1930s (Wellman, Case, Mengert, & Bradbury, 1931) and have continued periodically since that time. However, it seems appropriate to preface such a discussion with the problems inherent in these studies.

Large sample studies were initiated to look at a large number of children in order to examine which sounds were considered to be "mastered" at which age levels. To this end, they evaluated most of the speech sounds within a given native language. With a few exceptions (Irwin & Wong, 1983; Olmsted, 1971; Stoel-Gammon, 1985, 1987) these studies have used methods similar to articulation tests to collect their data: e.g., children were asked to name pictures, and certain sounds were then judged as being productionally "correct" or "incorrect."

With this type of procedure, specific problems arise. First, the fact that the child produces the sound "correctly" as a one-word response does not mean that the sound can also be produced "correctly" in natural speech conditions. Practitioners have always been aware of the often large articulatory discrepancies between single-word responses and the same sounds used in conversation. Second, the choice of pictures/words will certainly affect the production of the individual sounds within the word. Not only does the child's familiarity with the word play a role, but so do factors such as the length of the word, its structure, the stressed or unstressed position of the sound within the word, and the phonetic context in which the sound occurs. These factors help or hinder production. Therefore, strictly speaking, the only conclusion that can be drawn from cross-sectional studies is that the children could or could not produce that particular sound in that specific word.

The third point is a theoretical issue. As stated at the beginning, there has been an adoption of certain new concepts and terminology within the field of speech-language pathology. This chapter, for example, is called "Phonological Development," not "Speech Sound Development." With the inclusion of the terms *phonology* and *phonological development*, certain conceptual changes have been accepted. These cross-sectional studies are perhaps indicative of the inventory of speech sounds children typically possess at certain ages, but they are not a documentation of a particular child's phonological system. In other words, these studies do not examine how specific sounds function within the child's language system.

Specific methodological differences between various cross-sectional studies are also important factors when interpreting the results. These include the criteria used to determine whether the child has "mastered" a particular sound. Although this has been elaborated upon in several articles and books (e.g., Smit, 1986; Vihman, 1998), it is worth mentioning again. Table 8.2 provides a comparison between several of the larger cross-sectional studies.

Table 8.2 Mastery Levels for Speech Sound Development According to Several Studies

	Wellman et al. (1931)	Poole (1934)	Templin (1957)	Prather et al. (1975)	Arlt & Goodban (1976)	Smit (1993a)[1]
m	3	3½	3	2	3	2
n	3	4½	3	2	3	2
ŋ		4½	3	2	3	4
p	4	3½	3	2	3	2
b	3	3½	4	2;8	3	2
t	5	4½	6	2;8	3	2
d	5	4½	4	2;4	3	3
k	4	4½	4	2;4	3	2
g	4	4½	4	2;4	3	2
w	3	3½	3	2;8	3	2
j	4	4½	3½	2;4	not tested	3½
l	4	6½	6	3;4	4	5½
r	5	7½	4	3;4	5	7
h	3	3½	3	2	3	2
f	3	5½	3	2;4	3	3
v	5	6½	6	4	3½	4
s	5	7½	4½	3	4	6
z	5	7½	7	4	4	6
ʃ	not mastered by age 6	6½	4½	3;8	4½	3½
ʒ	6	6½	7	4	4	not tested
θ	not mastered by age 6	7½	6	4	5	5;6
ð	not mastered by age 6	6½	7	4	5	4½
tʃ	5		4½	3;8	4	3½
dʒ	not mastered by age 6		7	4	4	3½

Sources: Based on studies by Wellman, Case, Mengurt, & Bradbury (1931), Poole (1934), Templin (1957), Prather, Hedrick, & Kern (1975), Arlt & Goodban (1976), and Smit (1993a).

[1]For the Smit (1993a) study, mastery levels were not determined. For the purpose of this table, a sound has been considered mastered if the estimated percent acceptable use is approximately 75 percent.

Looking at age comparisons in Table 8.2, a difference in reported mastery of three years or more can be observed for some sounds. For example, note the difference between the ages of mastery for /s/ in the more recent Prather, Hedrick, and Kern (1975) in comparison to the older Poole (1934) study. The Poole investigation has a mastery age of 7½; years, while the Prather et al. investigation shows an age level of 3 years. A three-year difference can be found for /z/ acquisition when the Prather et al. data are compared to the Templin (1957) results. Again, Prather et al. assign a much earlier level of mastery. One question that is often asked in this context is, Does that mean children are now producing sounds "correctly" at an earlier age? Many of these differences are a consequence of the way "mastery" was defined. Poole, for instance, stated that 100 percent of the children must use the sound correctly in each of the positions tested. Prather et al. and Templin, on the other hand, set this level at 75 percent. In addition, rather than using the 75 percent cut-off level for all three positions (initial, medial, and final) as Templin had done, Prather et al. used only two positions (initial and final) for their calculations. This clearly changes the ages to which mastery can be assigned. A shift to earlier acquisition noted in the Prather study could be accounted for by these methodological changes. Also, as Smit (1986) points out, the Prather results are based on incomplete data sets, especially at the younger age groupings. Although Prather began with 21 subjects in each age group, several of these children did not respond to many of the words. Thus, at times only 8 to 12 subjects were used to calculate the norms. The children who did not respond to some words may have been avoiding them because they felt that they could not pronounce them "correctly." This, too, would alter the age norms.

Another way to view phonological acquisition is by using approximate age ranges for acquisition. Based on a variety of sources, Grunwell (1987) specified the sounds that might be expected at each stage. Figure 8.1 provides the sounds of American English divided between the age ranges of 1½ years of age to 4½ years and beyond.

If we were to try and summarize these results, the following could be offered:

Nasals: Nasals are very early developing sounds. Mastery age for approximately 75 percent of the children is before or around age 3. Typically, /m/ and /n/ are mastered before /ŋ/.

Stop-Plosives: Stop-plosives are early developing sounds. Mastery age for approximately 75 percent of the children is before or around age 3. Based on some of the studies, the stop-plosives /p/, /b/, /t/, and /d/ precede /k/ and /g/.

Glides: The glides /w/ and /j/ also appear early in the sound acquisition process. Mastery age for approximately 75 percent of the children is 3 to 4 years. The glide /w/ appears to be somewhat earlier in the acquisition process than /j/.

Fricatives: The /h/ appears very early, around the time of early stop-plosive development. Most studies demonstrate that /h/ is mastered by 75 percent of the children before or around age 3. /f/ is also an early developing fricative. Again, most of the studies demonstrate that most children (75 percent) have acquired /f/ by age 3. The voiced /v/ is clearly later; mastery level is from 4 to approximately 6

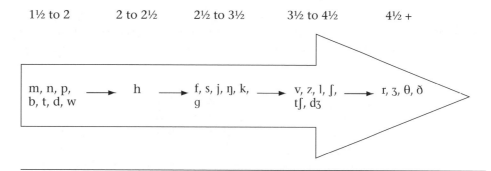

| 1½ to 2 | 2 to 2½ | 2½ to 3½ | 3½ to 4½ | 4½ + |

m, n, p, b, t, d, w → h → f, s, j, ŋ, k, g → v, z, l, ʃ, tʃ, dʒ → r, ʒ, θ, ð

Figure 8.1 Approximate Age Range of Phonological Development
Source: Based on Grunwell (1987).

years of age. The next fricative to develop is /ʃ/; due to its infrequency in American English, /ʒ/ is often not tested but is later than /ʃ/ in the acquisition process. These fricatives demonstrate mastery by most children (75%) around age 4. The rest of the fricatives are later developing sounds: /s/, /z/, /θ/, and /ð/. Mastery of these sounds may extend from 4 to 6 years of age.

Affricates: Most studies demonstrate that /tʃ/ and /dʒ/ develop approximately around the time of /ʃ/ and /ʒ/. Therefore, the affricates are typically mastered by most children around age 4.

Beginning Case Study

KATIE IN THE PHONOLOGY CLINIC

After looking at the overview of when different sounds should be mastered, Katie begins to sort things out. Paula's [t] for [k] substitution is one that developmentally should not be there. According to all that she has seen, /k/ is mastered by 4½ years old at the latest. However, Paula's r- and s-problems reflect later sounds in the acquisition process. She is not quite sure about Mikey's leaving off the ends of words, but his faulty [s] and [r] productions again coincide with later developing sounds. Coulton is still a dilemma. Although /f/ is an early fricative, Katie wonders about the fact that he substitutes [t] and [d] for several sounds. This seems like a different problem than just speech sound development.

FOCUS 3: *Why do the age results from the cross-sectional sound mastery studies vary?*

Several investigators (e.g., Irwin & Wong, 1983; Stoel-Gammon, 1985) have used spontaneous speech and/or longitudinal investigations to document phonological development. While spontaneous speech samples are in some respects better than the picture-naming tasks, several problems remain. Their use can also give us a biased picture. We actually probe only into a small portion of the child's conversational abilities and then generalize, assuming this is representative of the child's overall performance. Also, factors outside of our control might determine which words and sounds the child does produce and which ones are not articulated. As a result, the sample obtained will probably not contain all the sounds in that particular child's phonetic inventory.

Longitudinal data, on the other hand, can give us a real insight into the individual acquisition process, an important aspect missing in cross-sectional studies. The following discussion examines data from longitudinal studies on the consonant development in children.

Several longitudinal studies exist, but they report on either a single child or a small group of children (e.g., Leopold, 1947; Menn, 1971; Vihman et al., 1985). Therefore, the data cannot be readily generalized. However, Vihman and Greenlee (1987) used a longitudinal methodology to examine the phonological development of ten 3-year-old children with the following results:

1. Stops and other fricatives were substituted for /θ/ and /ð/ by all subjects.
2. Over half of the subjects also used substitutions for /r/ and /l/ sounds and replaced a palatal sound by an alveolar (/ʃ/ becomes /s/).
3. Two of the ten children demonstrated their own particular "style" of phonological acquisition.
4. On the average, 73 percent of the children's utterances were judged intelligible by three raters unfamiliar with the children. However, the range of intelligibility was broad, extending from 54 percent to 80 percent. As expected, children with fewer errors were more intelligible than those with multiple errors. Also, the children who used more complex sentences tended to be more difficult to understand.

Reflect on This: Clinical Application

USING CROSS-SECTIONAL MASTERY LEVEL CHARTS—YES OR NO?

This discussion has pointed out some of the problems with large cross-sectional studies that resulted in ages of sound mastery. Should these charts be completely discarded due to their inherent problems? Probably not. Sound mastery charts give useful information about the general ages and order speech sounds develop. Especially for beginning clinicians, they can provide a broad framework for comparison.

Clinicians should remember, however, that varying methodologies and criteria for sound mastery across investigations have produced a wide range of acquisition ages. Ages of mastery for some sounds often differ by three to four years. Based on the results of the Prather et al. (1975) study, a clinician could justify doing /s/ therapy with a 3-year-old, but according to the Poole (1934) investigation, a clinician should wait until 7½ years old to work on /s/. These sound mastery charts should never be the single deciding factor for intervention.

This last finding is significant. It documents the complex interaction between phonological development and the acquisition of the language system as a whole. The simultaneous acquisition of complex morphosyntactic and semantic relationships could well have an impact on the growth of the phonological system. It has been hypothesized that **phonological idioms** (Moskowitz, 1971) or **regression** (Leopold, 1947) occur as the child attempts to master other complexities of language. Both terms refer to accurate sound productions that are later replaced by inaccurate ones. When trying to deal with more complex morphosyntactic or semantic structures, the child's previously correct articulations appear to be lost, replaced by inaccurate sound productions.

Prosodic Feature Development

At the time when children begin to use two-word utterances, a further development in the usage of suprasegmentals occurs: **contrastive stress**. This term indicates that one syllable within a two-word utterance becomes prominent. The acquisition process seems to proceed in the following order. First, within the child's two-word utterance, a single prosodic pattern is maintained; the two words have a pause between them that becomes shorter and shorter. The next step appears to be the prosodic integration of the two words into one **tone-unit**. A tone-unit, or what is often called a sense-group, is an organizational unit imposed upon prosodic data (Crystal, 1986). Such a tone-unit conveys meaning beyond that which is implied by only the verbal production. When the two words become one tone-unit (i.e., without the pause between them and with one intonational contour), one of these words becomes more prominent than the other, usually louder and associated with an identifiable pitch movement (Crystal, 1986). At the end of this process, there exists a unifying rhythmic relationship between the two items; thus, pauses become less likely. The following developmental pattern could be observed:

Daddy (pause) eat
Daddy (pause shortens) eat
'Daddy 'eat (no pause, both stressed)
'Daddy eat (first word stressed)

The use of contrastive stress in the two-word stage may be used to establish contrastive meaning (Brown, 1973). It is assumed that the meaning of the combined one-tone utterance is different from the meaning of the two words in sequence. Later we see that this contrastive stress is used to signal differences in meaning with similar words. Thus, "<u>Daddy</u> eat" could indicate that "Daddy is eating," while "Daddy '<u>eat</u>" could indicate, perhaps, that "Daddy should sit down and eat."

The existing studies of prosodic feature development agree that the acquisition of intonation and stress begins at an early age. Adultlike intonational patterns are noted prior to the appearance of the first word, while the onset of stress patterns seems to occur clearly before the age of 2. However, true mastery of the whole prosodic feature system does not seem to take place until children are at least 12 years old (Atkinson-King, 1973; Malikouti-Drachman & Drachman, 1975).

The School-Age Child

By the time children enter school, their phonological development has progressed considerably. At age 5;0, most of them can converse freely with everyone and make themselves understood clearly to peers and adults alike. However, their pronunciation is still recognizably different from the adult norm. Phonologically, they still have a lot to learn. While their phonological inventory is nearly complete, this system must now be adapted to many more and different contexts, words, and situations. Certain phonological features are not mastered at this time. Later developing sounds are still frequently misarticulated, and some aspects of prosodic feature development are only beginning to be incorporated. The next section will serve as an overview of the phonological and prosodic features of the school-age child.

Segmental Form Development

Information on the development of the phonological system comes from quite different methodological backgrounds. Most of the information available is based on the results of articulation tests, i.e., based on responses to picture naming. Based on single-item pronunciation, most investigators agree that children complete their phonemic inventory by the age of 6;0 or, at the latest, 7;0. However, data from the Iowa-Nebraska Articulation Norms (Smit, 1993a) found dentalized /s/-productions in 10 percent of the 9-year-old children tested. Table 8.3 indicates the later developing sounds found in several cross-sectional studies.

One must keep in mind that most of these results are responses to single-word tasks. To assume, based on this type of task, that these sounds are now "learned" does not take into account the complexity of their use in naturalistic contexts, in new words and in conversational situations.

Consonant clusters can also be difficult to produce for the school-age child. The acquisition of clusters usually takes place anywhere from about age 3;6 to age 5;6. During this time, the child may demonstrate the reduction of the consonant cluster (omission of one of the consonants), lengthening of certain elements of the cluster (e.g., [s:no]), or epenthesis. In **epenthesis**, the child inserts a schwa vowel between two consonantal elements of a cluster, (e.g., [səno]). The Iowa-Nebraska data submitted by Smit (1993b) offer interesting insight into 27 different initial clusters. In this study, 1,049 children between the ages of 2;0 and 9;0 were screened using an articulation test format. The following summarizes these data:

1. On 14 of the 27 initial clusters tested, a small percentage of children in the 8;0- to 9;0-year-old group (N = 247; frequency of occurrence = approximately 2%) reduced two consonant clusters to a single element. These clusters included [pl], [kl], [gl], [sl], [tw], [kw], [tr], [dr], [fr], [sw], [sm], [sn], [st], and [sk].
2. The consonant clusters [br] and [θr] demonstrated a higher frequency of consonant cluster reduction (5–15%) for children from ages 5 to 9.
3. For the 5;6- to 7;0-year-olds, the consonant clusters that fell at 75 percent or below group accuracy included [sl], [br], [θr], [skw], [spr], [str], and [skr].

Table 8.3 Later Developing Sounds with Approximate Ages of Mastery

Sound	Age of Mastery	Source
[s]	4½; 4; 6	Templin (1957); Arlt & Goodban (1976); Smit (1993a)1
[z]	7½; 4; 6	Templin (1957); Arlt & Goodban (1976); Smit (1993a)
[r]	6; 5; 72	Templin (1957); Arlt & Goodban (1976); Smit (1993a)
[v]	6; 3½; 4	Templin (1957); Arlt & Goodban (1976); Smit (1993a)
[ʃ]	4½; 4½; 3½	Templin (1957); Arlt & Goodban (1976); Smit (1993a)
[ʒ]	6; 6½; 7	Templin (1957); Arlt & Goodban (1976); Prather et al. (1975)
[θ]	6; 5; 5½	Templin (1957); Arlt & Goodban (1976); Smit (1993a)
[ð]	7; 5; 4½	Templin (1957); Arlt & Goodban (1976); Smit (1993a)
[tʃ]	4½; 4; 3½	Templin (1957); Arlt & Goodban (1976); Smit (1993a)
[dʒ]	7; 4; 3½	Templin (1957); Arlt & Goodban (1976); Smit (1993a)

[1]For the Smit (1993a) data, mastery levels were not determined. For the purpose of this table, a sound has been considered mastered if the estimated percent acceptable use is approximately 75%.

[2]These data include /r/ in words such as "rope" and "rainbow" as well as central vowels with r-coloring and rhotic diphthongs as in "spider" or "beard." If just the data for the vowels are considered, then the 75% mastery-level age would be 3;6.

4. Epenthesis, or schwa insertion, in consonant clusters, occurs, depending on the consonant cluster, up to age 8;0 in over 5 percent of the children. The 9-year-olds exhibited schwa insertion rarely.

These data demonstrate that consonant cluster realizations are not adultlike for all children until approximately age 8. Table 8.4 is offered as an overview of the acquisition of consonant clusters as outlined by Smit (1993b). Although only the estimated percent of acceptable use is documented in her article, for the purpose of this table, mastery level was set at 75 percent. Unless otherwise noted, if an age range was given in the Smit (1993b) article, the earliest age in the range was used as the mastery level.

In addition, for school-age children, the timing of the sounds within consonant clusters is also not yet comparable to adult performance (Gilbert & Purves, 1977; Hawkins, 1979). When the temporal relationships between the elements of a cluster were compared for children and adults, it was found that differences, particularly in voice onset time, were still present at 8;0 years of age.

While this information indicates that phonological development extends past the age of 7, most of the available research has focused on the development of the phonological inventory. Unfortunately, other features of the phonological system are still relatively uncharted territory. For example, the development of allophonic variations in older children should

Table 8.4 Approximate Ages of Acquisition of Initial Consonant Clusters (Smit, 1993b)

Cluster	Mastery Age	Error Patterns Noted in 5 to 20% of the Children of That Age Group
tw	3;6	reduction of cluster to /t/ or /w/, substitution of /p,k,d/ for /t/ in cluster
kw	3.6	reduction of cluster to /k/ or /w/, substitution of /g/ for /k/
pl	5;6	reduction of cluster to /p/, substitution of /w/ for /l/
bl	5;6	reduction of cluster to /b/, substitution of /w/ for /l/
kl	5;6	reduction of cluster to /k/ or reduction to /t/, substitution of /w/ for /l/
gl	5;6	reduction of cluster to /g/, substitution of /w/ for /l/
fl	4;6	reduction of cluster to /f/, substitution of /w/ for /l/
sl	8;0	reduction of cluster to dentalized /s/, use of dentalized /s/ in cluster
pr	6;0	substitution of /w/ for /r/
br	7;0	reduction of cluster to /b/, substitution of /w/ for /r/
tr	6;0	substitution of /w/ for /r/, derhotacized /r/ production
dr	6;0	substitution of /w/ for /r/
kr	6;0	substitution of /w/ for /r/
gr	6;0	substitution of /w/ for /r/
fr	5;6	substitution of /w/ for /r/
θr	8;0	reduction of the cluster to a dentalized /s/, substitution of /w/ for /r/
sw	5;6	dentalized /s/ production
sm	5;0	dentalized /s/ production
sn	5;0	dentalized /s/ production
sp	5;6	dentalized /s/ production
st	5;0	dentalized /s/ production
sk	4;6	dentalized /s/ production
skw	5;0	dentalized /s/ production
spl	6;0	substitution of /w/ for /l/ in cluster, dentalized /s/ production
spr	8;0	dentalized /s/ production
str	8;0	dentalized /s/ production
skr	8;0	dentalized /s/ production

For the purpose of this table, mastery age was determined to be accurate production by 75% of the children. Since age ranges are given in the Smit (1993b) data (for example, 5;6 to 7;0), the lowest age in the range was used as the mastery age.

also be addressed. How do children learn the acceptable range of phonetic variation in different contexts within their speech community? Very little research has addressed this area of phonology. The variability of sound production and the learning of its acceptable allophonic limitations are decisively important tasks for the developing school-age child.

The intricate interrelation of normal phonological development with other areas of language growth, demands attention at this point in the child's development as well. The acquisition of vocabulary, for example, is a monumental task to be accomplished in a relatively short time. When children begin kindergarten, they are said to have an expressive vocabulary of approximately 2,200 words (Weiss & Lillywhite, 1981). New sound sequences occurring in words that will now be attained require, not only increased oral-motor control and improved timing skills, they also necessitate the internalization of new phonological rules. For instance, the conditions under which voiceless stops in English need to be aspirated or not might now become new achievements.

FOCUS 4: *Which sounds appear to be later developing sounds? How does the acquisition of consonant clusters fit into this acquisition process?*

Prosodic Feature Development

Very little documented research is available on the acquisition of prosodic features in the school-age child. Prosodic features in their variation of pitch, loudness, and duration can be used to signal attitudes and emotions; they can also assume grammatical function. For example, specific intonation patterns have to be employed to differentiate between statements and certain questions in English ("He is coming." ↘ versus "He is coming?" ↗). Contrasting stress realizations might signal different word classes ('con struct versus con 'struct). On the sentence level, the combined effects of higher pitch and increased loudness usually convey communicatively important modifications of basic meaning ("This is a 'pen." versus "'This is a pen.") This section examines the grammatical function of prosodic features in school-age children and their relationship to phonological development.

As previously noted, the child begins to use intonational patterns toward the end of the first year of life. As the child's grammatical abilities develop, new uses of intonation emerge. For example, the contrast between rising and falling pitch differentiates the two grammatical functions of a tag question in English: *asking*, as in "We're ready, aren't we?" ↗ and *telling*, as in "We're ready, aren't we!" ↘. Differences in intonation patterns like these appear to be learned during the child's third year (Crystal, 1987). However, the learning of intonation goes on for a long time. Studies report that children as old as 12 years were still acquiring some of the fundamental functions of English intonation, especially those for signaling grammatical contrasts (Cruttenden, 1985; Ianucci & Dodd, 1980). As reported by Crystal (1987), even teenagers have been shown to have difficulty understanding sentences where intonation and pausing are used to differentiate meanings. He used the example: "She dressed, and fed the baby" (indicating she dressed herself and then fed the baby) versus "She dressed and fed the baby" (indicating she dressed as well as fed the baby). Thus, while certain intonational features seem to be among the earliest phonological acquisitions, others may be some of the last.

Several studies have examined the use of *contrastive stress* both on the word level ('rec ord versus re 'cord) and on the sentence level (differentiating between whom Mary hit in the following sentences: "John hit Bill and then <u>Mary</u> hit him" versus "John hit Bill and then Mary hit <u>him</u>") (e.g.,

Atkinson-King, 1973; Chomsky, 1971; Hornby & Hass, 1970; Myers & Myers, 1983). Although the ages differ depending on the type and design of the research, results suggest that children are still learning certain aspects of contrastive stress up until the age of 13.

The acquisition of prosodic features is a gradual process that in some respects extends into the teens. It is closely connected to the new phonological, morphosyntactic, semantic, and pragmatic demands that are placed upon the developing child. As the complexity of the linguistic environment and the child's interaction with that environment increase, so do the subtle intricacies of each of these language levels.

Phonological Theories: Distinctive Feature, Natural Phonology, and Nonlinear Phonology

Children's acquisition of speech sounds has been documented for decades. At the same time, many different theories have been postulated that attempt to explain why and how children develop speech sounds in the manner that they do. Why is it that children, whether they are born in China, Spain, or in the United States develop the speech sounds of their native language in a rather orderly manner? And what is the mechanism that does not seem to function in the child with a speech sound disorder?

The following section will examine three different contemporary theories and how they interpret speech sound development. The first, distinctive feature theory, has served as the basis for many contemporary models. Although the original concept dates back to the 1930s, the use of distinctive features to explain contemporary models, such as the newer nonlinear theories, reflects its ongoing importance. The second theory, natural phonology, has gained wide recognition through its use of phonological processes to explain this acquisition process. The third approach, a nonlinear theory, examines this acquisition process from a completely different viewpoint. The following section will briefly examine how each of these theories explains the development of speech sounds in children.

Distinctive Features

The original distinctive feature theories hypothesized that the smallest constituent of language was not the phoneme, but rather the phoneme could be further divided into additional components. These units, which are smaller than sound segments, are considered to be "atomic" constituents of sound properties that cannot be broken down any more (Jakobson, 1949). **Distinctive features** are the smallest indivisible sound properties that establish phonemes. An inventory of distinctive features would demonstrate that some sounds are marked by the presence of this distinctive feature while other sounds lack this particular feature. A binary (+ and –) system was used to indicate the presence of a particular feature (+) versus the lack of that feature (–). The difficult part was establishing the different distinctive features that must be diverse enough to differentiate the various phonemes yet not be overwhelming in their number and characteristics. In addition, the original theories were devised to analyze not only the phonemes of American English but also those of all languages of the world. Not an easy task.

Therefore, many different distinctive features must be considered in order to arrive at those that distinguish between phonemes. First, consonants must be distinguished from vowels, voiced consonants from voiceless consonants, nasals from nonnasals, to mention just a few. To demonstrate how these distinctive features might be established, we can use the following approach.

/p/	/b/
is a consonant = + consonantal	is a consonant = + consonantal
is not a vowel = –vocalic	is not a vowel = –vocalic
is not voiced = –voiced	is voiced = + voiced

In this example, we arrive at + and – voicing as being the distinctive feature that distinguishes between /p/ and /b/. Now, if we expand a bit to consider the phoneme /m/, we find the following:

/p/	/b/	/m/
is a consonant = + consonantal	is a consonant = + consonantal	is a consonant = + consonantal
is not a vowel = – vocalic	is not a vowel = – vocalic	is not a vowel = –vocalic
is not voiced = –voiced	is voiced = + voiced	is voiced = + voiced
is not a nasal = – nasal	is not a nasal = –nasal	is a nasal = + nasal

Although + and – voicing distinguishes between /p/ and /b/, the only distinctive feature that differentiates /b/ from /m/ is nasality.

Over the years, many different distinctive feature systems have been developed (e.g., Jakobson, 1949; Jakobson & Halle, 1956; Ladefoged, 1971; Singh & Polen, 1972). Each had a somewhat different idea about which distinctive features were important when distinguishing between phonemes. Most of the distinctive feature systems were based on articulatory production features, but acoustic parameters have been used as well (Jakobson, Fant, & Halle, 1952). One of the most widely used systems is the one created by Chomsky and Halle (1968), which was an outgrowth of their book *The Sound Pattern of English*, often cited as the major work in this area. Chomsky and Halle divided the distinctive features into five different categories: (1) major class features, (2) cavity features, (3) manner of articulation features, (4) source features, and (5) prosodic features. Although prosodic features are named within this feature system, they are not further discussed. Therefore, the following discussion will elaborate on the first four categories of distinctive features.

MAJOR CLASS FEATURES. These features were established to characterize and distinguish between production possibilities that result in three sound classes that are essentially quite different, such as distinguishing vowels from consonants. These three categories are as follows:

1. **Sonorant.** An open vocal tract configuration promoting voicing. The principle of sonority and sonorants was discussed in Chapters 1 and 5.

American English vowels, nasals, approximants (glides and liquids), and /h/ belong to this category.

2. **Consonantal.** Sounds produced with a high degree of oral obstruction. American English stop-plosives, fricatives, affricates, nasals, and the central and lateral approximants /r/ and /l/ belong to this category. The semi-vowel approximants /w/ and /j/ as well as /h/ are considered – consonantal.

3. **Vocalic.** Sounds that are produced with a low degree of oral obstruction: The tongue is not higher than required for the vowel /i/ and /u/. American English vowels and the central and lateral approximants /r/ and /l/ are considered + vocalic.

CAVITY FEATURES. Cavity features reference active and passive articulators as distinctive features. Only those that are important to the classification of American English phonemes are included.

1. **Coronal.** Sounds produced with the apical/predorsal portion of the tongue elevated from its neutral position. American English consonants that are + coronal include /t, d, θ, ð, s, z, ʃ, ʒ, tʃ, dʒ, n, r, and l/.

2. **Anterior.** Sounds produced in the frontal region of the oral cavity with the alveolar ridge being the posterior border. American English labial, dental, and alveolar consonants are + anterior and include /p, b, t, d, θ, ð, f, v, s, z, m, n, and l/.

3. **Nasal.** Sounds produced with an open nasal passageway. The nasal consonants /m, n, and ŋ/ are + nasal.

4. **Lateral.** Sounds produced with lowered lateral edges of the tongue. The only American English consonant that is + in this category is /l/.

5. **High.** Sounds produced with as high tongue position. The high vowels /i, ɪ, u, and ʊ/ and the consonants /k, g, ʃ, ʒ, tʃ, dʒ, ŋ, w, and j/ are + high.

6. **Low.** Sounds produced with a low tongue position. The low vowels /æ, ɑ, and ɔ/ and the consonant /h/ are + low.

7. **Back.** Sounds produced with a retracted body of the tongue. The vowels /ɑ, ɔ, o, ʊ, u, and ʌ/ and the consonants /k, g, w, and ŋ/ are + back.

8. **Round.** Sounds produced with rounding of the lips. The rounded vowels /ɔ, o, ʊ, and u/ and the consonant /w/ are + round.

MANNER OF ARTICULATION. These features specify the way the airstream is modified by the active and passive articulators.

1. **Continuant.** Sounds produced without hindering the airstream by any blockages with the oral cavity. All vowels, the fricatives including /h/, and approximates /w, j, r, and l/ are + continuant.

2. **Delayed release.** Sounds produced with a slow release of a total obstruction within the oral cavity. This feature was created to account for the affricates that actually begin with – continuant and end with a + continuant portion. The affricates are + delayed release.

3. **Tense.** Sounds produced with greater muscular activity at the root of the tongue, which translates into more muscular tension and increased expiratory air pressure. This feature is often listed with tongue root features and appears to be rather controversial in its application (Yavaş, 1998). Vowels /i, e, ɑ, o, and u/ and the voiceless stop-plosives /p, t, and k/ are + tense.

SOURCE FEATURES. These features refer to specific laryngeal features. For American English only the two relevant features are included.

1. **Voiced.** Sounds produced with simultaneous vocal fold vibration. All American English vowels and the voiced consonants are + voiced.
2. **Strident.** Sounds that when produced have a characteristic noise component. Consonants that are + strident include /f, v, s, z, ʃ, ʒ, tʃ, and dʒ/.

Figure 8.2 and 8.3 are matrices of the consonants and vowels according to the Chomsky and Halle (1968) distinctive feature system. As you will note, the feature tense is included within the vowel matrix but not within the consonant matrix. While this feature is relevant for classifying vowels, it is not used typically to classify consonants of American English.

DISTINCTIVE FEATURES AND PHONOLOGICAL DEVELOPMENT. According to Jakobson (1941/1968), the order of development of the sound properties is based on a principle referred to as maximal contrast. Therefore, the child acquires features that have the greatest physiological contrast and then moves to finer distinctions. Thus, the gross motor contrasts are learned before the more refined, fine motor ones. This principle is not a new one, however; it dates back to at least Schultze's (1881/1971) position. However, Jakobson went a step beyond just using motor contrasts and included both acoustic and semantic contrasts. At each stage, the semantic (usually labeled as cognitive level), the acoustic, and motoric contrasts are bound together and maximal contrasts are established (Blache, 1978).

Figure 8.2 Distinctive Features of American English Consonants According to the Chomsky-Halle (1968) Distinctive Feature System

	p	b	t	d	k	g	θ	ð	f	v	s	z	ʃ	ʒ	tʃ	dʒ	m	n	ŋ	r	l	w	j	h
Sonorant	−	−	−	−	−	−	−	−	−	−	−	−	−	−	−	−	+	+	+	+	+	+	+	+
Consonantal	+	+	+	+	+	+	+	+	+	+	+	+	+	+	+	+	+	+	+	+	+	−	−	−
Vocalic	−	−	−	−	−	−	−	−	−	−	−	−	−	−	−	−	−	−	−	+	+	−	−	−
Coronal	−	−	+	+	−	−	+	+	−	−	+	+	+	+	+	+	−	+	−	+	+	−	−	−
Anterior	+	+	+	+	−	−	+	+	+	+	+	+	−	−	−	−	+	+	−	−	+	−	−	−
Nasal	−	−	−	−	−	−	−	−	−	−	−	−	−	−	−	−	+	+	+	−	−	−	−	−
Lateral	−	−	−	−	−	−	−	−	−	−	−	−	−	−	−	−	−	−	−	−	+	−	−	−
High	−	−	−	−	+	+	−	−	−	−	−	−	+	+	+	+	−	−	+	−	−	+	+	−
Low	−	−	−	−	−	−	−	−	−	−	−	−	−	−	−	−	−	−	−	−	−	−	−	+
Back	−	−	−	−	+	+	−	−	−	−	−	−	−	−	−	−	−	−	+	−	−	+	−	−
Round	−	−	−	−	−	−	−	−	−	−	−	−	−	−	−	−	−	−	−	−	−	+	−	−
Continuant	−	−	−	−	−	−	+	+	+	+	+	+	+	+	−	−	−	−	−	+	+	+	+	+
Delayed Release	−	−	−	−	−	−	−	−	−	−	−	−	−	−	+	+	−	−	−	−	−	−	−	−
Voiced	−	+	−	+	−	+	−	+	−	+	−	+	−	+	−	+	+	+	+	+	+	+	+	−
Strident	−	−	−	−	−	−	−	−	+	+	+	+	+	+	+	+	−	−	−	−	−	−	−	−

Figure 8.3 Distinctive Features of American English Vowels According to the Chomsky-Halle (1968) Distinctive Feature System

	i	ɪ	e	ɛ	æ	ɑ	ɔ	o	ʊ	u	ʌ
Consonantal	−	−	−	−	−	−	−	−	−	−	−
Vocalic	+	+	+	+	+	+	+	+	+	+	+
Coronal	−	−	−	−	−	−	−	−	−	−	−
Anterior	−	−	−	−	−	−	−	−	−	−	−
High	+	+	−	−	−	−	−	−	+	+	−
Low	−	−	−	−	+	+	+	−	−	−	−
Back	−	−	−	−	−	+	+	+	+	+	+
Round	−	−	−	−	−	−	+	+	+	+	−
Tense	+	−	+	−	−	+	−	+	−	+	−

The following is a brief overview of these stages and will focus on the development of consonants. The discussion of vowels remains a weak element of the distinctive feature theory, and it appears that true guidelines were never completely established (Blache, 1978). Wherever possible, the vowels have been included in the discussion:

First: *Consonantal versus vocalics* are established. Consonants that generally represent the consonantal class are the stop-plosives, which are produced more anteriorly, thus /p, b, t, and d/. Although any of these consonants could be used, /p/ is understood to be the most highly probable. It is paired with a wide, neutral vowel such /ɑ/ or /a/; an example of a word production would be /papɑ/. This provides maximal contrast, with the vowel being open and the consonant completely closed while providing the basic syllable structure.

Second: *Nasal versus nonnasal* contrasts are established. Any nasal consonants could be used at this stage together with the front stop-plosives; however, typically /m/ is contrasted to /p/. Articulatory maximal contrasts consist of velopharyngeal opening and closing and voicing versus devoicing. The semantic contrast was Jakobson's postulation that the terms for father and mother contain these sounds in various societies (Jakobson, 1971). This is indeed the case in American English, where [mɑmɑ] and [pɑpɑ] are used for these terms in the early developmental stages.

Third: Labial versus dental contrasts are established. In this stage, the labial, nonnasal, and nasal consonants /p, b, m/ are produced in opposition to a dental, nonnasal consonant and a dental, nasal consonant, /t, d, n/. Again, the vowel remains neutral. Thus, one possibility would be the opposition [pɑpɑ] versus [dɑdɑ] or [nɑnɑ].

Fourth: Narrow versus wide vowel contrasts are established. The narrow vowels correspond to the high vowels, where there is a narrow opening as the bulge of the tongue comes closer to the palate, while the wide vowels are those where the bulge of the tongue is in a low position. This leads to an opposition of /i, ɪ, u, ʊ/, and perhaps /e/ and /o/, to the low vowels /ɑ, a, ɔ, ɛ/. For maximal contrasts, the high front vowel /i/ or the high-back vowel /u/ would be contrasted to the low vowel /ɑ/ or /a/. This would generate expressions such as [pipi], [bibi], [mimi], [titi], [didi], [nini] or [pupu], [bubu], [tutu], [dudu], and [nunu]. Semantically, several of these expressions are common baby-talk expressions.

Fifth: Palatal versus velar vowel contrasts are established. Jakobson uses the expression *palatal vowels* to refer to what we are calling front vowels, and *velar* for back vowels. Therefore, at this stage the child contrasts front-to-back vowels and the low, neutral vowels. This establishes oppositions such as [pipi], [papa], and [pupu] or [bibi], [dada], and [nunu]. The extreme points of the vowel quadrilateral are now present and contrasted, high-front vowels to high-back vowels and low, neutral vowels.

Sixth: Velar versus nonvelar consonant contrasts are established. In this stage, front tongue sounds are contrasted to back tongue sounds. Thus, /p/ and /t/ are now contrasted to /k/. The front and back tongue positions are also contrasted in phonemes such as /w/, /j/, /l/, and /r/.

Seventh: Intermediate vowels are now established. The child now starts to use intermediate vowels under the assumption that front vowels precede back vowels of the same height. Therefore, the child will acquire /e/ before /o/ and /ɛ/ before /ɔ/.

Eighth: Voiced versus voiceless contrasts are established. The child now further differentiates, using both voiced and voiceless contrasts if they were not present earlier.

Ninth: Continued versus interrupted consonant contrasts are now established. This stage separates the stop-plosives from the fricatives. Thus /p, t, and k/ are contrasted to /f, s, and ʃ/, for example.

Tenth: Strident versus nonstrident consonant contrasts are established. Here the strident /s/ and /z/ are contrasted to the nonstrident /θ/ and /ð/.

Although distinctive features are not typically used in contemporary assessment and intervention, their clinical application was attempted in the 1970s and 1980s. Two possibilities were utilized. First, distinctive feature analysis was used to contrast the features of the target sound to the substitutions displayed by the child. The end product was a list of distinctive features that could show whether the error and target sounds shared common features, and if specific error patterns existed. The child was then taught to differentiate between the presence and absence of these differentiating distinctive features. Typically, the presence or absence of a distinctive feature was chosen based on its high frequency of occurrence in the child's error patterns. Minimal pair work, with two sounds representing the presence (+) or absence (–) of that feature, were used to demonstrate the concept to the child. It was hypothesized that these (+) and (–) features would generalize to other consonants.

The second possibility used the developmental model that was just presented. For example, Blache (1989) outlines a therapy protocol based on this acquisition process. He notes the sounds in error and then uses minimal pairs to establish higher level distinctive feature contrasts. For example, if the child substitutes [t] and [d] for [θ] and [ð], he would use minimal

Reflect on This: Clinical Application

The following is a portion of the results from Nick, age 6½. This is an example of how distinctive features could be analyzed according to Jakobson's developmental theory (1941/1968) and Blache's (1989) therapy guidelines.

Word	Production	Distinctive Feature Breakdown (Blache, 1989)
house	[haʊθ]	strident vs nonstrident
cup	[tʌp]	velar vs. nonvelar
gun	[dʌn]	velar vs. nonvelar
shovel	[ʃʌbəl]	continued vs. interrupted
vacuum	[bækjum]	continued vs. interrupted
vase	[beɪθ]	continued vs. interrupted
that	[dæt]	continued vs. interrupted
bath	[bæt]	continued vs. interrupted
feather	[fɛdɚ]	continued vs. interrupted

There are three distinctive feature contrasts that impact this child's phonological system: strident versus nonstrident, velar versus nonvelar, and continued versus interrupted. The velar–nonvelar contrast should appear earlier in the acquisition process; therefore, minimal pairs such as tea–key, tape–cape, or ten–Ken could be used. One could assume that other velar–nonvelar contrasts could also be targeted that might generalize, such as win–wing, run–rung, or Ron–wrong.

pairs to contrast continuant versus interrupted sounds. However, if [θ] and [ð] are used as substitutions for [s] and [z], then he would work on the strident system.

FOCUS 5: *What are distinctive features? How do distinctive features explain the development of the child's phonological system?*

Natural Phonology

Natural phonology was specifically designed to explain the development of the child's phonological system. The theory postulates that the patterns of speech are governed by an innate, universal set of phonological processes. Thus, all children are born with the capacity to use the same system of processes. Phonological processes, as natural processes, are easier for the child to produce and are substituted for sounds, sound classes, or sound sequences when the child's motor capacities do not yet allow their standard realization. These innate, universal natural phonological processes are all operating as each child attempts to use and organize its phonological system. Therefore, all children begin with innate speech patterns but must progress to the language-specific system that characterizes their native language. Phonological processes are used to constantly revise existing differences between the innate patterns and the standard "adult" pronunciation. The theory points out prominent developmental steps children go through until the goal of adult phonology is reached in the child's adolescent years. On the other hand, disordered phonology is seen as an inability to realize this "natural" process of goal-oriented adaptive change.

NATURAL PHONOLOGY AND PHONOLOGICAL DEVELOPMENT. Natural phonology assumes that the child's innate phonological system is continuously revised in the direction of the adult phonological system. Stampe (1979) proposed mechanisms to account for these changes. These mechanisms reflect properties of the innate phonological system as well as the universal difficulties children display in the acquisition of the adult sound system. One of these mechanisms is suppression. *Suppression* refers to the child's ability to eliminate one or more phonological processes as he or she moves from the innate speech patterns to the adult norm production. Therefore, a previously used phonological process is no longer used by the child.

A concept central to natural phonology is that of phonological processes. Since phonological processes are so central to the workings of natural phonology, including the clinical application of these principles, some of the more common processes are listed on the following pages.

PHONOLOGICAL PROCESSES. Although many different processes have been identified in the speech of normally developing children and those with phonological disorders, only a few occur with any regularity. Those processes that are common in the speech development of children across languages are called **natural processes**.

Phonological processes are categorized according to syllable structure processes, substitution processes, and assimilatory processes. Syllable structure processes describe those changes that affect the structure of the syllable. Substitution processes are used for those sound modifications in which one sound class is replaced by another. Assimilatory processes denote specific types of articulatory adjustments in which a sound becomes similar to, or is influenced by, a neighboring sound in a word. The following is a list of phonological processes that are frequently used by normally developing children. An explanation is given as well as the approximate age of suppression of the process.

SYLLABLE STRUCTURE CHANGES. Syllable structure processes are manifestations of the general tendency of young children to reduce words to basic CV structures. They become evident between the ages of 1;6 and 4;0, at a time when there is a rapid growth in vocabulary and the onset of two-word utterances (Ingram, 1989b).

> **Reduplication:** The replacement of a syllable or part of a syllable by a repetition of the preceding syllable.

> Example: "water" [wɑtɚ] is articulated [wɑwɑ], "doggie" [dɑgi] becomes [dɑdɑ]

Reduplication is an early syllable structure process. Ingram (1989b) notes that it is a common process during the child's first-fifty-word stage. There was no evidence of this process in the youngest group of children (1;6 to 1;9) in the Preisser, Hodson, and Paden (1988) study.

Weak syllable deletion or **unstressed syllable deletion:** The omission of an unstressed syllable.

Example: "banana" [bənænə] is reduced to [nænə], "potato" [pəteɪto] is reduced to [teɪto].

Unstressed syllable deletion, sometimes called weak syllable deletion, lasts until approximately 4 years of age (Ingram, 1989b). This is also confirmed by Grunwell's (1987) data. However, Preisser et al. (1988) noted that most of the children appeared to have suppressed this process around their second birthday. (Only 3% of the 20 children over age 2;2 demonstrated unstressed syllable deletion.)

Final consonant deletion: The omission of a syllable-arresting consonant.

Example: "ball" [bɑl] is reduced to [bɑ], "coat" [koʊt] is reduced to [koʊ].

Final consonant deletion is a relatively early process. Preisser et al. (1988) state that it was extremely rare in the utterances of the subjects in the 2;2 to 2;5 age group. Ingram (1989b) and Grunwell (1987) note the disappearance of this process around age 3.

Cluster reduction: The articulatory simplification of consonant clusters by omitting one consonant (in two-consonant clusters) or one or two consonants (in three-consonant clusters).

Example: "spoon" [spun] becomes [pun], "street" [strit] becomes [trit]

Cluster reduction is a syllable structure process that lasts for a relatively long time. Haelsig and Madison (1986) noted cluster reductions that still occurred in 5-year-old children, while Roberts, Burchinal, and Footo (1990) evidenced rare instances of this process in their 8-year-old children. In the Smit (1993b) study, there was some evidence of cluster reduction in the 8;0- to 9;0-year-old children for specific initial consonant clusters (approximately 1–4% of the 247 children for primarily three-consonant clusters).

Epenthesis: The insertion of a sound segment into a word, thereby changing its syllable structure. The intrusive sound can be a vowel as well as a consonant, but most often it is restricted to a schwa insertion between two consonants.

Example: "please" [pliz] becomes [pəliz], "bread" [brɛd] becomes [bərɛd].

Epenthesis seems to be a process that can occur in children between the ages of 2;6 and 8;0, according to Smit (1993b) and Smit and colleagues (Smit, Hand, Freilinger, Bernthal, & Bird, 1990).

SUBSTITUTION PROCESSES. Substitution processes are the substitution of one speech sound for another. There are many different substitution process; some are suppressed relatively early, others much later. The following substitution processes are divided into those in which the change occurs relative to (1) the active and passive articulators, (2) the manner of articulation, and (3) voicing.

Changes in active and passive articulators

Fronting: Sound substitutions in which the active and/or passive articulators are more anteriorly located for the production than the target sound.

Prominent examples are *velar fronting* (t/k substitution) and *palatal fronting* (s/ʃ substitution). Palatal fronting may also occur in affricate productions, [tʃ] → [ts] and [dʒ] → [dz].

Example: "coat" [koʊt] becomes [toʊt], "ship" [ʃɪp] becomes [sɪp], "cheese" [tʃiz] becomes [tsiz].

Lowe, Knutson, and Monson (1985) found velar fronting to be more prevalent than palatal fronting. They also found that fronting rarely occurred after the age of 3;6. Based on the Smit (1993a) data, both velar fronting and palatal fronting were still noted until approximately age 5;0, but the frequency of occurrence was very limited (below 5% of the 186 children).

Labialization: The replacement of a nonlabial sound by a labial one.

Example: "thumb" [θʌm] is realized as [fʌm].

According to Lowe (1996), 75 percent of the children used for the standardization of the ALPHA (*Assessment Link Between Phonology and Articulation*, rev. ed.) suppressed this process by age 6;0.

Alveolarization: The change of nonalveolar sounds, mostly interdental and labio-dental sounds, into alveolar ones.

Example: "fig" [fɪg] is realized as [sɪg], "those" [ðoʊz] is realized as [zoʊz].

Lowe (1996) notes suppression of this process by 75 percent of the children tested at age 5;0.

Changes in manner of articulation

Stopping: Most frequently, the replacement of fricatives and affricates by stops.

"sun" [sʌn] becomes [tʌn], "feet" [fit] becomes [pit]

Due to the fact that fricatives and affricates are acquired at different ages, stopping is not a unified process but should be broken down into the individual sounds for which this process is employed. Table 8.5 summarizes the ages at which stopping is suppressed for the different fricative sounds.

Table 8.5 Age of Suppression of Stopping

[f]	10–15% occurrence in 2;0- to 3;0-year-olds, rare (less than 3%) in 3½-year-olds
[v]	5–15% occurrence in 4- to 4½-year-olds, rarely noted later
[s]	around 3;0 years of age, after that distortions predominate
[z]	between 3;6 and 4;0, after that distortions predominate
[ʃ]	less than 10% in 3½-year-olds, after that distortions are more frequent
[tʃ]	10–15% occurrence in 3½-year-olds
[dʒ]	5–15% occurrence in 3½- to 4-year-olds
[θ]	5–15% occurrence in 3½-year-olds, rarely noted later
[ð]	5–15% occurrence in 4½-year-olds, rarely noted later

Source: Summarized from Smit (1993a).

Beginning Case Study

KATIE IN THE PHONOLOGY CLINIC

Katie notes that Mikey, who is leaving off the end consonants of words, is still using final consonant deletion. This is a process that should be suppressed by 3 years of age, clearly something that should be addressed. Coulton's errors are the stopping of fricative consonants. This phonological process would account for all the substitutions that make his speech unintelligible. This is also a process that should be suppressed at his age. If she could get Coulton to understand the difference between stops and fricatives, this hopefully will generalize to his phonological system.

Affrication: The replacement of fricatives by homorganic affricates.

Example: "shoe" [ʃu] is produced as [tʃu].

Lowe (1996) notes that this process is suppressed by 75 percent of the children tested by age 3;0.

Deaffrication: The production of affricates as homorganic fricatives.

Example: "cheese" [tʃiz] realized as [ʃiz], "juice" [dʒus] is realized as [ʒus].

This process extends somewhat longer than affrication. According to Lowe (1996), 75 percent of the children he tested suppressed this process by age 4;0.

Denasalization: The replacement of nasals by homorganic stops.

Example: "noon" [nun] changed to [dud], "meet" [mit] produced as [bit].

Smit (1993b) notes that this was the most common error for [m] and [n] but is used only occasionally in 2-year-olds (fewer than 10%).

Gliding of liquids/fricatives: The replacement of liquids or fricatives by glides.

Example: "red" [rɛd] is produced as [wɛd], "shoe" [ʃu] becomes [ju].

Gliding of [r] and [l] seems to extend beyond 5;0 years of age (Grunwell, 1987; Smit, 1993a) and can be infrequently found even in the speech of children as old as 7 (Roberts et al. 1990; Smit, 1993a).

Vowelization (vocalization): The replacement of syllabic liquids and nasals, foremost [l], [r], and [n], by vowels.

Example: "table" [teɪbəl] becomes [teɪbo]; "ladder" [lædɚ] is pronounced as [lædʊ].

Lowe (1996) noted vowelization until approximately 4;6 years of age. At that time, 75 percent of the children tested suppressed this process.

Derhotacization: The loss of r-coloring in central vowels with r-coloring [ɝ] and [ɚ].

Examples: "better" [bɛtɚ] becomes [bɛtə], and "word" [wɝd] becomes [wɜd].

Smit (1993a) reports that 90 percent of the children suppressed this process by age 4;0.

Changes in voicing

Voicing: The replacement of a voiced for a voiceless sound.

Example: "two" [tu] is pronounced [du].

Devoicing: The replacement of a voiceless for a normally voiced sound.

Example: "beet" [bit] is pronounced as [pit].

Context-sensitive voicing changes are typically suppressed around age 3;0 (Grunwell, 1987). Initial voicing and final devoicing are later. Initial voicing was not seen in 85 percent of the children tested by Khan and Lewis (2002) at age 6;0, while final devoicing was suppressed by 85 percent of the children by age 5;0.

ASSIMILATION PROCESSES. There are many different assimilation processes that occur in the speech of children. Children within early stages of their speech development tend to utilize assimilation processes in systematic ways. Assimilation processes were discussed in some detail in Chapter 7; however, there are typical assimilations that occur in the speech of young children.

One of the most frequently occurring assimilatory processes is velar harmony (Smith, 1973). Prominent examples:

[gɑg] for "dog"
[keɪk] for "take"
[kɑk] for "talk"

However, regressive assimilation processes are not limited to velar consonants. Smith (1973) reported similar regressive assimilations in which labials influenced preceding nonlabial consonants and consonant clusters. Among his examples:

[bebu] for "table"
[bɔp] for "stop"

Nasalization was also occasionally used in which a continuant would become nasal if preceded by a nasal consonant.

[nɔ͡ini] for "noisy"
[mɛn] for "smell"

Although not all children display these types of assimilation processes, they may be present in the speech of 1½- to 2-year-olds. If they persist beyond 3 years of age, they constitute a danger sign for a disordered phonological system (Grunwell, 1987).

According to natural phonology, phonological processes are recognizable steps in the gradual articulatory adjustment of children's speech to the respective adult standard. That implies a chronology of phonological processes, i.e., specific ages in which the process could be operating and when the process should be suppressed (Grunwell, 1981, 1987; Vihman, 1984). As useful as a chronology of normative data might seem for clinical purposes, tables of established age norms can easily be misleading. Individual variation and contextual conditions may play a large role in the use and suppression of phonological processes.

To summarize, the theory of natural phonology assumes an innate phonological system that is progressively revised during childhood until it corresponds with the adult phonological system. Phonological processes are developmentally conditioned simplifications in the realization of the standard phonological system. These simplifications are gradually overcome, and the phonological processes become suppressed.

FOCUS 6: *What is natural phonology? What role do phonological processes play in this model?*

The next section will discuss briefly the nonlinear or multilinear approach to the analysis of speech sounds of children. These theories are a radical departure from earlier theories. First, basic information will be given to guide the student to an understanding of these contemporary approaches.

Nonlinear Theories

To understand the nonlinear approaches to phonology, it is first necessary to conceptualize what has been termed *surface level* and *underlying* representations. The actual productions of speech, which are obtained using tape recording and phonetic transcription, represent the surface-level representation, or the surface-level forms. They are the actualities of speech

Reflect on this: Clinical Application

DIAGNOSTIC IMPLICATIONS OF PHONOLOGICAL PROCESS SUPPRESSION

Approximate ages of suppression have been provided for several common phonological processes. This information can be helpful during our diagnostic assessment. The following phonological processes were identified in Clint, age 3;6.

Word	Production	Phonological Process
house	[haʊ]	final consonant deletion
cup	[kʌ]	final consonant deletion
gun	[gʌ]	final consonant deletion
shovel	[ʃʌbəl]	stopping of [v]
vacuum	[bækju]	stopping of [v], final consonant deletion
vase	[beɪ]	stopping of [v], final consonant deletion
scratching	[krætʃɪŋ]	consonant cluster reduction
skunk	[kʌŋk]	consonant cluster reduction
star	[tɑɚ]	consonant cluster reduction
jumping	[dʌmpɪŋ]	stopping of [dʒ]
jelly	[dɛli]	stopping of [dʒ]
jeep	[dip]	stopping of [dʒ]
that	[dæt]	stopping of [ð]
bath	[bæt]	stopping of [θ]
feather	[fɛdɚ]	stopping of [ð]

Similar processes were also noted in conversational speech.

Which of the noted processes should be suppressed by age 3;6? Final consonant deletion is usually suppressed by around age 3;0, while stopping of [v], [θ], [ð], and [dʒ] extend to age 3;6 or beyond. Consonant cluster reduction is also a process that is suppressed at a relatively late age. Based on these results, the only process that might cause concern at this age would be final consonant deletion. Again, discretion must be exercised when using these approximate ages of suppression as the sole criterion for determining the necessity for intervention.

production. Newer phonologies expanded on this concept to include what has been called the underlying representation. The underlying representation or form is a purely theoretical concept that is thought to represent a mental reality behind the way people use language (Crystal, 1987). Underlying forms exemplify the person's language competency as one aspect of his or her cognitive capabilities.

Thus, newer models assume two levels of speech sound possibilities: an abstract underlying representation and the actualities of speech sound production called surface forms.

Underlying forms
also serve as points
of orientation to
describe regularities
of speech reality as
they relate to other
areas of language,
notably morphology
and syntax. This
principle was first
developed by Noam
Chomsky (1957) in
his concept of gen-
erative phonology. It
has served as the
basis of phonologi-
cal theories since
that time. Although
natural phonology is
also based on sur-
face forms and
underlying represen-
tations, it is not
considered a nonlin-
ear approach.

Phonological theories, including natural phonology, were based on the understanding that all speech segments are arranged in a sequential order. Consequently, underlying representations and surface forms consisted of a string of discrete elements. For example, the sentence "He's cool" is a sequence of segments that begins with [h] and ends with [l]. All segments in between follow each other in a specific order to convey a particular message. Such an assumption that all meaning-distinguishing sound segments are serially arranged characterizes all **linear phonologies.** Linear phonologies can be characterized by the following features:

1. Emphasis is on the linear, sequential arrangement of segments.
2. All segments have equal value and all features are equal, thus, no one segment has control over other units.
3. The systematic changes that occur apply only to the segmental level.

However, linear phonologies with sound segments as central analytical units fail to recognize and describe larger linguistic units. Linear phonologies also do not account for the possibility that there could be a hierarchical interaction between segments and other linguistic units. **Nonlinear phonologies,** or what have been called **nonsegmental** or **multilinear phonologies,** attempt to account for these factors.

In contemporary nonlinear phonologies, the linear representation of phonemes plays a subordinate role. Segments are seen as being governed by more complex linguistic dimensions, for example, stress, intonation, metrical, and rhythmical linguistic factors. These theories explore the hierarchical relationships among units of various sizes. Therefore, rather than a linear view of equally valued segments (in a left-to-right horizontal sequence), a hierarchy of factors is hypothesized affecting segmental units. Rather than a static sequence of segments of equal value (linear phonology), a dynamic system of features, ranked one above the other, is proposed (nonlinear phonology). For example, syllable structure may affect the segmental level. A child may demonstrate the following pattern:

win	[wɪn]	winner	[wɪ.ɚ]
dog	[dɑg]	doggie	[dɑ.i]
big	[bɪg]	bigger	[bɪ.ɚ]

The child deletes the consonant in the second syllable in a multisyllabic word; however, this consonant deletion does not occur in one-syllable words. The number of syllables in a word may interact and affect the segmental level. In this example, the number of syllables has priority over the segmental level; it determines the segmental features.

Another example of a factor that may affect the segmental level is stress. Children have a tendency to delete segments in unstressed syllables. For example:

ba'nana → [næne]

po'tato → [teɪto]

'telephone → [tɛfoʊn]

In these examples, the syllable stress affects the segmental level; word stress has priority over the segmental level. "Instead of a single, linear representation (one unit followed by another with none having any superiority or control over other units), they [nonlinear phonologies] allow a description of underlying relationships that would permit one level of unit to be governed by another" (Schwartz, 1992, p. 271).

There are many different types of nonlinear phonologies. Several new theories have been advanced, while others have been modified. All nonlinear phonologies are based on the hierarchical interaction between different linguistic units. Many of these models use a tiered representation in which the tiers interact with one another. The higher level features dominate more than one other feature and serve as a link between the features. These tiers play a role in how the nonlinear models view the development of the phonemic system in children.

FOCUS 7: *What are the basic differences between linear and nonlinear phonologies?*

NONLINEAR PHONOLOGY AND PHONOLOGICAL DEVELOPMENT. Nonlinear phonologies represent clearly a departure from the linear models. To exemplify this, a contrast will be made between the child's development of its phonological system according to natural phonology (Stampe, 1979) and one nonlinear model (Bernhardt & Stemberger, 1998)

First, let's compare the acquisition process analyzed from the viewpoint of natural phonology. The child's use of phonological processes represents surface-form mismatches between the child's and the adult's norm productions. Therefore, if the child says [to͡up] for "soap," we say that there is a mismatch in the form: The child has used the natural process of stopping. As the child's phonological system becomes more developed, this process is suppressed resulting in a norm production of [so͡up]. However, as a portion of this theory, it is assumed that the child's underlying representation was adultlike. Therefore, although the child says [to͡up], the child's underlying system is said to be fully intact, i.e., the child has the same understanding of the /s/ phoneme as an adult does. One problem with this explanation was that it was highly abstract and lacked empirical data to support the claims about the child's underlying adultlike representation. For example, if the child always produces [t] for [s], what indication do we have that the child's underlying representation is one that matches the adult's? Even if the child can discriminate between /t/ and /s/, that only indicates that some sort of differentiation has occurred, not that the child actually utilizes the same discrimination categories that adults use. In addition, phonological processes do not explain why certain substitution processes occur and others do not. Velar fronting is a common phonological process. However, why are velar consonants replaced by alveolars and not bilabials? For this there is no explanation in the natural phonology construct.

This specific nonlinear phonological theory accounts for the developmental process in a different manner. First, the child is viewed as coming to the language-learning process with a "set of universally determined templates with regard to segmental properties" (Yavaş, 1998, p. 277). Therefore, mismatches could indicate that the child has not yet internalized the adultlike underlying representation. In this nonlinear approach, underlying representations can be formulated that are consistent with the child's production while not contradicting properties of the target system. A look at the selected features of one of the nonlinear approaches, feature geometry, will be helpful for the following discussion. Figure 8.4 is a representation of the tiers of this nonlinear model. It should be noted that not all features are presented from the original model but only those that apply to this discussion. Root, laryngeal, and place are classified as nodes; the rest are denoted as features.

The following brief explanation is offered for the nodes and features:

Root Highest level node, therefore earliest in the acquisition process. Marked by the features lateral (in this case /l/), nasal (/m, n, ŋ/), continuant (vowels, glides /w/, /j/, liquids /l/, /r/, and the fricatives), consonantal (stops, affricates, nasals, fricatives, and laterals), sonorant (vowels, glides, liquids /r/ and /l/, /h/, and nasals).

Laryngeal Next highest level node, therefore somewhat after the root node in the acquisition process. The feature + laryngeal consists of those sounds that are produced with vocal fold vibration, i.e., vowels and voiced consonants.

Place The lowest level node, thus latest in the acquisition process. Contains the features labial (/m, p, b, f, v/), coronal (t, d, n, s, z, ʃ, ʒ, θ, ð, tʃ, dʒ, r, l), and dorsal (k, g, ŋ, w, j, and dark l/).

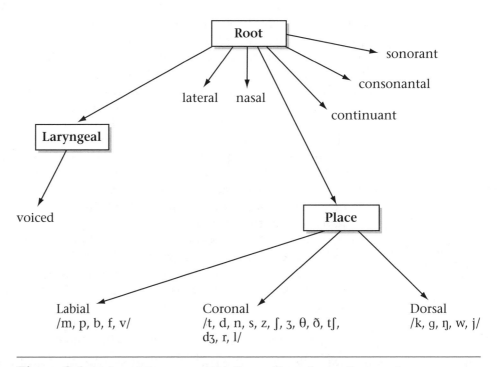

Figure 8.4 Selected Features of Nonlinear Phonology—Feature Geometry
Source: Adapted from Bernhardt & Stemberger (1998). To simplify the material, not all the original features have been listed. Only those relevant to the discussion are included.

According to feature geometry, when features are not contrastive in the child's production, it is stated that the underlying representation is *underspecified.*

If a child replaces [k] with [t], then features distinguishing between /k/ and /t/ are underspecified (in this case *dorsal* and *coronal* are not contrastive, therefore, these features are underspecified). In the absence of phonemic contrasts in the child's system and the subsequent lack of an underlying specification, so-called *default features* are formulated. These default features are used to explain the error patterns. The child who replaces all [k] productions with [t] but can produce [p] and [b], for example, demonstrates that there is no contrast between nonlabial stop-plosives. Therefore, labial stop-plosives (/p/ and /b/) are represented, but the dorsal and coronal features have no underlying representation; they are underspecified. However, /t/ is seen as the default feature. When either /t/ or /k/ is needed, /t/ is supplied as the default. In the course of development, the child's underlying underspecified features give way to more specified representations, which create a match between the child's phonological system and the target system.

Second, this nonlinear model can represent the general order of the acquisition of features. Thus, it is structured so that those higher level nodes and features are developmentally earlier than those that are lower or more deeply embedded on the tier, such as coronal, labial, and dorsal place features. As children develop, their phonological mismatches are typically related to features that are lower on the tiers. Therefore, according to this framework, early distinctions should develop between nasal versus non-nasal and voiced versus voiceless contrasts. Looking at the developmental patterns of children, we see that these are indeed some of the earliest contrasts: /p/, /b/, and /m/, for example.

In addition, common processes, i.e., those that typically occur in the development of children's phonological systems versus idiosyncratic or unusual processes, can be accounted for by using this system's tiered representation. Velar fronting (/t/ replaces /k/) is a common process that involves changes in a lower level tier (coronal replaces dorsal). On the other hand, an idiosyncratic or unusual process, such as liquid stopping (/d/ replaces /r/), affects a higher level tier. This can be explained by noting that both /d/ and /r/ are located within the coronal feature under the place node. Therefore, the coronal feature is not underspecified. They are both voiced consonants, so voiced (under the laryngeal node) is not underspecified. However, if we look at the features of the root node, we find that the consonantal feature (which contains /d/) and the sonorant feature (which contains /r/) are not used contrastively. According to the implications of this nonlinear approach, these two "substitutions" would indicate something quite different in the development of the child's phonological system.

Nonlinear phonology is an innovative way to look at phonological development. Although certain hierarchical features and specific theories are still being debated, it has much to offer within the framework of a developing phonological system. For more information on phonological development and nonlinear phonology, the reader is advised to turn to the *Handbook of Phonological Development from the Perspective of Constraint-Based Nonlinear Phonology* by Bernhardt and Stemberger (1998).

Case Study

The following consonant clusters were noted in Gary, age 7;0:

Word	Production	Word	Production
slide	[slaɪd]	clown	[klaʊn]
string	[stwɪŋ]	grapes	[gweɪpθ]
spoon	[spun]	presents	[pwɛzənts]
skunk	[skʌŋk]	umbrella	[əmbwɛlə]
three	[θwi]	swing	[swɪŋ]
scratch	[skrætʃ]	frog	[fwɑg]
flag	[flæg]	bread	[bwɛd]
blocks	[blɑks]	brush	[bwʌʃ]
truck	[twʌk]	crayons	[kreɪɔns]
drum	[dwʌm]	squirrel	[skwɝ˞əl]

Smit (1993b) reports that the following consonant clusters were still inaccurate in the speech of 5;6- to 7;0-year-olds to a fairly high degree (approximately 25% of the time): [sl], [br], [θr], [skw], [spr], [str], and [skr]. Other consonant cluster difficulties were noted only in a very small percentage of children.

How do the results from Gary compare to those found by Smit (1993b)? Should one worry about the consonant cluster difficulties demonstrated by this child?

Summary

FOCUS 1: *What are the prelinguistic stages? What are the features and the approximate ages for each stage?*

Stage 1: Reflexive crying and vegetative sounds (birth to 2 months)

Reflexive vocalizations include cries, coughs, grunts, and burps that seem to be automatic responses reflecting the physical state of the infant. Vegetative sounds may be divided into grunts and sighs that are associated with activity and clicks and other noises, for example, that are associated with feeding.

Stage 2: Cooing and laughter (2 to 4 months)

During this stage, cooing or gooing sounds are produced during comfortable states. Although these sounds are sometimes referred to as vowel-like, they also contain brief periods of consonantal elements that are produced at the back of the mouth. From 12 weeks onward, a decrease in the frequency of occurrence of crying is noted, and most infants' primitive vegetative sounds start to disappear. At 16 weeks sustained laughter emerges.

Stage 3: Vocal play (4 to 6 months)

Although there is some overlap between Stages 2 and 3, the distinguishing characteristics of Stage 3 include longer series of segments and the production of prolonged vowel- or consonant-like steady states. It is during this stage that the infant often produces extreme variations in loudness and pitch. Transitions between the segments are much slower than is the case with children or adults. In contrast to Stage 2, Stage 3 vowels demonstrate more variation in tongue height and position.

Stage 4: Canonical babbling (6 months and older)

Although canonical babbling usually begins around 6 months of age, most children continue babbling into the time when they say their first words. This stage is divided into two types of babbling behavior: reduplicated and nonreduplicated, or variegated, babbling. Smooth transitions can now be noted between vowel and consonant productions.

Stage 5: Jargon stage (10 months and older)

This babbling stage overlaps with the first meaningful words. The jargon stage is characterized by strings of babbled utterances that are modulated by primarily intonation, rhythm, and pausing. It sounds as if the child is actually attempting sentences but without actual words, since many jargon vocalizations are delivered with eye contact, gestures, and intonation patterns that resemble statements or questions.

FOCUS 2: *Which types of syllable shapes, vowels, and consonants predominate the first-fifty-word stage?*

Certain syllable types clearly predominate the first-fifty-word stage. These are CV, VC, and CVC syllables. When CVCV syllables are present, they are full or partial syllable reduplications.

There is a wide range of variability among individual subjects in the first-fifty-word stage. If one wants to generalize, then the marked use of voiced labial (/m, b/) and coronal-alveolar stops and nasals (/n, d/) has to be underlined; however, postdorsal-velar sounds are also present. With the exception of affricates, all manners of articulation are represented in these initial consonant productions. The first vowel is typically /a/ or /ɑ/, followed by /u/ and/or /i/.

FOCUS 3: *Why do the age results from the cross-sectional sound mastery studies vary?*

These differences are a consequence of the way "mastery" was defined. The methodology used in the Poole (1934) study, for instance, stated that 100 percent of the children must use the sound correctly in each of the positions tested. Prather et al. (1975) and Templin (1957), on the other hand, set this level at 75 percent. In addition, rather than using the 75 percent cut-off level for all three positions (initial, medial, and final) as Templin had done, Prather et al. used only two positions (initial and final) for their calculations. This clearly changes the ages to which mastery can be assigned. A shift to earlier acquisition noted in the Prather study could be accounted for by these methodological changes. Also, the Prather results are based on incomplete data sets, especially at the younger age groupings. Although Prather began with 21 subjects in each age group, several of these children did not respond to many of the words. Thus, at times only 8 to 12 subjects were used to calculate the norms. The children who did not respond to some words may have been avoiding them because they felt that they could not pronounce them "correctly." This, too, would alter the age norms.

FOCUS 4: *Which sounds appear to be later developing sounds? How does the acquisition of consonant clusters fit into this acquisition process?*

The following sounds seem to be the latest to develop:

[s] (4½–6), [z] (4–7½), [r] (5–7), [v] (3½–6), [ʃ] (3½–4½), [ʒ] (6½–7), [θ] (5–6), [ð] (5–7), [tʃ] (3½–4½), [dʒ] (3½–7)

Consonant clusters also prove difficult for the school-age child. According to some research, a small percentage of children are still having difficulties with some aspects of consonant clusters until age 8.

FOCUS 5: *What are distinctive features? How do distinctive features explain the development of the child's phonological system?*

Distinctive features are the smallest indivisible sound properties that establish phonemes. An inventory of distinctive features would demonstrate that some sounds are marked by the presence of this distinctive feature, while other sounds lack this particular feature. A binary (+ and –) system was used to indicate the presence of a particular feature (+) versus the lack of that feature (–).

According to Jakobson (1941/1968), the order of development of the sound properties is based on a principle referred to as maximal contrast. Therefore, the child acquires features that have the greatest physiological contrast and then moves to finer distinctions. Thus, the gross motor contrasts are learned before the more refined, fine motor ones. This principle is not a new one, however; it dates back to at least Schultze's (1880/1971) position. However, Jakobson went a step beyond just using motor contrasts and included both acoustic and semantic contrasts. At each stage, the semantic (usually labeled as *cognitive level*), acoustic, and motoric contrasts are bound together and are maximal in character.

FOCUS 6: *What is natural phonology? What role do phonological processes play in this model?*

Natural phonology is a theory that postulates that the patterns of speech are governed by an innate, universal set of phonological processes. Thus, all children are born with the capacity to use the same system of processes. Phonological processes, as natural processes, are easier for the child to produce and are substituted for sounds, sound classes, or sound sequences when the child's motor capacities do not yet allow their standard realization. These phonological processes are all operating as each child attempts to use and organize its phonological system. Therefore, all children begin with innate speech patterns but must progress to the language-specific system that characterizes their native language. Phonological processes are used to constantly revise existing differences between the innate patterns and the standard, "adult" pronunciation. The theory points out prominent developmental steps children go through until the goal of adult phonology is reached in the child's adolescent years.

Stampe (1979) proposed mechanisms to account for these changes. These mechanisms reflect properties of the innate phonological system as well as the universal difficulties children display in the acquisition of the adult sound system. One of these mechanisms is suppression. *Suppression* refers to the child's ability to eliminate one or more phonological processes as they move from the innate speech patterns to the adult norm production. Therefore, a previously used phonological process is no longer used by the child.

 FOCUS 7: *What are the basic differences between linear and nonlinear phonologies?*

Linear phonologies can be characterized by the following features:

1. Emphasis is on the linear, sequential arrangement of segments.
2. All segments have equal value, and all features are equal, thus, no one segment has control over other units.
3. The systematic changes that occur apply only to the segmental level.

However, linear phonologies with sound segments as central analytical units fail to recognize and describe larger linguistic units. Linear phonologies also do not account for the possibility that there could be a hierarchical interaction between segments and other linguistic units.

In contemporary nonlinear phonologies, the linear representation of phonemes plays a subordinate role. Segments are seen as being governed by more complex linguistic dimensions, such as stress, intonation, and metrical and rhythmical linguistic factors. These theories explore the hierarchical relationships among units of various sizes. Therefore, rather than a linear view of equally valued segments (in a left to right horizontal sequence), a hierarchy of factors is hypothesized affecting segmental units. Rather than a static sequence of segments of equal value (linear phonology), a dynamic system of features, ranked one above the other, is proposed (nonlinear phonology). All nonlinear phonologies are based on the hierarchical interactions of different linguistic units. Many of these models use a tiered representation in which the tiers interact with one another. The higher level features dominate more than one other feature and serve as a link between the features. These tiers play a role in how the nonlinear models view the development of the phonemic system in children.

Further Readings

Ball, M., & Kent, R. (1997). *The new phonologies: Developments in clinical linguistics.* San Diego: Singular.

Bernhardt, B., & Stoel-Gammon, C. (1994). Nonlinear phonology: Introduction and clinical application: Tutorial. *Journal of Speech and Hearing Research, 37,* pp. 123–143.

Ingram, D. (1976). *Phonological disability in children.* New York: Elsevier.

Key Concepts

affrication p. 266
alveolarization p. 265
canonical babbling p. 239
cavity features p. 258
cluster reduction p. 264
contrastive stress p. 251
cooing and laughter stage p. 238
deaffrication p. 266
denasalization p. 266
derhotacization p. 267
devoicing p. 267
districtive features p. 256
epenthesis p. 252
final consonant deletion p. 264
first word p. 241
fronting p. 265
gliding of liquids/fricatives p. 267
jargon stage p. 240
labialization p. 265
linear phonologies p. 270
major class features p. 257
multilinear phonologies p. 270
manner of articulation p. 258
natural processes p. 263
nonlinear phonologies p. 270

nonreduplicated babbling p. 239
nonsegmental phonologies p. 270
phonetic variability p. 242
phonetically consistent forms p. 242
phonological idioms p. 251
prelinguistic behavior p. 237
protowords p. 242
quasi-words p. 242
reduplicated babbling p. 239
reduplication p. 263
reflexive crying and vegetative sounds p. 238
reflexive vocalizations p. 238
regression p. 251
source features p. 259
stopping p. 265
tone-unit p. 251
unstressed syllable deletion p. 264
variegated babbling p. 239
vegetative sounds p. 238
vocables p. 242
vocal play stage p. 238
voicing p. 267
vowelization (vocalization) p. 267
weak syllable deletion p. 264

Think Critically

1. Give three word examples demonstrating velar fronting and three demonstrating palatal fronting. Write the words and the substitutions in phonetic transcription.

2. The following are the results of an articulation test from Ryan, age 6;6.

horse	[hoɚθ]	pig	[pɪg]	chair	[tʃɛɚ]
wagon	[wægən]	cup	[kʌp]	watch	[wɑʃ]
monkey	[mʌŋki]	swinging	[s̬wɪŋɪŋ]	thumb	[fʌm]
comb	[koʊm]	table	[teɪbəl]	mouth	[maʊf]
fork	[foɚk]	cat	[kæt]	shoe	[tsu]
knife	[naɪf]	ladder	[læɾɚ]	fish	[fɪts]
cow	[kaʊ]	ball	[bɑl]	zipper	[ðɪpɚ]
cake	[keɪk]	plane	[pweɪn]	nose	[noʊθ]
baby	[beɪbi]	cold	[koʊd]	sun	[θʌn]

Identify the sound substitutions Ryan uses.

3. Based on the Smit (1993a, b) data from pages 247 and 257, identify which sounds and consonant clusters Ryan should be producing at his age.

4. Identify the phonological processes that Ryan uses.

5. Identify which phonological processes are age appropriate and which should be suppressed at this time.

Test Yourself

1. If a child says [bæftəb] for "bathtub," this is an example of which phonological process?

   a. palatal fronting

   b. stopping

   c. labialization

   d. alveolarization

2. Which one of the following is not a syllable structure process?

   a. reduplication

   b. weak syllable deletion

   c. consonant cluster reduction

   d. consonant cluster substitution

3. *Prelinguistic behavior* refers to

   a. the sounds used in the initial words of the child.

   b. the acoustic analysis of the infant's cries.

   c. all vocalizations prior to the first word.

   d. the study of the gestures used prior to the first word.

4. During which prelinguistic stage does the child begin to communicate to adults through imitation games with vocal productions?

   a. Stage 2: Cooing and laughter

   b. Stage 3: Vocal play

   c. Stage 4: Canonical babbling

   d. Stage 5: Jargon stage

5. During which prelinguistic stage does the child produce strings of utterances that are modulated primarily by intonation, rhythm, and pausing?

   a. Stage 2: Cooing and laughter

   b. Stage 3: Vocal play

   c. Stage 4: Canonical babbling

   d. Stage 5: Jargon stage

6. Which one of the following is not a characteristic of the first-fifty-word stage?

   a. frequent use of consonant clusters

   b. phonetic variability

   c. limited use of syllable structures

   d. limited use of varied segmental productions

7. Often the results of large cross-sectional studies of sound mastery demonstrate differing results. This is due to the
   a. differing methodologies employed.
   b. type of children who were used in the research.
   c. type of articulation test that was used.
   d. age of the investigation: older investigations show later mastery ages.

8. If a child at age 3;0 says [sæm] for "Sam," but at age 3;6 says [θæm] for "Sam," this is known as
   a. avoidance.
   b. epenthesis.
   c. regression.
   d. final-consonant deletion.

9. Which one of the following syllable structure processes is suppressed at a later age?
   a. reduplication
   b. final-consonant deletion
   c. weak syllable deletion
   d. consonant cluster reduction

10. Which one of the following fricatives is not among the later developing sounds?
   a. /f/
   b. /v/
   c. /s/
   d. /z/

1. c   2. d   3. c   4. c   5. d   6. a   7. a   8. c   9. d   10. a

For additional information, go to www.phonologicaldisorders.com

CHAPTER 9

Phonetic and Phonemic Analysis

CLINICAL APPLICATION

Chapter Highlights

- What are some of the advantages and disadvantages of using an articulation test?
- What is stimulability testing, and how should it be used in our diagnosis?
- What are the advantages and disadvantages of using spontaneous speech sampling in our diagnosis?
- What is a phonological inventory? What are phonological contrasts?
- What is an independent analysis?
- How are syllables categorized?

Chapter Application: Case Study

 Herb has two children on his caseload who both have phonological disorders. One is Jane, a 4-year-old child with Down syndrome who has a limited word inventory. The second child, Dee, is fairly unintelligible and has many sound errors. In addition, Dee's vowels seem to be distorted, and Herb notices that she does not use some of the vowels of American English in words. Herb is wondering how to assess and document these children's two very different problems. An articulation test is an option, but it is probably not possible to get results from Jane. He also notices that most of the articulation tests do not test vowels, which he would like to evaluate with Dee. In addition, Dee seems to be able to produce single, isolated words much better than when she is just talking in conversation. What type of measures can he use to assess the consonants and vowels of both of these children? Are there additional measures that he could use before he establishes a treatment plan?

How and when children develop their speech sound system is one important aspect when assessing articulation and phonological disorders in the preschool and school-age population. Speech sound development involves a necessary time span in order for children to acquire adultlike speech sound forms. As seen in the previous chapter, some sounds are considered "early," indicating that children acquire adequate speech sound form for these sounds at a relatively young age. Other sounds are considered "later," indicating that they require a much longer time until all their production features can be realized.

This understanding of a particular time span for speech sound acquisition is built into several measures that we use to assess children with possible phonological disorders. For example, articulation testing provides us with this type of data. Other measures, such as spontaneous speech sampling, are used to supplement our testing, giving us an understanding of the child's articulation in a more natural conversational setting. Both of these measures utilize phonetic transcription to document the child's production possibilities. First, this chapter will introduce the basic procedures that we use for articulation testing and spontaneous speech sampling. The advantages and disadvantages of these types of assessment tools will be discussed. Documenting the child's articulation based on these procedures is an important portion of our phonetic assessment. However, we would also like to know about the child's phonemic system, the way that this child organizes and uses phonemes as meaning-differentiating units. The second portion of this chapter will demonstrate how we can analyze our phonetic data to examine the phonemic system of our clients. Phonemic inventory, phonemic contrasts, syllable structure, and the distribution of phonemes will be introduced as possibilities to examine an individual's phonological system. These two types of procedures, phonetic testing and phonemic analysis, will guide us as we assess the speech capabilities of our clients.

Articulation Testing

Articulation tests are typically designed to elicit spontaneous naming based on the presentation of pictures. Most consonants of General American English are tested at the beginning, the end, and somewhere in the middle of a word. Articulation tests are often referred to as citation-form testing. *Citation-form* refers to the spoken form of a word produced in isolation, as distinguished from the form it would have when produced in conversational speech.

There are several advantages to using a citation-form articulation test. First, these tests are relatively easy to give and score. The child is shown a series of pictures, which he or she is asked to identify. The clinician then notes the responses of the child on a score form. Second, the results provide the clinician with a quantifiable list of sound productions that were not articulated in an adult-norm manner. Thus, correct and incorrect productions can be listed and documented. This is clearly relevant to the assessment process. Third, several of the tests provide standard, norm-referenced scores. These scores allow the clinician to compare the individual client's performance with the performance of other children of a similar age. Thus, the scores are correlated to the previously noted time span for the development of speech sounds in children. It can then be determined if the child has age-appropriate errors or not. In addition, these standard scores can be used to document the client's need for, and progress in, therapy.

There are, however, also several problems inherent in citation-form articulation tests. A citation-form articulation test examines sound articulation in selected isolated words. However, eliciting sounds based on single-word responses can never give adequate information on the client's production realities in connected speech. Sound articulation within selected words may not be representative of the child's ability to use a particular sound in an adultlike manner under natural speech conditions.

In addition, articulation tests do not give enough information about the client's phonological system. Articulation tests are measures of speech sound production; they are phonetic tests. As such, they were never meant to provide enough assessment data for a phonological analysis. Although some single-word measures are now labeled tests of phonology, they differ only in the means in which the single speech sounds are analyzed.

Articulation tests do not test all sounds in all the contexts in which they occur in American English. For example, most do not examine vowel productions and are limited in the consonant clusters that are examined. Finally, the sounds that are tested are not in comparable phonetic contexts; that is, they are not context-controlled. For example, the sounds surrounding the tested consonants are different from word to word. The words used also vary in respect to their length and phonetic complexity. This presents the child with a task that changes in production difficulty from word to word. Table 9.1 is a list of the more commonly used articula-

Table 9.1   Examples of Articulation Tests

Name	Age Range	Word Positions Tested	Scores Provided	Comments
Arizona 3: Arizona Articulation Proficiency Scale (3rd ed.), by J. Fudala 2000, Los Angeles: Western Psychological Services	1;6 to 18;11 years	Initial- and final-word positions	Standardized, gives standard score, Z-score, percentile, speech intelligibility values, and level of articulatory impairment	Gives weighted scores for each consonant. Tests vowels.
Assessment Link Between Phonology and Articulation—Revised, by R. Lowe, 1996. Mifflinville, PA: Speech and Language Resources	3;0 to 8;11 years	Initial- and final-word positions	Standardized, gives standard scores, percentile ranks	Several different analyses are provided in the manual. Gives analysis form that can be used to document phonological processes, vowel errors, and consonant clusters.
Bankson Bernthal Test of Phonology, by N. Bankson & J. Bernthal, 1990, Austin: Pro-Ed	3 to 6 years	Initial- and final-word positions	Standardized, gives standard score, percentile rank, and standard error of measurement	Provides various ways to analyze results. Phonological processes included.

(continues)

Table 9.1   Examples of Articulation Test (*continued*)

Name	Age Range	Word Positions Tested	Scores Provided	Comments
Clinical Assessment of Articulation & Phonology, 2002, by W. Secord & J. Donohue, Greenville, SC: Super Duper Publications	2;6 to 8;11 years	Initial- and final-word positions	Standardized, gives standard score, percentile rank, and age equivalency	Tests sounds in sentences and provides phonological processes. Error difference score can provide information on single word versus sound in sentence inventory.
Fisher-Logemann Test of Articulation Competence, by H. Fisher & J. Logemann, 1971, Boston: Houghton Mifflin	3 years to adult	Analyzes according to prevocalic, intervocalic, and post-vocalic positions	Not standardized, provides a distinctive feature analysis	Consonants analyzed according to place, manner, and voicing. Analyzes vowels.
Goldman-Fristoe 2 Test of Articulation (2nd ed.), by R. Goldman, & M. Fristoe, 2000, Circle Pines, MN: American Guidance Service	2 to 16+ years	Initial-, medial-, and final-word positions	Standardized, gives standard score, percentile rank, and a confidence interval can be calculated	Can be used with the Khan-Lewis (L. Khan & N. Lewis, 1986, Circle Pines, MN: American Guidance Service) to assess phonological processes.
HAPP-3 Hodson Assessment of Phonological Patterns (3rd ed.), by B. Hodson, 2004, Austin: Pro-Ed	Preschool	Initial-, medial-, and final-word positions	Standardized, gives percentile rank and severity rating	Assesses phonological processes, can be used as a direct link to the cycles approach.
Photo Articulation Test: PAT-3 (3rd ed.), by S. Lippke, S. Dickey, J. Selmar, & A. Soder, 1997, Danville, IL: Interstate Printers and Publishers	3 to 12 years	Initial-, medial-, and final-word positions	Standardized, gives standard scores, age equivalents, and percentiles	Uses actual photographs to test sounds. Tests vowels and diphthongs.
Smit-Hand Articulation and Phonology Evaluation, 1997, by A. Smit & L. Hand, Los Angeles: Western Psychological Services	3 to 9 years	Initial- and final-word positions	Standardized, gives percentiles and z-scores, manual provides normative data on phonological processes	Both an independent analysis (phonetic inventory, syllable structures) and a relational analysis (phoneme-by-phoneme analysis compared to adult norm, phonological processes) are provided.

| Structured Photographic Articulation Test II, 2001, by J. Dawson & P. Tattersall, DeKalb, IL: Janelle Publications | 3 to 9 years | Initial- and final-word positions | Standardized, gives standard scores, percentile ranks, and test age equivalents for the consonant inventory | Consonants can be elicited in a story. Stimulability, vowel productions, complex blends, phonological processes and various other measures are provided. |

This list is not exhaustive but is only meant to provide some examples of more recent tests that are commonly used.

tion tests. It includes several variables that are important to a clinician; such as the age range tested, whether the sounds are tested in initial-, medial- and final-word positions, and if the test is standardized.

Articulation tests, like all standardized tests, are selected *probes* into rather limited aspects of an individual's total abilities. Therefore, an articulation test examines only a very small portion of that child's articulatory behavior, i.e., it explores the child's performance with particular test items, on a certain day, in a unique testing situation. To generalize from such limited results and assume that this probe represents a reliable measure of the client's articulatory abilities would be an obvious mistake.

 FOCUS 1: *What are some of the advantages and disadvantages of using an articulation test?*

Organizing Articulation Test Results: Describing the Error

Most articulation tests include a form that can be used to record the client's responses. By completing this form, the clinician obtains information about the accuracy of the sound articulation and the position of this sound within the test word. Each articulation test gives directions on how to record accurate and inaccurate sound realizations. To describe sound errors, at least three different *scoring systems* are available (Shriberg & Kent, 2003). The following scoring systems are available to choose from:

1. *Two-way scoring.* A choice is made between "right," an adult-norm articulation of the sound in question, and "wrong," a production that falls outside these parameters. Two-way scoring can be used effectively to give feedback to the client and to document therapy progress. However, because of its limitations and its inability to render any usable information about the kind of nonstandard articulation, the two-way scoring system is inappropriate for the scoring of articulation test results. This type of scoring is demonstrated in Table 9.2, which shows the results of a therapy session with Rodney on August 21.

2. *Five-way scoring.* This system uses a classification based on the type of error. "Correct" productions constitute one category. The other four categories are (a) *deletion* or *omission*, i.e., a sound is deleted completely; (b) *substitution*, a sound is replaced by another sound; (c) *distortion*, the target

Table 9.2 Response Form for Two-Way Scoring

Date 8/21/07

Client's Name __Rodney__   Therapist __Dana__

Target Sound __[s]__   Target Behavior __[θ]__

RESPONSE	1	2	3	4	5	6	7	8	9	10
soup	+	+	+	+	+	+	+			
seil	+	+	+	+	+					
sɪn	+	+	+	+	+	+				
sɪstɚ	+ +	+ +	+ +	+ −	~ −	+ +				
sɪli	+	+	+	+	+	+				

sound is approximated but not close enough to be considered a correct realization; and (d) *addition*, a sound or sounds are added to the intended sound. The five-way scoring system is commonly suggested in the manuals of articulation tests. However, this system has several inherent problems.

First, most articulation tests do not define, or give examples of, what is considered a correct articulation. There are many dialectal and contextual variations that could result in a somewhat different but entirely acceptable pronunciation. For example, the alveolar flap [ɾ] is a common pronunciation for [d] in "ladder." Should this variation be considered "correct" if the medial d-sound is being tested? Clinicians should be aware of these common variations and how they could impact their scoring. Second, the category of *deletion or omission* may include the presence, rather

Reflect on This: Clinical Application

PHONETIC TRANSCRIPTION USED IN AN ARTICULATION TEST

Daniel, Age 4;3

1. pie   [pa]
2. puppy   [bʌpi]
3. cup   [kʌp˺]
4. boy   [pɔɪ]
5. baby   [beɪpi]
6. tub   [tʌb]
7. music   [muzət]
8. hammer   [hæmə]
9. broom   [bwum]
10. nose   [noʊz]

Words are examples from the Weiss Comprehensive Articulation Test (Weiss, 1980).

than the absence, of a sound. Normally, deletion implies that a sound segment has been eliminated, as in [mu] for "moon," for example. However, Van Riper and Irwin (1958) include glottal stops, unvoiced articulatory placements, and short exhalations under omissions as well. If the production of [wæʔən] for "wagon" is considered, according to these authors, the [g] would be classified as a deletion. Actually, it would be more accurate to label this as a substitution of a glottal stop for a [g]. This ambiguous definition of deletion can detract from the accuracy of the results when analyzing sound realizations. Figure 9.1 shows the five-way scoring system as described by some articulation tests.

Figure 9.1　　Five-Way Scoring of Articulation Tests

Examples based on different ways to score different productions of the word "tree"

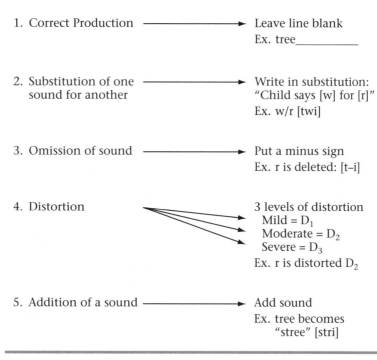

1. Correct Production ⟶ Leave line blank
Ex. tree_____

2. Substitution of one sound for another ⟶ Write in substitution:
"Child says [w] for [r]"
Ex. w/r [twi]

3. Omission of sound ⟶ Put a minus sign
Ex. r is deleted: [t–i]

4. Distortion ⟶ 3 levels of distortion
Mild = D_1
Moderate = D_2
Severe = D_3
Ex. r is distorted D_2

5. Addition of a sound ⟶ Add sound
Ex. tree becomes "stree" [stri]

Examples based on different ways to score different productions of the word "tree"

3. *Phonetic transcription.* This system describes the speech behavior. The goal of any phonetic transcription is to represent spoken language by written symbols as accurately as possible. Of the three systems, phonetic transcription requires the highest degree of clinical skill. The goal is not to judge specific misarticulations but to describe them as accurately as possible. Phonetic transcription has several advantages over the other two systems: (a) It is far more precise, (b) it gives more information about the misarticulation, which is helpful both diagnostically and therapeutically, and (c) among professionals it is the most universally accepted way to communicate information about articulatory features. This system should be used for the analyses of both citation-form articulation tests and spontaneous speech samples. The clinical applications provide examples of how phonetic transcription can be used on an articulation test and in a spontaneous speech sample.

Stimulability Testing

Stimulability testing refers to the client's ability to produce the correct articulation of a misarticulated sound when some kind of "stimulation" is provided by the clinician. Many variations in this procedure exist, but commonly the clinician asks the client to "watch and listen to me, and then you try to say it exactly like I did." An isolated sound is first attempted. If a norm articulation is achieved, then the sound is placed within a syllable and, subsequently, in a word context. If, after two to (maximally) five attempts the client cannot produce a standard production of the error sound, the procedure is discontinued (Diedrich, 1983).

For many clinicians, stimulability testing is a standard procedure concluding the administration of an articulation test. It provides a measure of consistency of a client's performance on two different tasks: the spontaneous naming of a picture and the imitation of a speech model provided by the clinician. This information is very helpful in appraising the articulatory capabilities of a client (see Bleile, 2002; Hodson, Scherz, & Strattman, 2002; Khan, 2002; Lof, 2002; Miccio, 2002; Tyler & Tolbert, 2002).

Children's stimulability to produce a particular sound or sounds has been used to determine therapy goals and to predict which children might benefit more from therapy. In respect to therapy goals, it was suggested that sounds that were more stimulable would be easier to work on in therapy; therefore, highly stimulable sounds would be targeted first (Rvachew & Nowak, 2001). When used as a means to predict which children might benefit from therapy, high stimulability was correlated with more rapid success in therapy (Miccio, Elbert, & Forrest, 1999). It was also proposed that high stimulability might mean that children were on the verge of acquiring the sounds and would not even need therapeutic intervention (Khan, 2002). Although stimulability testing seems to be one type of data collected by most clinicians, its effect on treatment targets is still questionable. In her article on treatment efficacy, Gierut (1998) points out that two studies (Klein, Lederer, & Cortese, 1991; Powell, Elbert, & Dinnsen, 1991) have documented that targeting nonstimulable sounds prompted change in those sounds and other untreated stimulable sounds. In comparison, treatment of a stimulable sound did not necessarily lead to changes in untreated stimu-

Table 9.3 Example of Stimulability Testing

Sound	Syllable Level	Word Level	Sentence Level
[s] ✓	Initial + Medial + Final +	— — —	
[ʃ] —	Initial — Medial — Final —		
[θ] ✓	Initial + Medial + Final +	— — —	
	Initial Medial Final		
	Initial Medial Final		

lable or nonstimulable sounds. Gierut concludes that treatment of nonstimulable sounds may be more efficient than treatment of stimulable sounds due to the widespread change that seems to occur. However, another study (Rvachew, Rafaat, & Martin, 1999) noted lack of treatment progress on nonstimulable sounds when compared to stimulable ones.

As a portion of the data collected in a client's appraisal, stimulability testing gives useful information. However, stimulability testing should not be the only source when deciding whether a client receives services or which therapy sequence to choose. Table 9.3 provides an example of how stimulability testing could be documented.

FOCUS 2: *What is stimulability testing and how should it be used in our diagnosis?*

Spontaneous Speech Sample

Over the years, numerous authors have documented the differences that exist in children's speech when single-word responses, termed *citing*, are compared to spontaneous speech, *talking* (e.g., Andrews & Fey, 1986; Hoffman, Schuckers, & Daniloff, 1989; Klein, 1984). However, assessment and treatment protocols continue to be based primarily on the results of single-word articulation tests. Some may argue that they don't have time to complete the transcription and analysis of a spontaneous speech sample even though these samples can serve a multiplicity of functions. For example, conversational speech samples can also provide additional information about the language, voice, and prosodic capabilities of the client. In addition, a conversational sample could provide specific semantic, morphosyntactical, and pragmatic analyses that supplement language testing when required. The conversational speech sample should not be seen as an option but as a necessity for every evaluation.

Although any conversational speech sample is more representative of a client's production capabilities than a one-word sample, the type of situation also plays a role. Several authors have found an increase or decrease in errors depending on the required production task. First, more complex linguistic contents generally cause an increase in misarticulations (Panagos & Prelock, 1982). Second, different communicative needs can also influence production accuracy. For example, Menyuk (1980) noted the improvement of speech patterns in five children when they were trying to relate information that was important to them.

To obtain the most representative sample, clinicians should carefully select a *variety of talking situations*. This could include a description of pictures, storytelling, describing the function of objects, or problem solving in addition to a normal conversation about school or the last vacation. Varying communicative situations could also include conversations with siblings, parents, or classmates before or after the diagnostic session. None of these talking events needs to be lengthy; however, the variety will certainly aid in documenting the client's production realities.

Beginning Case Study

HERB, TWO CHILDREN WITH PHONOLOGICAL DISORDERS

Herb thinks that it would be a good idea to test Dee with an articulation test and use a spontaneous speech sample to document not only the vowels that she uses but also the discrepancy between her production of sounds on single words and in conversational speech. He will have to structure the conversational sample very carefully, as Dee often becomes unintelligible if she is just talking.

Reflect on This: Clinical Application

The following is an example of a portion of a spontaneous speech sample produced by Charlene, age 3;2.

Hi, this is Charlene.	[haɪ dɪt ɪd jɑ̈əlin]
I played with daddy.	[aɪ pleɪd wɪt dædi]
I watched Huey.	[aɪ wʌt jui]
Yukon and Sady are puppies.	[jukan æn jeɪdi ɑ̈ə pʌpid]
I get them dog food.	[aɪ gɪd dɛm dɑ wud]
You have to put it in the water.	[ju hæ tə ʊt ɪt ɪn də wadə]
Put warm (water) on it.	[pʊt wʊm an ɪt]
And the other one can eat it.	[æn jə nʌdə wʌn kæn it ɪt]

FOCUS 3: *What are the advantages and disadvantages of using spontaneous speech sampling in our diagnosis?*

This section examined how we could document the phonetic production features of vowels and consonants. We have been introduced to articulation testing, stimulability measures, and spontaneous speech sampling as means to document these features. In this next section, the focus will change. Emphasis will now be placed on some basic principles that will be useful when analyzing the phonemic system of children and adults.

Phonology studies the sound systems of languages. The basic unit of phonology is the phoneme, which can be analyzed within the sound system in several different ways. A basic analysis includes, first, the inventory of phonemes—i.e., which phonemes are contained within that language—and second, the distribution of phonemes—i.e., how these phonemes are arranged within that language. In addition, syllable structures and syllable constraints would be a portion of our analysis. These variables are the focus of this next section. Each area of the phonemic analysis will be defined, and clinical examples provided. These basic principles form the foundation of a phonological analysis and will be instrumental in our work with children and adults with speech disorders.

Phonemic Analysis: Phonemic Inventory and Contrasts

The field of phonology examines the phoneme in several different ways. First, the repertoire or inventory of phonemes is documented. Thus, the **phonemic inventory** includes all the vowels and consonants an individual uses as contrastive phonemes. We would find that most adult native speakers of American English demonstrate a complete inventory of vowels and consonants. However, based on the dialect of the speaker, a slightly different set of vowels may be noted. As discussed in a previous chapter, speakers in the Midwest typically use the vowel [ɑ] in words such as "thought" or "tall," whereas speakers of Eastern American English may use the vowel [a]. On the other hand, very young children may demonstrate a smaller number of phonemes. As children mature, this inventory consistently grows until it matches that of the adults. Also, children with phonological disorders very often have a limited phonemic inventory. Although most vowels are typically present, the number of consonants may be restricted.

When examining the phonemic inventory, it might be helpful to have a matrix that could be used to keep track of the vowels and consonants that are utilized. The following is offered as a possibility for recording vowels and consonants: One simply could circle the noted sounds that were used by the individual. The matrix in Figure 9.2 is organized by manner of articulation across the vertical axis and the passive articulator along the horizontal axis. Thus, the following order is given from left to right: stop-plosives, nasals, fricatives, affricates, approximants. The passive articulator is ordered from top to bottom as labial/dental, alveolar, postalveolar/prepalatal, mediopalatal, velar, and glottal.

A similar matrix for vowels could also be established. In Figure 9.3, front-to-back vowels are along the horizontal axis, and high-to-low vowels

Figure 9.2 Matrix for Recording Consonants

p	b	m	θ	ð			w	
			f	v				
t	d	n	s	z			l	
			ʃ	ʒ	tʃ	dʒ		
							j	r
k	g	ŋ						
			h					

Figure 9.3 Matrix for Recording Vowels

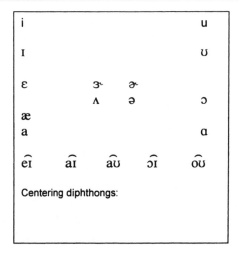

across the vertical axis. Diphthongs are recorded at the bottom. Centering diphthongs can also be written in at the bottom.

As important as the inventory is in our analysis, the use of phonemic contrasts is also an essential variable. **Phonemic contrasts** refer to the ability of an individual to use phonemes contrastively to differentiate meaning. Therefore, if two or more phonemes are represented by the same sound production, then the contrastive phonemic function has not been maintained. For example, if a child produces [w] for [w], [r], and [l] ("rip," "lip," and "whip" all sound like "whip"), then the child is not using the necessary phonemic contrasts of American English. Children with phonological disorders often demonstrate difficulties with specific phonemic contrasts. Phonemic inventory and contrasts are two related variables that form the basis of a phonemic analysis. Out of necessity, a limited inventory will reduce the number of possible phonemic contrasts.

To examine how the sound inventory and contrasts can be used clinically, the following sample from an adult speaker of Midwest American English dialect will be contrasted to a speaker from the East.

Reflect on This: Clinical Application

The following sentences were spoken by a college student from Ohio and represent a Midwest American dialect.

He needs to park the car in the garage.   [hi nidz tə pɑɚ̯k ðə kɑɚ̯ ɪn ðə gərɑʒ]

I want to go shopping downtown.   [aɪ wʌnt tə goʊ ʃapən daʊntaʊn]

She has new sneakers and jeans.   [ʃi hæz nu snikɚz n̩ dʒinz]

Pete and Linda are coming to the party.   [pit n̩ lɪndə ɑɚ̯ kʌmən tu ðə pɑɚ̯ti]

Robin left her pocketbook at the market.   [rabən lɛft hɝ pakətbʊk æt ðə mɑɚ̯kət]

If we use the consonant and vowel matrixes, then we would find the following:

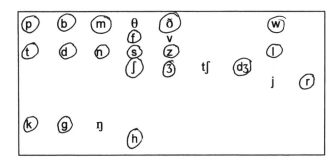

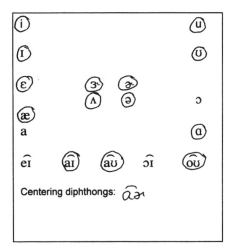

In summarizing the inventory, we will find the following:

Consonants: /p, b, t, d, k, g, m, n, ð, f, s, z, ʃ, ʒ, h, dʒ, w, l, r/

Vowels: /i, ɪ, ɛ, æ, ɝ, ɚ, ʌ, ə, u, ʊ, ei͡, ai͡, oʊ͡, au͡, ɑɚ͡/

Note: The following transcriptions would be considered "normal" in informal Standard English pronunciation: to [tə], shopping [ʃapə̠n], and [n̩], coming [kʌmə̠n].

If you compare the vowels and consonants in the transcription to those normally seen in American English, you will first find that not all vowels and consonants have been used. For example, the consonants /tʃ/ and /j/ are not part of the conversation, and /ŋ/ in its informal variation is pronounced as [n] in words such as *shopping* or *coming*. On the other hand, certain vowels and consonants appear frequently. This is a product of our speech sample and probably an important feature for a clinician when dealing with a spontaneous speech sample: It is very difficult to obtain all of the consonants and vowels represented in American English. That is one of the reasons that material is often used, such as single word articulation tests, in which most, if not all, of the consonants of American English are represented.

Now let's look at the same sentences produced by an adult speaker of Eastern American Dialect.

Reflect on This: Clinical Application

He needs to park the car in the garage.	[hi nidz tə pak ðə ka ɪn ðə gəraʒ]
I want to go shopping downtown.	[aɪ wʌnt tə goʊ ʃapən dantan]
She has new sneakers and jeans.	[ʃi hæz nu snikaz n̩ dʒinz]
Pete and Linda are coming to the party.	[pit n̩ lɪndə a kamən tu ðə pati]
Robin left her pocketbook at the market.	[rabən lɛft ha pakətbʊk æt ðə makət]

If we use the consonant and vowel matrixes, then we would find the following:

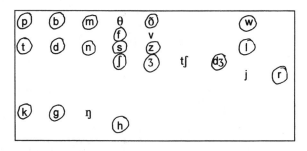

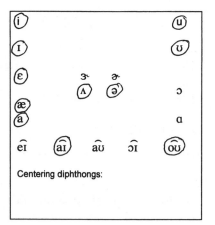

Centering diphthongs:

If we analyze the inventory, we find the following:

Consonants: /p, b, t, d, k, g, m, n, ð, f, s, z, ʃ, ʒ, h, dʒ, w, l, r/

Vowels: /i, ɪ, ɛ, æ, a, ʌ, ə, u, ʊ, a͡ɪ, o͡ʊ/

Note: The following transcriptions would again be considered "normal" in informal Standard English pronunciation: to [tə], shopping [ʃapən], and [n̩], coming [kʌmən].

If we compare the vowels and consonants of the Midwest versus the Eastern dialect, we will find that there is some comparability; the number of consonants is fairly similar. However, the vowels are different for the two speakers. If we compare the vowels, we will find the following:

Word Example	Midwest Dialect	Eastern Dialect
park	[pa͡ɚk]	[pak]
car	[ka͡ɚ]	[ka]
downtown	[da͡ʊnta͡ʊn]	[dantan]
sneakers	[snikɚz]	[snikaz]
are	[a͡ɚ]	[a]
party	[pa͡ɚti]	[pati]
Robin	[rabən]	[rabən]
her	[hɝ]	[ha]
pocketbook	[pakətbʊk]	[pakətbʊk]
market	[ma͡ɚkɜt]	[makət]

Based on the differences in the vowel inventory between the two different speakers, certain comparisons could be made.

For this speaker of Eastern dialect:

1. The central vowel with r-coloring [ɝ] and the centering diphthong [a͡ɚ] are produced as [a].
2. The low back vowel [ɑ] is produced as a low front vowel [a].
3. The diphthong [a͡ʊ] is produced as a monophthong [a].

Based on these comparisons, what can be said about the phonemic contrasts used by these speakers? In other words, are there any phonemes that are not used contrastively? Going through the list above, we see that central vowels with r-coloring, the centering diphthong [a͡ɚ], the low back vowel [ɑ], and the diphthong [a͡ʊ] can all be pronounced as [a] in the speaker representing Eastern dialect. Thus, there are no production contrasts between [a͡ɚ], [ɑ], [a͡ʊ], and [a]. The second step would be to determine if this lack of differentiation in production indeed signals a phonemic contrast in American English. As noted in Chapter 3, [a], [ɑ], and [ɔ] are considered allophonic variations of a single phoneme. If one produces a word such as "bought" as [bat], [bɑt], or [bɔt], it does not change the meaning. Therefore, a phonemic contrast does not exist between [a], [ɑ], and [ɔ]. However, this is not the case with the diphthong [a͡ʊ] and [a]. For example, the words "louse" [la͡ʊs] and "loss" [las] demonstrate that [a͡ʊ] and [a] function as meaning differentiating units. This is also the case with the central vowel [ɝ], the centering diphthong [ɑɚ], and [a]. The words "cart" ([kɑɚt]), "curt" ([kɝt]), and "caught" ([kat]) attest to these sounds being meaning-differentiating phonemes. Thus, although the inventories established by the two speakers for consonants were identical, the vowel inventories and contrasts showed definite differences between the two different dialect speakers.

Phonemic inventories and resulting contrasts can be one way to establish differences between two speakers. As speech-language therapists, we often compare the phonemic inventory and contrasts of a specific child to what we know to be the established adult features. Typically, we will use an articulation test and spontaneous speech to gather this information.

Reflect on This: Clinical Application

The following results are from the Arizona Articulation Proficiency Scale (2nd ed.) (Fudala & Reynolds, 1994) and are based on the productions of a 5;2, female child, Charlene.

horse	[hɔɚt]	pig	[pɪg]	chair	[tʃɛɚ]
wagon	[wægən]	cup	[kʌp]	watch	[watʃ]
monkey	[mʌŋki]	swinging	[wɪŋɪn]	thumb	[tʌm]
comb	[koʊm]	table	[teɪbəl]	mouth	[maʊt]
fork	[tɔɚk]	cat	[kæt]	shoe	[tu]
knife	[naɪt]	ladder	[lædɚ]	fish	[wɪt]
cow	[kaʊ]	ball	[bal]	zipper	[dɪpɚ]
cake	[keɪk]	plane	[pweɪn]	nose	[noʊd]
baby	[beɪbi]	cold	[koʊld]	sun	[tʌn]
bathtub	[tʌb]	jumping	[dʌmpən]	house	[haʊt]
nine	[naɪn]	TV	[tivi]	steps	[tɛp]
train	[tweɪn]	stove	[toʊ]	nest	[nɛt]
gun	[gʌn]	ring	[wɪŋ]	books	[bʊk]
dog	[dag]	tree	[twi]	car	[kaɚ]
yellow	[wɛloʊ]	green	[gwin]	ear	[ɪɚ]
doll	[dal]	that	[dæt]		
bird	[bɝd]	whistle	[wɪtəl]		
carrots	[kɛɚət]				

If we use the consonant and vowel matrixes, then we would find the following:

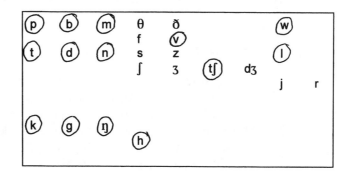

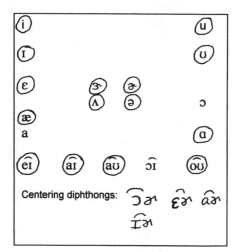

When we analyze the consonant and vowel inventories, the following can be noted:

Consonants: Stop-plosives /p, b, t, d, k, g/

Nasals /m, n, ŋ/

Fricatives /v, h/, no other fricatives (all fricatives tested except for ʒ)

Affricates /tʃ/ (dʒ tested)

Approximants /w, l/

Vowels: Front vowels /i, ɪ, ɛ, æ/

Back vowels /u, ʊ, ɑ/

Central vowels /ʌ, ə, ɝ, ɚ/

Diphthongs /eɪ, aʊ, aɪ, oʊ/ (ɔɪ not tested)

Centering diphthongs /ɔɚ, ɛɚ, ɑɚ, ɪɚ/

In summarizing Charlene's inventory, we find that her vowel system is complete; however, her consonant inventory is limited. Although all stop-plosives and nasals are present, she has virtually no fricatives, the voiced affricate /dʒ/ is not included, and the approximants /r/ and /j/ are also missing.

Based on this rather limited inventory, we would expect that the phonemic contrasts would show differences when compared to the adult norm. If we summarize, we find the following:

1. /s/ is produced as [t] (see "horse," "whistle"), except in consonant combinations, where the [s] is deleted (see "books," "steps," for example).
2. /z/ is produced as [d] (see "zipper" or "nose").
3. /f/ if produced as [t] (see "knife" and "fork").
4. /r/ is produced as [w] (see "ring" and "tree").
5. /θ/ is produced as [t] (see "thumb").
6. /ð/ is produced as [d] (see "that").
7. /v/ is omitted (see "stove").
8. /dʒ/ is produced as [d] (see "jumping").
9. /ʃ/ is produced as [t] (see "shoe"); [ʒ] was not tested.
10. /j/ is produced as [w] (see "yellow").

Based on these comparisons, what can be said about the phonemic contrasts used by this child? In other words, are there any phonemes that are not used contrastively? For the sounds tested, we find that /z/, /ð/, and /dʒ/ are all produced as [d]. Therefore, the contrasts between these phonemes are not apparent based on the child's articulation of the tested words. Also, /s/, /f/, /θ/, and /ʃ/ are all articulated as [t]; /r/ and /j/ are replaced by /w/. In American English, the contrasts between these phonemes are meaning-differentiating ones, as can be noted in words such as "sin," "fin," "thin," "shin," and "tin" (/s/, /f/, /θ/, and /ʃ/ are all articulated as [t]); "seize," "seethe," and "siege" (/z/, /ð/, and /dʒ/ are all produced as [d]); or "rot," "yacht," and "watt" (/r/ and /j/ are replaced by [w]).

Therefore, an examination of the inventory and contrasts produced by this child reveals a limited inventory and the elimination of several meaning-differentiating phonemic contrasts. This information would be important when establishing a diagnosis and possible treatment protocol and should be a portion of a comprehensive phonemic analysis.

For this last example, the child's inventory and contrasts were compared to the adult system; i.e., the expected adult inventory was used as a basis for comparison. This is referred to as a **contrastive** or **relational analysis.** The child's productions are identified from an adult point of view. This viewpoint compares the child's output with the adult form to establish those elements that must be changed for the child's phonology to be more like that of an adult. However, a relational analysis may not be the best or the only way to examine a child's phonological system. The next portion will describe a different analysis procedure known as an independent analysis.

 FOCUS 4: *What is a phonological inventory? What are phonological contrasts?*

Independent Analysis

An **independent analysis** evaluates the child's phonological system independently of the adult target form. Thus, no comparison is made between the two, but rather the child's inventory is established: Vowels and consonants that are evidenced in the speech of the child are documented and analyzed. An independent analysis may be our choice for several different reasons. First, the age of the child may dictate this procedure. An independent analysis would be our choice, such as with very young children who are still in the prelinguistic stage of development or those with emerging phonological systems. At this stage in the child's development, a comparison to the adult norm would not be productive; we would not expect the child to have a complete inventory. Second, the developmental level of the child may dictate this procedure. Even somewhat older children who have very limited phonemic inventories may be good candidates for such an analysis. This would include children who, due to their limited inventory, are considered unintelligible. Again, at this stage a comparison to the adult system would probably not be useful. At this stage of the child's development, more information can be gained by seeing which sounds are present. The child's inventory must be expanded before comparisons to the adult model can be made.

Although a comparison will not be made to the adult form, we could use the consonant and vowel matrixes to categorize the sounds in Andrea's inventory.

Reflect on This: Clinical Application

To examine how an independent analysis could be used clinically, the following transcription is provided of a 16-month-old child, Andrea. Andrea has some words but also uses one- and two-syllable babbles. Intended words are noted; other babbled verbalizations are also supplied.

Word	Production	Other Verbalizations
Mom	[mamə]	[pɑ], [ʌb]
Daddy	[dædæ]	[ɛ.ɛ], [æ]
ball	[ba]	[ʌdə], [ʌbə]
bubbles	[bʌbə]	[aʊbə], [ɛ]
out	[aʊ]	[ʌdəb], [na]
dog	[dɔ]	[nabə], [ʌ.ʌ]
no	[noʊ]	[nʌ], [ɔ]

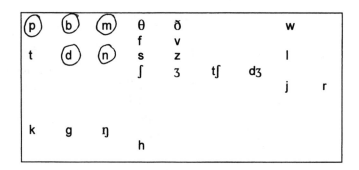

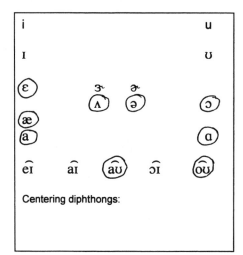

Centering diphthongs:

The following vowels and consonants can be found in Andrea's inventory:

Consonant inventory: /p, b, d, m, n/

Vowel inventory: /ɛ, æ, a, ɑ, ɔ, ə, ʌ, aʊ͡, oʊ͡/

We could summarize the findings as follows: Andrea has mid-front, low-front, mid- and low-back vowels, and central vowels without r-coloring. She has two diphthongs that she uses in words and while babbling. Consonants include bilabial and coronal-alveolar nasals and stop-plosives.

For an independent analysis, the inventory is used as a means to document which sounds are within the child's repertoire. It is not used contrastively with the adult target but rather as a baseline measure to show the present status and where expansion could occur. However, as you look at this example, you might have wanted to know more about the syllable structure, i.e., how many syllables the child does use in one utterance and which types of syllables can be observed. Syllable length and syllable structure are also important variables in our phonemic analysis. The next section will look at the various types of syllables and their structure, relating this information to the analysis of speech in children and adults.

Beginning Case Study

HERB, TWO CHILDREN WITH PHONOLOGICAL DISORDERS

An independent analysis would be a good idea for Jane, the 4-year-old child with Down syndrome. She is just developing her phonemic system, and although she verbalizes a lot, she has a limited number of real words that she uses. An independent analysis would give Herb a good idea about the various vowels and consonants that she is actually producing. In addition, an independent analysis could be carried out in a more naturalistic setting. Herb is sure that Jane would not be able to sit through an articulation test nor probably respond to the pictures in a consistent manner.

FOCUS 5: *What is an independent analysis?*

Syllable Structure

The syllable is important for a number of reasons. It is clearly a fundamental unit of structure. If we are asked to break words down into component parts, then syllables seem to be more natural divisions than sounds. Speakers of languages that do not have a written form, such as many of the Native American languages, will characteristically use syllable and not sound divisions if they are asked to analyze a word into its component parts. They may even resist the notion that any further breakdown is possible (Ladefoged, 2006). Syllabification is also used as a means to analyze words by young children prior to reading and writing. It is only after children are exposed to letters and writing that they begin to understand that words can be divided into sounds. Thus, syllables appear to be basic structural forms.

Counting the number of syllables in a word is a relatively easy task. Even the number of syllables in extremely long words such as "supercalifragilisticexpialidocious," which appears in the Oxford English Dictionary, can easily be counted. The more difficult task becomes where each specific syllable begins and ends. Is it "su-per-<u>cal</u>-i" or "su per-<u>ca</u>-li," for example? If one thinks about rules for syllabification, then one might arrive at the conclusion that the dictionary might be helpful. The dictionary does demonstrate how you divide up words. However, the dictionary is only a good source for providing *written* syllabification rules. For example, we learn from the dictionary that "running" is to be divided "run-ning" or "summer" as "sum-mer." These examples point out the differences between the written and the *spoken* syllable. When speaking, we would not repeat the [n] or [m]; i.e., we do not say [rʌn.nɪŋ] or [sʌm.mɚ]. The divisions [rʌ.nɪŋ] and [sʌ.mɚ] would be more probable during normal speech. As helpful as a dictionary might be for providing the rules that divide the written word, it is not a good source for syllabification of the spoken word. As a matter of fact, a dictionary of rules for boundaries of spoken syllables does not exist. Although several authors have provided guidelines for spoken syllable divisions, it must always be kept in mind that these are just guidelines and not hard and fast rules. See Table 9.4 for some guidelines for spoken syllabification.

Structurally, the syllable can be divided into three parts: peak, onset, and coda (Sloat, Taylor, & Hoard, 1978). The **peak** is the most prominent, acoustically most intense part of the syllable. A peak may stand alone as in the first syllable of the word "a-lone," or it can be surrounded by other sounds as in "stand" or "clean." Although vowels are more prevalent as syllable peaks, in many languages, including American English, consonants can function as syllable peaks as well. This is exemplified by "button" ([bʌtn̩]) or "bottle" ([bɑtl̩]). Consonants that serve as syllable peaks are called *syllabic consonants.*

The **onset** of a syllable consists of all the segments prior to the peak, while the **coda** is made up of all the sound segments of a syllable following the peak. In American English, both onset and coda are not necessary for a syllable. For example, in the word "a-way," the first syllable does not have an onset or a coda, and the second syllable does not contain a coda. The number of segments that can be contained in an onset or a coda is regulated by the rules of that particular language. In American English, onsets can consist of one to three segments (<u>s</u>ing, <u>st</u>ing, <u>str</u>ing), and codas can have from one to four consonants (si<u>t</u>, si<u>ts</u>, sea<u>rched</u>, si<u>xths</u>). Segments that occur as onsets of a syllable are termed **syllable initiating** segments, while those that are coda of a syllable are labeled **syllable terminating** sounds.

Table 9.4 Guidelines for Spoken Syllabification of Multisyllabic Words

1. Compound words are divided according to their lexical structure.

   Examples: dog-house, bath-tub, green-house

2. Single consonant *sounds* within a word are typically considered part of the following syllable. The exception to this is the "ng" sound [ŋ], which is considered the end sound of the first syllable.

   Examples: fa-ther, ta-ble, su-mmer, ru-nning, to-ma-to *but* ring-ing *or* sing-ing

3. A sequence of two consonant sounds within a word is divided C-C except when the two consonants are acceptable combinations that could occur at the beginning of a syllable.

   Examples: fin-ger, win-dow, in-ven-tor, *but* te-le-graph. The /gr/ combination is an acceptable one in American English.

4. A sequence of three consonant sounds within a word is divided C-CC unless this results in an unacceptable combination of sounds.

   Examples: un-spoiled, pen-guin *but* Ox-ford (The division C-CC would yield k-sf, which is not an acceptable combination in American English; thus, the word is divided ks-f.)

Sources: French (1988); Grunwell (1986); Yavaş (1998).

Another way of categorizing a syllable is to refer to the onset and the rhyme. The **rhyme** consists of the nucleus plus the coda of a syllable, if a coda is present. Thus, for the words "hat," "cat," and "bat," the rhyme is "at" ([æt]). However, for the words "bee," "see," and "me," the rhyme is [i].

Syllables are also categorized according to the presence or absence of a coda. Syllables that do not contain a coda are called **unchecked** or **open syllables**. Syllables that do have codas are called **checked** or **closed syllables**. In the word "baby," both syllables are open (unchecked) syllables, while in "doghouse" both syllables are closed (checked).

FOCUS 6: *How are syllables categorized?*

Distribution of Phonemes

Phonemes can also be analyzed according to their arrangement within a particular language. This arrangement is rule-governed based on the language. Thus, the **distribution** of phonemes refers to the rule-governed patterns of sounds and syllables within a particular language. This can also be referred to as the **distribution requirement** of a particular language or the **phonotactic constraints**. Both terms refer to the restrictions on word and

Reflect on This: Clinical Application

OPEN VERSUS CLOSED SYLLABLES IN THE DEVELOPMENT OF CHILDREN

Many children seem to begin the process of language development with just open syllables that are consonant-vowel (CV) or just vowel (V) in structure (Velleman, 1998). However, 2-year-olds do produce closed syllables in CVC structures at least part of the time (Stoel-Gammon, 1987). Several authors have noted that in the language development of children closed syllables in one-syllable words seem to co-occur with the production of two-syllable words (Demuth & Fee, 1995; Fee, 1996). Children with phonological disorders often have problems with closed syllables. The presence of open syllables may persist much longer than would normally be expected for their age.

The following examples are from Leroy, who was 4 years, 9 months, of age at the time of testing. Leroy was in therapy for his speech difficulties.

nose [no͡ʊ]	frog [frɑ]
coat [ko͡ʊ]	car [kɑ]
door [do͡ʊ]	bird [bɝ]
girl [gɝ]	rabbit [ræbɪ]

Note that Leroy can produce r-sounds, which are considered to be rather late sounds developmentally. At the same time, he persists in the production of open syllables.

syllable shapes relative to which types of phonemes can occur in which word positions. For example, in American English certain phonemes can only occur at the beginning of a word or syllable, while others are found only at the end of a word or syllable. Two phonemes that are only syllable initiating are /h/ and /w/, while /ŋ/ can only terminate a syllable in American English. Words such as "hen" and "a-hoy" or "when" and "a-way" attest to the phonotactic constraints of /h/ and /w/. Although words can be written with the *letters* "w" or "h" at the end of a word, such as "low" or "sigh," these are letter and not sound occurrences. The word *low* is said typically as [loʊ] and *sigh* as [saɪ]. Also "sing" or "sing-ing" demonstrate the distribution requirement of /ŋ/ that it occur at the end of the syllable.

The distribution requirements also dictate how many phonemes can be combined together at the beginning and end of syllables and the particular ones that can be combined. As noted in the previous section, we find that in American English only three consonants are allowed at the beginning of a syllable and up to four at the end. Also, certain consonant combinations are permitted at the beginnings and ends of syllables. The combination /ps/ is not one that can begin a syllable, but it does end syllables, such as in "stops" or "claps." In addition, phonotactic constraints apply to the combinations that can actually occur in American English. The /s/ phoneme can occur in many combinations: /sp/ in "spoon," /sl/ in "sled," /st/ in "sting," /sw/ in "swing," and /sk/ in "skunk." However, the combination /sr/ is not possible in American English. There is a phonotactic constraint on combining /s/ + /r/.

The distribution of consonants and phonotactic constraints become important if we are conducting a phonemic analysis. For a linguist studying a new language, for example, this would play a role in understanding the phonemic system and its function. It is also a critical factor when analyzing the disordered phonological system of children and adults. Not unlike the linguist, who is trying to comprehend how the phonemic system functions within a new unknown language, we are trying to figure out the function of the phonemic system that is displayed by the individual with a speech-disorder. Although the system displayed by a phonologically disordered child or adult may at first seem somewhat chaotic and unsystematic, for that individual it is a functional entity. It becomes our task to figure out that particular system. By understanding the distribution and phonotactic constraints employed by our clients, we can be more goal directed in our intervention process.

Distribution and phonotactic constraints can be applied to an independent or a relational analysis. The distribution of phonemes is analyzed by noting the segments relative to their occurrence as syllable-initiating or syllable-terminating sounds. Thus, if a child says [boʊ] for "boat" but [toʊ] for "toe," we could say that the child uses /b/ and /t/ to initiate syllables, but in this limited sample, /t/ is not used terminating a syllable. Phonotactic constraints would apply to the restrictions that are noted in the use of sound segments. For the previous example, the phonotactic constraints would note the fact that /t/ is not used as a terminating phoneme (which is typically the case in American English) and that the child does not seem to use final consonants; the child only produces open syllables.

The matrixes that were used previously could be adapted to note the distribution of sounds. Thus, two charts would be included: one for syllable-initiating and one for syllable-terminating consonants (see Figure 9.4).

Reflect on This: Clinical Application

INDEPENDENT ANALYSIS

The following is an example of how distribution and phonotactic constraints can be used within an independent analysis. Bonnie is a 2-year-old Down syndrome child who is being followed in the early intervention program. These words and babbles were gathered by the speech-language therapist and by Bonnie's mother.

yes	[jɛ]	pig	[pɪ]
mom	[mʌm]	dad	[dæd]
hi	[hɑ]	bye	[bɑ]
grandpa	[dapa]	duck	[dʌk]
truck	[tʌk]	bike	[baɪ͡]
hug	[hʌk]	dollie	[dɑdi]
look	[lʌk]	bug	[bʌk]

Additional babbles:

[ho͡ʊ]	[dɪdɪ]	[bubo͡ʊ]	[pu]
[bap]	[pubi]	[o͡ʊ]	[jaja]
[lala]	[tadi]	[tʌtʌ]	[tu]
[hæhæ]	[mo͡ʊmo͡ʊ]	[næni]	[nab]

If we summarize the previous information from this chapter and add distribution and phonotactic constraints to the analysis, the following areas relative to a phonemic analysis can be documented for Bonnie:

- Vowel inventory
- Consonant inventory
- Syllable shapes
- Distribution
- Phonotactic constraints

Figure 9.4 Matrixes for Syllable Initiating and Terminating Consonants

---

Syllable-Initiating Consonants	**Syllable-Terminating Consonants**

p b m θ ð   w
        f v
t d n s z   l
        ʃ ʒ tʃ dʒ
                  j r
k g
 	
     h
	p b m θ ð
	        f v
	t d n s z l
	        ʃ ʒ tʃ dʒ
	k g ŋ

As noted below, the matrices can be used to examine both the inventory and the distribution of phonemes.

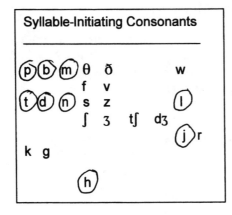

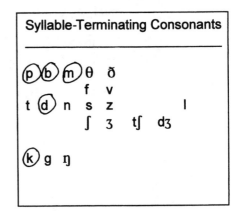

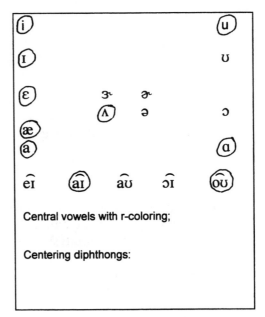

Central vowels with r-coloring;

Centering diphthongs:

The following summarizes the matrixes and adds syllable shapes and phonotactic constraints:

Consonant inventory: /p, b, t, d, k, m, n, h, l, j/

Vowel inventory: /i, ɪ, ɛ, æ, a, u, ɑ, ʌ, aɪ̑, oʊ̑/

Syllable shapes: CV, V, CVCV, CVC

Distribution: Syllable-initiating segments: /p, b, t, d, m, n, h, l, j/
Syllable-terminating segments: /p, b, d, k, m/

Phonotactic constraints: The segment /l/ is noted as only syllable initiating, while /k/ is noted as only syllable terminating. (If we wanted to further examine /k/, we could state that it only occurs after the vowel /ʌ/.) We would not expect /j/ and /h/ to appear in the syllable-terminating position, as the phonotactic constraints of American English dictate the exclusion of these sounds as syllable codas.

The inventory, syllable shapes, distribution, and phonotactic constraints give us information about the child's current status and possibilities for expanding the child's phonological system. We could try to elicit the sounds that appear to be syllable initiating but not terminating, such as /n, t, l/, as syllable codas. On the other hand, /k/ appears only as a coda and could possibly be expanded to syllable-initiating positions. Syllable shapes show a dominance of CVCV structures. Expansion of CVC and possibly VC syllables may be helpful in the acquisition of final-consonant productions. Thus, this information becomes a valuable source for planning our intervention strategies.

Case Study

RELATIONAL ANALYSIS

The following small sample of words is from Jenna, a 5½-year-old child with a phonological disorder:

broom	[bwum]	flag	[fwæ]
hammer	[hæmə]	drum	[twʌm]
sandwich	[tæmɪʃ]	rabbit	[wæbɪ]
finger	[fɪŋə]	feather	[fɛdə]
vacuum	[bæku]	skunk	[tʌŋk]
stove	[toʊb]	zipper	[dɪpə]
thumb	[tʌm]	car	[kɑə]
balloon	[bɑlu]	swing	[fwɪŋ]
string	[twɪŋ]	music	[mudɪ]
zoo	[du]	orange	[ɔwɪn]
lamp	[læm]	spoon	[pun]
ring	[wɪŋ]	clown	[taʊn]
green	[dwin]	plane	[pweɪn]
yellow	[jɛwoʊ]	bird	[bɝd]
nine	[naɪn]	table	[teɪbo]
sheep	[dip]	brush	[bwʌʃ]

As can be seen from Jenna's sample, there are also consonant clusters that are produced. For the purpose at hand, each cluster will divided into its two component parts and listed, for example, for *broom* [bwum], both [b] and [w] will be listed as syllable-initiating consonants. However, all consonant clusters will also be noted at the bottom of the matrix.

If the matrixes are used to document the inventory and distribution of consonants and vowels, the following is noted:

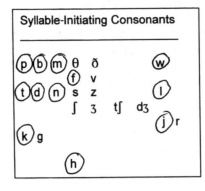

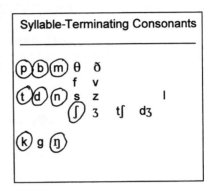

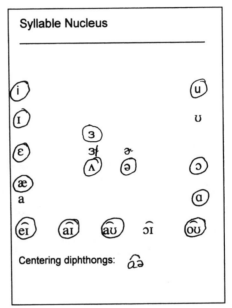

Consonant clusters: *broom* /br/ becomes → [bw], *stove* /st/ → [t], *string* /str/ → [tw], *green* /gr/ → [dr], *flag* /fl/ → [fw], *drum* /dr/ → [tw], *skunk* /sk/ → [t], *swing* /sw/ → [fw], *spoon* /sp/ → [p], *clown* /kl/ → [t], *plane* /pl/ → [pw], *brush* /br/ → [bw].

The following summarizes the matrixes and adds syllable shapes and phonotactic constraints:

Vowel inventory: Front vowels: /i, ɪ, ɛ, æ/

Back vowels: /u, ɔ, ɑ/

Central vowels: /ə, ʌ, ɜ/

Diphthongs: /a͡ʊ, e͡ɪ, o͡ʊ, a͡ɪ/

Centering diphthong: a͡ə

The vowel /ʊ/ was not tested.

Consonant inventory:	Stop-plosives: /p, b, t, d, k/
	Nasals: /m, n, ŋ/
	Fricatives: /h, f, ʃ/. The fricative /ʒ/ was not tested.
	Affricates: none
	Approximants: /w, l, j/
Distribution:	Syllable-initiating /p, b, t, d, k, m, n, f, h, w, l, j/
	Syllable-terminating /p, b, t, d, k, m, n, ŋ, ʃ/
Syllable shapes:	CV, CVC, CCV, CCVC, CVCV, VCVC, CVCC, CVCVC. Jenna has a tendency to change CVCVC syllables to CVCV (see *balloon*, *rabbit*, and *music*) and also reduces a CCVC to a CCV (see *flag*). In addition, when two consonants come together as syllable onsets or codas, she occasionally reduces the CC to a C syllable (see *lamp*, *clown*, *spoon*, *orange*).

Phonotactic constraints:

1. Syllable-initiating /ʃ/ is produced as [d]; however, the child does appear to have an accurate /ʃ/ in the syllable-terminating position (see *brush*).
2. The /l/ demonstrates variability in its accuracy relative to onset and coda positions. It is occasionally accurate as syllable onset (see *lamp* or *balloon*); however, /l/ is not used accurately as a syllable coda.

If we wanted to further summarize, the following can be noted:

1. Syllable-initiating /r/ and r-clusters are produced as [w]. Also, vowels with r-coloring demonstrate a loss of the characteristic r-quality.
2. Both /θ/ and /s/ are articulated as [t], while /ð/ and /z/ show [d] substitutions. In addition, /v/ is replaced by [b]. Thus, this child does have a tendency to replace certain fricatives with stop-plosives.
3. In the syllable-onset position, /l/ is occasionally replaced by [w].

It should be noted that the list of words that was used has its limitations. Certain sounds such as [dʒ], were not tested in both onset and coda positions; other sounds were not tested at all such as [ʒ]. However, by documenting the inventory, distribution, syllable shapes, and phonotactic constraints on these rather limited results, we have a fairly good picture of which sounds Jenna can produce, which ones she does not seem to have in her inventory at all, and which sounds appear to demonstrate production variability. In addition, the constraints on certain syllable structures can be noted.

Summary

FOCUS 1: *What are some of the advantages and disadvantages of using an articulation test?*

Advantages: First, these tests are relatively easy to give and score. The child is shown a series of pictures that he or she is asked to identify. The clinician then notes the responses of the child on a score form.

Second, the results provide the clinician with a quantifiable list of sound productions that were not articulated in an adult-norm manner. Correct and incorrect productions can be listed and documented.

Third, several of the tests provide standard, norm-referenced scores. These scores allow the clinician to compare the individual client's performance with the performance of other children of a similar age. Thus, the scores are correlated to the time span for the development of speech sounds in children. It can then be determined if the child has age-appropriate errors or not. In addition, these standard scores can be used to document the client's need for, and progress in, therapy.

Disadvantages: First, a citation-form articulation test examines sound articulation in selected isolated words. However, eliciting sounds based on single-word responses can never give adequate information on the client's production realities in connected speech. Sound articulation within selected words may not be representative of the child's ability to use a particular sound in an adultlike manner under natural speech conditions.

Second, articulation tests do not give enough information about the client's phonological system. Articulation tests are measures of speech sound production; they are phonetic tests. As such, they were never meant to provide enough assessment data for a phonological analysis. Although some single-word measures are now labeled tests of phonology, they differ only in the means in which the single speech sounds are analyzed.

Third, articulation tests do not test all sounds in all the contexts in which they occur in American English. For example, most do not examine vowel productions and are limited in the consonant clusters that are examined.

Fourth, the sounds that are tested are not in comparable phonetic contexts; i.e., they are not context controlled. For example, the sounds surrounding the tested consonants are different from word to word. The words used also vary in respect to their length and phonetic complexity.

Fifth, an articulation test examines only a very small portion of that child's articulatory behavior; i.e., it explores the child's performance with particular test items, on a certain day, in a unique testing situation. To generalize from such limited results and assume that this probe represents a reliable measure of the client's articulatory abilities would be a mistake.

FOCUS 2: *What is stimulability testing and how should it be used in our diagnosis?*

Stimulability testing refers to the client's ability to produce the correct articulation of a misarticulated sound when some kind of "stimulation" is provided by the clinician. Many variations in this procedure exist, but commonly the clinician asks the client to "watch and listen to me, and then you try to say it exactly like I did." An isolated sound is first attempted. If a norm articulation is achieved, then the sound is placed within a syllable and, subsequently, a word context. If, after two to (maximally) five attempts, the client cannot produce a standard production of the error sound, the procedure is discontinued.

Research surrounding stimulability measures and their relationship to treatment outcomes has been controversial. Some studies have documented that targeting nonstimulable sounds prompted change in those sounds and other untreated stimulable sounds. In comparison, treatment of a stimulable sound did not necessarily lead to changes in untreated stimulable or nonstimulable sounds. However, another study noted lack of treatment progress on nonstimulable sounds when compared to stimulable ones.

As a portion of the data collected in a client's appraisal, stimulability testing gives useful information. However, stimulability testing should not be the only source when deciding whether a client receives services or which therapy sequence to choose.

FOCUS 3: *What are the advantages and disadvantages of using spontaneous speech sampling in our diagnosis?*

Advantages: First, over the years numerous authors have documented the differences that exist in children's speech when single-word responses, termed *citing*, are compared to spontaneous speech, *talking*. Therefore, spontaneous speech samples give information about how a child uses speech sounds in a more naturalistic setting.

Second, conversational speech samples can also provide additional information about the language, voice, and prosodic capabilities of the client. In addition, a conversational sample could provide specific semantic, morphosyntactical, and pragmatic analyses that supplement language testing when required.

Disadvantages: First, although any conversational speech sample is more representative of a client's production capabilities than a one-word sample, the type of situation also plays a role. Several authors have found an increase or decrease in errors depending on the required production task. First, more complex linguistic contents generally cause an increase in misarticulation. Second, different communicative needs can also influence production accuracy. For example, a research study found improvement of speech patterns in five children when they were trying to relate information that was important to them.

Third, children will probably use only a small repertoire of sounds within the speech sample. This will depend on the topic, the length of the sample, and whether the child avoids certain sounds due to the child's own knowledge that she or he has difficulties with certain words.

FOCUS 4: *What is a phonemic inventory? What are phonological contrasts?*

The phonemic inventory includes all the vowels and consonants an individual uses as contrastive phonemes. Very young children may demonstrate a relatively small inventory of phonemes. As children mature, this inventory consistently grows until it matches that of the adults. Also, children with phonological disorders very often have a limited phonemic inventory. Although most vowels are typically present, the number of consonants may be restricted.

Phonemic contrasts refer to the ability of an individual to use phonemes contrastively to differentiate meaning. Therefore, if two or more phonemes are represented by the same sound production, then the contrastive phonemic function has not been maintained.

FOCUS 5: *What is an independent analysis?*

An independent analysis evaluates the child's phonological system independently of the adult target form. Thus, no comparison is made between the two, but rather the child's inventory is established; vowels and consonants that are evidenced in the speech of the child are documented and analyzed.

An independent analysis would be our choice, for example, with very young children who are still in the early stages of development or those with emerging phonological systems. At this stage in the child's development, a comparison to the adult norm would not be productive; we would not expect the child to have a complete inventory.

FOCUS 6: *How are syllables categorized?*

Structurally the syllable can be divided into three parts: peak, onset, and coda. The peak is the most prominent, acoustically most intense part of the syllable. A peak may stand alone as in the first syllable of the word "a-go," or it can be surrounded by other sounds, as in "broom" or "tenth." Although vowels are more prevalent as syllable peaks, consonants can function as syllable peaks as well. Consonants that serve as syllable peaks are called *syllabic consonants*. The onset of a syllable consists of all the segments prior to the peak, while the coda is made up of all the sound segments of a syllable following the peak. In American English, both onset and coda are not necessary for a syllable. For example, in the word "a-lone," the first syllable does not have an onset or a coda. Segments that occur as onsets of a syllable are termed *syllable-initiating segments*, while those that are coda of a syllable are labeled *syllable-terminating sounds*.

Another way of categorizing a syllable is to refer to the onset and the rhyme. The rhyme consists of the nucleus and the coda if a coda is present. Thus, for the words "hat," "cat," and "bat" the rhyme is "at" (/æt/). However, for the words "bee," "see," and "me," the rhyme is /i/.

Syllables are also categorized according to the presence or absence of a coda. Syllables that do not contain a coda are called open or unchecked syllables. Syllables that do have codas are called closed or checked syllables. In the word "baby," both syllables are open (unchecked) syllables, while in "doghouse" both syllables are closed (checked).

Further Readings

Bauman-Waengler, J. (2008). *Articulatory and phonological impairments: A clinical focus. (3rd ed.).* Boston: Pearson: Allyn and Bacon.

Velleman, S. (1998). *Making phonology functional: What do I do first?* Woburn, MA: Butterworth-Heinemann.

Williams, L. (2003). *Speech disorders: Resource guide for preschool children.* Clifton Park, NY: Thomson Delmar Learning.

Key Concepts

checked syllables p. 303
closed syllables p. 303
coda p. 302
contrastive analysis p. 298
distribution p. 303
distribution requirement p. 303
independent analysis p. 299
onset p. 302
open syllables p. 303
peak p. 302

phonemic contrasts p. 292
phonemic inventory p. 291
phonotactic constraints p. 303
relational analysis p. 298
rhyme p. 303
stimulability testing p. 288
syllable initiating p. 302
syllable terminating p. 302
unchecked syllables p. 303

Think Critically

1. Find three words for each of the following syllable structures: (a) no coda, (b) no onset, (c) one onset and one coda element, and (d) two onsets and two coda elements.

2. The following is a transcription of a speech sample of Dawn, a 24-month-old child.

Word	*Production*
Mom	[mɑmə]
Daddy	[dædæ]
ball	[ba]
bubbles	[bʌbə]
out	[aʊ̂]
dog	[dɔ]
no	[noʊ̂]
bathtub	[ʌdəb]
teddy	[tɛti]
bottle	[bɑtoʊ̂]
milk	[mɪk]

Determine the consonant and vowel inventories. What type of syllable shapes does Dawn use?

3. Make a list of one-syllable words that you could use to test all the consonants of American English in the onset syllable position. Transcribe the words.

4. Make a list of one-syllable words that you could use to test the consonants of American English in the coda syllable position. Transcribe the words.

Test Yourself

1. There are many reasons why a spontaneous speech sample should be completed as part of a comprehensive evaluation. Which one of the following is not one of those reasons?

   a. a spontaneous speech sample demonstrates the differences that exist between citing and talking

   b. a spontaneous speech sample provides a typical measure of speech performance

   c. a spontaneous speech sample aids in determining the stimulability of the error sounds

   d. a spontaneous speech sample might be useful in determining language, voice, and/or prosodic capabilities of the client

2. This type of scoring demonstrates the highest level of accuracy and should be used when scoring an articulation test:

   a. two-way scoring

   b. five-way scoring

   c. phonetic transcription

3. Why is stimulability testing important?

   a. because it can absolutely predict which error sounds will improve in therapy

   b. because it can tell you at which level to start in therapy (isolated-sound, syllable, or word level, for example)

   c. because it can predict which children do not need therapy

   d. because it provides the clinician with a measure of the child's consistency on two different tasks

4. What is an independent analysis?

   a. the child's productions are considered but not compared to the adult-norm model

   b. the clinician does an independent assessment without the aid or intervention of the caregivers

   c. the child's speech sound productions are considered, but independent from other language areas

   d. the clinician utilizes informal assessment procedures, independent from standardized assessment tools

5. What type of information is collected for an independent analysis?

   a. the inventory of syllable shapes

   b. the inventory of speech sounds

c. the use of any constraints on sounds relative to their syllable structure

d. all of the above

6. Constraints on sound sequences refers to

a. a reduced inventory of consonants.

b. a reduced inventory of vowels.

c. any sounds or patterns that are used exclusively in certain words or syllable structure positions.

d. the exclusive use of a certain type of syllable structure.

7. Which one of the following terms refers to analyzing where the norm and aberrant productions occur within a word?

a. inventory of speech sounds

b. distribution of speech sounds

c. sound constraints

d. syllable constraints

8. The regular pronunciation of the word "window" has which type of syllable shape?

a. CVCV

b. CVCVC

c. CVCCV

d. CVCCVC

9. Which one of the following terms refers to analyzing which type of syllables occur within a word?

a. inventory of speech sounds

b. distribution of speech sounds

c. sound constraints

d. syllable inventory

10. This type of scoring is the one that classifies sounds according to omissions, distortions, substitutions, and additions.

a. two-way scoring

b. five-way scoring

c. phonetic transcription

Answers 1. c   2. c.   3. d   4. a   5. d   6. c   7. b   8. c   9. d   10. b

For additional information, go to www.phonologicaldisorders.com

Transcription Workbook

Preface to the Workbook

This workbook is organized to systematically introduce students to the vowel and consonant symbols of the International Phonetic Alphabet. Each module builds upon the next module, and exercises progress from relatively easy identification exercises to more complex transcription work. The transcription exercises use both audio and video clips of adults as well as children. The workbook starts with a module on sound–letter correspondence followed by a module identifying stress in two-syllable words. The identification and later transcription of stressed syllables progresses through each of the following modules. The final module of the workbook introduces short, spontaneous speech samples of children, followed by audio and video clips of the results of an articulation test given to a child with a speech disorders.

This workbook and the accompanying textbook are foreseen as beginning-level tools for freshmen and sophomore classes in phonetic transcription. To that end, the module on diacritics contains several identification exercises where the student is asked to fill in the appropriate diacritic marker. However, the actual listening section, where the student will be transcribing, targets only the more commonly used diacritics.

The author realizes that each instructor, student, or learner of phonetic transcription has his or her own particular way of transcribing certain sounds. For example, the diphthongs in words such as "cake" or "throw" can be transcribed in various ways. One can also see different types of transcription for the centering diphthongs in words such as "horse" or "farm." The author has chosen one particular way of transcribing these sounds that seemed commonly acceptable and useful. However, students should check with their instructor to see how she or he would like them to transcribe these and other sounds.

Additional information, additions, and corrections can be found at www.phonologicaldisorders.com.

Module 1—Letters Versus Sounds

Sometimes there is a correspondence between the number of letters in a word and the number of sounds. For example, the word "top" contains three letters and three sounds. Often, though, there is not a correspondence between the letters in a word and the sounds. For example, "caught" has six letters but only 3 sounds.

Helpful Hints

1. Vowels in one-syllable words are counted as 1 sound. Thus, the vowels in "c<u>a</u>ke," "t<u>oy</u>," "b<u>i</u>te," and "c<u>oa</u>t" are counted as one vowel. However, vowel sounds that have a syllable break between them, such as "L<u>ou</u>–<u>ie</u>" or "ph<u>oo</u>–<u>ey</u>" are always counted as two vowels.
2. An r-sound at the beginning of a word is counted as one sound. For example, "r" at the beginning of the word as in "rat" or "rope" is 1

sound. Central vowels with r-coloring, such as "b<u>ir</u>d" or "s<u>ir</u>," are considered to be 1 sound. Although in the words "b<u>ore</u>d" or "b<u>eer</u>" two phonetic symbols are used, 1 sound is usually counted (see Chapter 4). Central vowels with r-coloring and centering diphthongs will be counted as one sound even though two phonetic transcription markers are used. Listen to the number of syllables: If there are two syllables with two adjacent vowels, then this would count as 2 sounds.

3. There are sounds that are spelled with two letters even though they are actually only 1 sound. Examples include the "sh" in "shoe," "ch" in "check," and "ng" in "wing." In each of these words, two letters represent 1 sound.

4. There are also sounds that are spelled with one letter but are actually 2 sounds. The "x" in "box" is an example.

5. Some words are spelled with double letters, such as "running" and "sitting." However, if you say the word slowly, then you realize that the "n" and "t" are produced only one time.

Exercises

1.1

Say the following words:

		1	2
radio	After the "d" sound, are there 1 or 2 sounds?	☐ 1	☒ 2
purr	Do the letters "urr" represent 1 or 2 sounds?	☒ 1	☐ 2
more	Do the letters "ore" represent 1 or 2 sounds?	☒ 1	☐ 2
wax	Does the letter "x" represent 1 or 2 sounds?	☐ 1	☒ 2
watch	Do the letters "tch" represent 1 or 2 sounds?	☒ 1	☐ 2
bought	Do the letters "ough" represent 1 or 2 sounds?	☒ 1	☐ 2

1.2

In the following list, there are only three words that contain 3 sounds. Underline those three words:

how   did   the   tiny   goat   eat   all   those   flowers

In the following list, there are only four words that contain 4 sounds. Underline those four words:

can   the   girls   find   the   books   they   lost

In the following list, there are five words that contain 5 sounds. Underline those five words:

she   wants   Mindy and Nancy to go shopping on Tuesday

1.3

Put the words into the list according to the number of sounds they contain. At the end, all the lists should contain the same number of words.

2 sounds	3 sounds	4 sounds	5 sounds
her	Gail	broke	sandy
the	chain	dunes	running
up	tall	yellow	pretty

~~Gail~~   broke   ~~her~~   yellow   pretty   chain
~~running~~   up   ~~the~~   ~~tall~~   ~~sandy~~   dunes

1.4

How many sounds does the word "not" have?   ❏ 2   ☒ 3   ❏ 4
How many sounds does the word "fish" have?   ❏ 2   ☒ 3   ❏ 4
How many sounds does the word "lift" have?   ❏ 2   ❏ 3   ☒ 4
How many sounds does the word "thought" have?   ☒ 3   ❏ 4   ❏ 5
How many sounds does the word "boat" have?   ☒ 3   ❏ 4   ❏ 5

1.5

Do "top" and "hat" have the same number of sounds?   ❏ yes   ❏ no
Do "soap" and "box" have the same number of sounds?   ❏ yes   ❏ no
Do "window" and "curtain" have the same number of sounds?   ❏ yes   ❏ no
Do "better" and "worse" have the same number of sounds?   ❏ yes   ❏ no
Do "ketchup" and "burger" have the same number of sounds?   ❏ yes   ❏ no

1.6

Which one of the following words does not have 3 sounds?

❏ shop   ❏ hat   ❏ laugh   ❏ stop

Which one of the following words does not have 4 sounds?

❏ well   ❏ claws   ❏ heavy   ❏ wind

Which one of the following words does not have 5 sounds?

❏ crazy   ❏ friend   ❏ cactus   ❏ faucet

1.7

How many sounds does the word "you" have?   ❏ 2   ❏ 3   ❏ 4
How many sounds does the word "ring" have?   ❏ 2   ❏ 3   ❏ 4
How many sounds does the word "bread" have?   ❏ 2   ❏ 3   ❏ 4
How many sounds does the word "hello" have?   ❏ 3   ❏ 4   ❏ 5
How many sounds does the word "pocket" have?   ❏ 3   ❏ 4   ❏ 5

1.8

Do "post" and "thief" have the same number of sounds?	❏ yes	❏ no
Do "see" and "toe" have the same number of sounds?	❏ yes	❏ no
Do "crash" and "climb" have the same number of sounds?	❏ yes	❏ no
Do "study" and "books" have the same number of sounds?	❏ yes	❏ no
Do "thoughtless" and "boxes" have the same number of sounds?	❏ yes	❏ no

1.9

Which one of the following words does not have 3 sounds?

❏ snow   ❏ she   ❏ leap   ❏ ax

Which one of the following words does not have 4 sounds?

❏ fleas   ❏ hold   ❏ champ   ❏ watch

Which one of the following words does not have 5 sounds?

❏ lovely   ❏ clever   ❏ strong   ❏ Peter

1.10

How many sounds does the word "look" have?	❏ 2	❏ 3	❏ 4
How many sounds does the word "shoe" have?	❏ 2	❏ 3	❏ 4
How many sounds does the word "missed" have?	❏ 2	❏ 3	❏ 4
How many sounds does the word "sell" have?	❏ 3	❏ 4	❏ 5
How many sounds does the word "beast" have?	❏ 3	❏ 4	❏ 5

1.11

Do "sell" and "sauce" have the same number of sounds?	❏ yes	❏ no
Do "league" and "clock" have the same number of sounds?	❏ yes	❏ no
Do "cat" and "yacht" have the same number of sounds?	❏ yes	❏ no
Do "heat" and "rice" have the same number of sounds?	❏ yes	❏ no
Do "friend" and "crazy" have the same number of sounds?	❏ yes	❏ no

1.12

Which one of the following words does not have 3 sounds?

❏ find   ❏ heat   ❏ caught   ❏ rough

Which one of the following words does not have 4 sounds?

❏ cream   ❏ sleep   ❏ this   ❏ trees

Which one of the following words does not have 5 sounds?

❑ eggnog   ❑ fries   ❑ salad   ❑ pizza

✓ *Listen to the Examples in Module 1.*

1.1 LISTEN

Listen to the following words and choose the correct number of sounds (not letters) that you hear:

gone	❑ 3	❑ 4	❑ 5
skate	❑ 3	❑ 4	❑ 5
judge	❑ 3	❑ 4	❑ 5
Fiat	❑ 3	❑ 4	❑ 5
street	❑ 3	❑ 4	❑ 5
sleepy	❑ 3	❑ 4	❑ 5
Max	❑ 3	❑ 4	❑ 5
clever	❑ 4	❑ 5	❑ 6
burp	❑ 3	❑ 4	❑ 5
berry	❑ 3	❑ 4	❑ 5
her	❑ 2	❑ 3	❑ 4
water	❑ 4	❑ 5	❑ 6
stars	❑ 4	❑ 5	❑ 6
farmer	❑ 4	❑ 5	❑ 6
burst	❑ 4	❑ 5	❑ 6

1.2 LISTEN TO THE FOLLOWING WORDS AND WRITE THE NUMBER OF SOUNDS YOU HEAR IN EACH.

1. shock _____
2. window _____
3. think _____
4. cleaner _____
5. taxi _____
6. bathroom _____
7. chicken _____
8. rooster _____
9. bathing _____
10. taco _____
11. assume _____
12. laundry _____

13. bridges _____
14. creamy _____
15. willow _____
16. slippery _____
17. rodeo _____
18. chocolate _____
19. celebrate _____
20. butterfly _____
21. calendar _____
22. hummingbird _____
23. element _____
24. burning man _____

25. curious _____ 31. waterfall _____

26. damages _____ 32. lollipop _____

27. period _____ 33. surgery _____

28. clarify _____ 34. turpentine _____

29. satisfy _____ 35. percolate _____

30. listening _____

Module 2—Stressed Versus Unstressed Syllables: An Introduction

A stressed syllable is produced by (1) pushing more air out of the lungs, as (2) an increase in respiratory activity when compared to an unstressed syllable, and (3) an increase in laryngeal activity. From a listener's point of view a stressed syllable is often (but not always) **louder**—more intense—than an unstressed syllable. Stressed syllables are also usually, but not always, produced with a higher pitch. Also, the vowels within the stressed syllable are normally longer in duration.

 Helpful Hints

1. Many of the words in American English are stressed on the first syllable. Words such as "wagon," "happy," and "coffee" are all stressed on the first syllable.
2. If you are having difficulty hearing which syllable is stressed, try varying the loudness from one syllable to the next. One syllable should sound "better"—more accurate—when it is louder. That will be the stressed syllable.

The diacritic marker for stressing is a line above and in front of the stressed syllable. Look at the following examples with the stressed marker.

'bo ttom—This word is typically stressed on the first syllable.

a 'way—This word is typically stressed on the second syllable.

'ye llow—This word is typically stressed on the first syllable.

a 'hoy—This word is typically stressed on the second syllable.

Exercises

2.1

Say the following words, which have stress on the first syllable:

button   paper   typing   study   listen   ready   teacher

Cross out the one word in the following list that does not have stress on the first syllable.

cutting   letter   ~~exam~~   reader   pencil   tablet   package

Say the following words, which have stress on the second syllable:

undress   undo   adjourn   applaud   enclose   above   ago

Cross out the one word in the following list that does not have stress on the second syllable.

embrace   garage   offend   observe   cocoon   college   agree

2.2

For certain words, the meaning is changed depending on whether the word is stressed on the first or second syllable. Consider the following sentences:

She lost her <u>com</u>pact in the car.

The car was very com<u>pact</u>.

In the first sentence, the word "compact" is used as a noun. Here the stress is on the first syllable. In the second sentence, the word is used as an adjective. The stress is on the second syllable.

   Listen as you say the words that are in bold in the following sentences. Underline the stressed syllable for each.

The **<u>con</u>sole** of the car was dirty.

He wanted to **con<u>sole</u>** her.

The football player just signed a lucrative **<u>con</u>tract**.

Will he **con<u>tract</u>** the virus?

The redhead was the **<u>ob</u>ject** of his affection.

He didn't **ob<u>ject</u>** to anything she did.

He was **con<u>tent</u>** to watch TV.

The **<u>con</u>tent** of the book was not good.

He got his parking **<u>per</u>mit**.

It would **per<u>mit</u>** him to park anywhere on campus.

2.3

Say the following words, and write each one into the correct column. Which words are stressed on the first syllable, and which ones on the second syllable?

Stressed on First Syllable	Stressed on Second Syllable
✓ christmas	advice
✓ finger	baboon
✓ campus	bamboo
✓ listen	discuss
✓ letter	return
✓ midnight	roulette
shower	routine

Christmas	campus	bamboo
finger	listen	routine
advice	discuss	midnight
baboon	return	roulette
shower	letter	

2.4

Say the words in the following columns. Underline the words that are *not* in the correct column.

Stress on First Syllable	Stress on Second Syllable
humor	unhook
charcoal	harpoon
concern	enough
pirate	forward
perhaps	survive
weather	flower

2.5

Circle the one word that is not usually stressed on the first syllable.

football   camper   chowder   willow   alarm   ladder   pastry

Circle the one word that is not usually stressed on the second syllable.

event   excite   illness   impose   insert   invite   involve

Four of the following words are normally produced with stress on the second syllable. Circle these four.

angry   again   winner   exist   bizarre   bigger   bacon

diver   elope

Four of the following words are normally produced with stress on the first syllable. Circle these four.

forgot   ballet   winter   global   expand   coffee   before

garden

2.6

Say the following words, and put a stress marker (') in front of the stressed syllable.

de mand   de ˈmand

den tist

dis cuss

an gel

Mon day

co llect

la goon

en grave

bi gger

bin go

be lieve

in sure

in jure

mea sure

co llapse

a wake

2.7

Say the following words, and write each word into the correct column.

Stress on First Syllable	Stress on Second Syllable

logo   gossip   concoct   admire   antique

awesome   campaign   hamster

2.8

Underline the word that does not fit the stress pattern of the other words.

List 1:   balloon   bassoon   buffoon   buffet   bacon
List 2:   canoe   cocoon   college   cassette   collapse
List 3:   patrol   police   polite   paper   pollute
List 4:   secret   season   severe   senile   seashore

2.9

Take the stressed syllable of each of the following words to make a sentence.

pursue   awaits   fortune   billboard   butler   billfold

became   lately

2.10

Say the following words and write in the blanks whether the word is stressed on the first or the second syllable.

1. lately	_____	16. sunny	_____
2. robot	_____	17. respect	_____
3. glasses	_____	18. foreign	_____
4. disturb	_____	19. perspire	_____
5. closet	_____	20. predict	_____
6. turkey	_____	21. social	_____
7. repair	_____	22. suppose	_____
8. alike	_____	23. lovely	_____
9. open	_____	24. afraid	_____
10. request	_____	25. decoy	_____
11. focus	_____	26. parade	_____
12. option	_____	27. return	_____
13. observe	_____	28. halter	_____
14. crossing	_____	29. collide	_____
15. release	_____	30. jersey	_____

 Listen to the Examples in Module 2.

2.1 LISTEN

Listen to the following words, and mark whether they are stressed on the first or second syllable:

reader	❏ Stressed on first syllable	❏ Stressed on second syllable
region	❏ Stressed on first syllable	❏ Stressed on second syllable
forget	❏ Stressed on first syllable	❏ Stressed on second syllable
margin	❏ Stressed on first syllable	❏ Stressed on second syllable
erase	❏ Stressed on first syllable	❏ Stressed on second syllable

applause	❑ Stressed on first syllable	❑ Stressed on second syllable
surprise	❑ Stressed on first syllable	❑ Stressed on second syllable
absorb	❑ Stressed on first syllable	❑ Stressed on second syllable
question	❑ Stressed on first syllable	❑ Stressed on second syllable
abroad	❑ Stressed on first syllable	❑ Stressed on second syllable

2.2 LISTEN

Listen to the following words, and put the stress marker (') before the stressed syllable.

ac quaint	be lieve
gi raffe	com pact
gar den	con tract
un til	per mit
com pare	

2.3 LISTEN

Listen to the following words and put the stress marker (') before the stressed syllable.

1. ladder	21. peanut
2. scratching	22. either
3. allow	23. ocean
4. shadow	24. retire
5. over	25. burger
6. insect	26. parade
7. restful	27. many
8. challenge	28. perspire
9. receive	29. above
10. running	30. liquid
11. acquaint	31. ashamed
12. withdraw	32. survey
13. sugar	33. forget
14. locus	34. erupt
15. under	35. compete
16. beneath	36. again
17. pizza	37. around
18. prepare	38. detail
19. endure	39. chauffeur
20. forgive	40. cyclone

Module 3—Introducing the Vowels /i/, /ɑ/, and /u/ and Variations of /ɑ/: /ɔ/ and /a/

This exercise introduces the IPA transcription of three vowels of American English: /i/, /ɑ/, and /u/. In addition, the vowels /ɔ/ and /a/ will be contrasted to /ɑ/. These beginning exercises with /ɑ/, /ɔ/, and /a/ will provide simple contrasts so that the student begins to hear and see differences in vowel productions. At the end of the module, stressing exercises will again be provided.

The first vowel, /i/, represents the vowel sound as typically pronounced in the words "<u>ea</u>t," "m<u>ee</u>t," "k<u>ey</u>," and "l<u>ea</u>ve." It is a high-front vowel, indicating that the body of the tongue is relatively close to the palate and forward in the mouth.

In General American English, the second vowel /ɑ/ is used in the words "h<u>o</u>t," "m<u>o</u>p," "cl<u>o</u>ck," and "d<u>o</u>g." The vowel /ɑ/ is a low-back vowel; thus, the body of the tongue is farther away from the palate, and the slight bulge in the tongue is more toward the back of the mouth. When producing this vowel, the jaw is lowered, and there is not any lip rounding

The third vowel, /u/, is typically heard in words such as "m<u>oo</u>n," "h<u>oo</u>p," "d<u>u</u>ne," and "st<u>ew</u>." It is a high-back vowel, indicating that the tongue body is relatively close to the palate, and the bulge in the body of the tongue is toward the back of the mouth. The /u/ vowel is produced with lip rounding.

The vowels /ɔ/ and /a/ are allophonic variations of /ɑ/. Thus, in dialects of General American English, /ɔ/ and /a/ can replace /ɑ/ without any change in the meaning of the word.

/ɔ/ is a (lower) mid-back vowel that is not used by some speakers, used only occasionally by others. Its use appears to be related to the respective dialect of the speaker. Therefore, distinguishing between /ɑ/ and /ɔ/ productions is difficult for many speakers. During production of /ɔ/, the lips are somewhat rounded and protruded. This is not the case when producing /a/ or /ɑ/.

/a/ is a low-front vowel sounding somewhere between /æ/ and /ɑ/. /a/ is dialect dependent; e.g., one can often hear this vowel in speakers of the New England area.

Words with /i/ vowels: deep, bead, each, ski

Words with /ɑ/ vowels: stop, shot, box, flock

Words with /u/ vowels: boot, blue, glue, shoe

Helpful Hints

1. The vowel /i/ can be spelled in a number of ways. The most common spellings are "e" as in "me," "ee" as in "feet," "ea" as in "bean," and "e - e" as in "scene." Less common spellings may include "ei"

("receive"), "ie" ("believe"), "ey" ("key"), and "eo" ("people"). However, one should be careful with spellings and listen to the vowel quality. Many words can be spelled in the abovementioned ways but are not pronounced with /i/. For example, "l<u>eo</u>pard," "b<u>eau</u>tiful," "l<u>ie</u>," and "m<u>ea</u>dow" have these spellings but do not contain /i/ vowels.

2. The vowel /ɑ/ is often spelled with "o," as in "lock" or "cot." However, it can be spelled many different ways, such as "a" in "talk," "ea" as in "heart," or "ua" as in "guard."

3. There are many different ways to spell the /u/ vowel. Common ones include "oo" ("boot"), "u" ("duly"), "u - e" ("dude"), and "o" ("do"). However, other spellings include "oe" as in "shoe," "ew" as in "stew," "ui" as in "fruit," "ou" as in "group," and "ough" as in "through." Again, one should listen to the vowel quality, as similar spellings may not represent /u/.

Exercises

3.1

One of the words in the following list does not typically contain /i/. Cross out the word that is not usually pronounced with /i/.

heat   dream   leap   (lip)   cheek   beat   seat

One of the words in the following list does not typically contain the /ɑ/. Cross out the word that is not usually pronounced with the /ɑ/.

rob   nod   talk   (call)   doll   lap   shot

One of the words in the following list does not typically contain /u/. Cross out the word that is not usually pronounced with /u/.

flew   (cut)   goof   snoop   cube   gloom   duke

3.2

Put the following words into the correct list. When done, each of the lists should contain an equal number of words.

/i/	/ɑ/	/u/
league	top	tune
beep	blonde	hoop
east	odd	juice
cheese	chop	cool

~~top~~ ~~blond~~ ~~league~~ ~~tune~~ ~~beep~~ ~~east~~ ~~odd~~ ~~hoop~~ ~~chop~~ ~~juice~~ ~~cheese~~ ~~cool~~

3.3

Transcribe the vowel sounds /i/, /ɑ/, or /u/ in the following words:

Eve	/iv/
bead	/bid/
dot	/dat/
deed	/did/
shock	/shak/
dude	/dud/
mood	/mud/
jeans	/jins/
knew	/nuw/
lodge	/ladg/
job	/jab/
suit	/sut/
neat	/nɨt/
root	/rut/
loss	/laws/

3.4 STRESS REVIEW

Say the following words. Underline the stressed syllable in each. Transcribe the vowel sound in the stressed syllable.

cooler	/kulǝr/
meatball	/mit/
hockey	/nak/
peeking	/pik/
season	/si/
lobby	/lab/
waffle	/waf/
losing	/lus/
shopper	/shap/
tuba	/tu/
recruit	/krut/
ruin	/ru/
retrieve	/triv/
upon	/an/
beater	/bit/

al<u>oo</u>f	/luf/
<u>R</u>obert	/ra/
sal<u>u</u>te	/lut/
m<u>ea</u>ger	/mi/
app<u>ea</u>l	/pil/
<u>g</u>ooey	/gu/
<u>b</u>ody	/ba/
l<u>o</u>cket	/la/
<u>s</u>eason	/si/
al<u>ong</u>	/la r/
acute	
t<u>o</u>pic	/ta/
un<u>tr</u>ue	/tru/

3.5

Underline the words that typically contain the /i/.

<u>heat</u>   hat   hit   hope   <u>keep</u>   ship   <u>team</u>   <u>bean</u>   mill

Underline the words that typically contain /ɑ/.

hat   <u>hot</u>   map   <u>mop</u>   <u>lot</u>   lap   <u>love</u>   <u>rock</u>   rat

Underline the words that typically contain /u/.

<u>soon</u>   sun   gun   <u>wood</u>   <u>clue</u>   <u>shoe</u>   luck   <u>flu</u>

3.6

Put the following words together with the appropriate vowel sound:

/i/	/ɑ/	/u/

you   each   dock   boss   beak   food
new   east   doll   fox   loose   tooth

3.7

How many words contain /i/ in the following list?

on   sun   keen   meal   tip   niece   sheet   ❏ 2   ❏ 3   ❏ 4

How many words contain /ɑ/ in the following list?

pond   rope   soap   cape   lag   rod   rode   ❏ 2   ❏ 3   ❏ 4

How many words contain /u/ in the following list?

two   ton   threw   prune   club   wood   bruise   ❏ 2   ❏ 3   ❏ 4

3.8

From the pair of words, underline the ones that contain either an /i/, /ɑ/, or /u/ vowel.

peak–pick

wrote–rot

wheel–will

full–fool

knock–nook

eat–it

brook–broom

ship–sheep

pull–pool

cop–cope

3.9

Look at the transcription of the vowel sounds in the following words. According to typical pronunciation, which ones are correct ☺ and which ones are incorrect ☹?

troop	/u/	☺	☹
roof	/ɑ/	☺	☹
stop	/ɑ/	☺	☹
lean	/i/	☺	☹
lodge	/u/	☺	☹
peach	/i/	☺	☹
wheat	/ɑ/	☺	☹
soothe	/u/	☺	☹
youth	/ɑ/	☺	☹
solve	/ɑ/	☺	☹

3.10

Underline the words that are typically produced with /i/ in the stressed syllable.

easel   diesel   kitten   neon   equip   chimney   appeal   offend

Underline the words that are typically produced with /ɑ/ in the stressed syllable.

olive   body   matter   convince   hostage   comma   lower   upon

Underline the words that are typically produced with /u/ in the stressed syllable.

doodle   losing   untrue   dusky   jumper   bully   aloof   football

Listen to the Examples in Module 3.

Listen to the following words, and transcribe the vowel sound.

3.1 LISTEN

1. si
2. du
3. rɑb
4. map
5. fild
6. hu
7. nɑd
8. hit
9. frut
10. _____

3.2 LISTEN

Listen to Melissa, who is 6 years old. Transcribe the vowels in the words that she says.

1. ʀe
2. múv
3. jɑg
4. hup
5. skul
6. lɑk
7. ni
8. kɑb
9. gus

10. tɔlk
11. sniz
12. bæp
13. tim
14. pand
15. hæp
16. min
17. bʌt
18. tuth
19. tu
20. bɑt

3.3 LISTEN

Listen to the following words, and transcribe the vowel in the stressed syllable.

eagle _____

dollar _____

rooster _____

truly _____

copy _____

rocket _____

chewy _____

undo _____

lobby _____

retreat _____

3.4 LISTEN

The following exercises contrast /ɔ/, /ɑ/, and /a/. They can be done later in the program if that seems more appropriate. Consult your instructor as to the sequence of these particular listening exercises.

Contrasting /ɔ/ to /ɑ/ Each of the vowels is transcribed after the word. Do you hear the differences? Remember that /ɔ/ is a rounded vowel. Watch the video to see which of the vowels in the pair has lip rounding.

caught	[ɔ]	cot	[ɑ]
hock	[ɑ]	hawk	[ɔ]
lawn	[ɔ]	lawn	[ɑ]
frog	[ɔ]	frog	[ɑ]
all	[ɑ]	all	[ɔ]
Don	[ɑ]	dawn	[ɔ]
bought	[ɔ]	bought	[ɑ]

Now you try to transcribe the vowels of the last three word pairs:

dog _____   dog _____
stall _____   stall _____
talk _____   talk _____

3.5 LISTEN

Contrasting /ɑ/ to /a/   Each of the vowels is transcribed after the word. Can you hear the difference?

hot	[ɑ]	hot	[a]
stop	[ɑ]	stop	[a]
lock	[a]	lock	[ɑ]
moss	[ɑ]	moss	[a]
tall	[a]	tall	[ɑ]
on	[ɑ]	on	[a]
talk	[a]	talk	[ɑ]
rob	[ɑ]	rob	[a]

Try to transcribe the vowels in the last three word pairs.

hot _____   hot _____
cough _____   cough _____
Tod _____   Tod _____

3.6 TRANSCRIBE THE FOLLOWING VOWELS WITH [i], [ɑ], [u], [a], OR [ɔ]

1. sleep _____	11. bomb _____	21. tune _____
2. stall _____	12. law _____	22. sheep _____
3. brief _____	13. caught _____	23. beach _____
4. spot _____	14. loop _____	24. spoon _____
5. toss _____	15. leap _____	25. sock _____
6. rock _____	16. clean _____	26. knee _____
7. stock _____	17. reach _____	27. thought _____
8. mean _____	18. shoe _____	28. loon _____
9. teach _____	19. laws _____	29. jaws _____
10. rot _____	20. cop _____	30. sauce _____

Module 4—Introducing the Stop-Plosives

This module introduces the stop-plosives /p, /b/, /t/, /d/, /k/, and /g/.

The first pair, /p/ and /b/, are bilabial stop-plosives. *Bilabial* indicates that the upper and lower lips come together to produce the sounds. While /p/ is voiceless, produced without any vocal fold vibration, /b/ is voiced.

The second pair, /t/ and /d/, are coronal-alveolar stop-plosives. The corona or edges of the tongue come in contact with the alveolar ridge. /t/ is voiceless in this pair, while /d/ is voiced.

The third set, /k/ and /g/, are postdorsal-velar stop-plosives. *Postdorsal* indicates the posterior portion of the tongue, while *velar* refers to the soft palate or velum. Therefore, to produce these sounds, the posterior portion of the tongue makes contact with the soft palate. /k/ is voiceless, while /g/ is voiced.

Helpful Hints

1. In American English, there is a relatively high correspondence between the letters "p" and "b" and /p/ and /b/. However, there are a few exceptions. The letters "ph" can sound like /p/ as in the word "shepherd," and infrequently "gh" is pronounced as /p/ in, for example, "hiccough." The letters "p" and "b" can be silent, as in "receipt" and "comb."
2. There is also a high correspondence between the letters "t" and "d" and /t/ and /d/. Some words, however, may be spelled with "d" but actually be pronounced /t/. Examples include the "ed" ending in "stopped," "hopped," and "clapped."
3. /k/ can be spelled with "k" as in "keep" or "key." However, orthographically it is often signified by "c" (as in "cat" or "coat"), "ck" (as in "back" or "lock"), "ch" (as in "school" or "scholar"), and even "q" (in the words "queen" or "quit"). On the other hand, there is a relatively high degree of correspondence between the letter "g" and /g/ as in "girl" or "green." Both the letters "k" and "g" can be silent, as in "knee," "gnome," "night," and "caught."

Exercises

4.1

Say the following words. Do you hear the stop-plosive /p/ or /b/ at the beginning, middle, or end of the word or not at all? Underline the correct answer.

pill	beginning	middle	end	not at all
apple	beginning	middle	end	not at all

cellophane	beginning	middle	end	not at all
mop	beginning	middle	end	not at all
soap	beginning	middle	end	not at all
jumping	beginning	middle	end	not at all
oboe	beginning	middle	end	not at all
thumb	beginning	middle	end	not at all

4.2

Say the following words. Do you hear the stop-plosives /t/ or /d/ at the beginning, middle, or end of the word or not at all?

dove	beginning	middle	end	not at all
hit	beginning	middle	end	not at all
showed	beginning	middle	end	not at all
tease	beginning	middle	end	not at all
board	beginning	middle	end	not at all
thigh	beginning	middle	end	not at all
toe	beginning	middle	end	not at all
ado	beginning	middle	end	not at all

4.3

Say the following words. Do you hear the stop-plosives /k/ or /g/ at the beginning, middle, or end of the word or not at all?

come	beginning	middle	end	not at all
knife	beginning	middle	end	not at all
sigh	beginning	middle	end	not at all
egg	beginning	middle	end	not at all
ago	beginning	middle	end	not at all
lucky	beginning	middle	end	not at all
gnaw	beginning	middle	end	not at all
shock	beginning	middle	end	not at all

4.4

Underline the words in the following list that have stop-plosives at the beginning, middle, or end of the words.

bean–mean	gopher–knower
dune–noon	collar–dollar
pill–sill	catch–fetch
read–seed	acer–baker
knee–feet	should–could

4.5

The following words are written in phonetic transcription. Write in the words that they represent.

[du] _____   [it] _____
[but] _____   [kup] _____
[kip] _____   [bɑt] _____
[kɑp] _____   [tɑk] _____
[pik] _____   [ki] _____

Listen to the Examples in Module 4.

4.1 LISTEN

The following words contain the stop-plosives /p/, /b/, /t/, /d/, /k/, and /g/ with the vowels /i/, /ɑ/, and /u/. Transcribe the entire word.

1. _____
2. _____
3. _____
4. _____
5. _____
6. _____
7. _____
8. _____
9. _____
10. _____
11. _____
12. _____
13. _____
14. _____
15. _____

4.2 LISTEN

Listen to Sandy, who is 6 years old. All words contain the stop-plosives and the vowel /i/, /u/, or /ɑ/. Transcribe the words that she says.

1. _____
2. _____
3. _____
4. _____
5. _____
6. _____

7. _____

8. _____

9. _____

10. _____

11. _____

12. _____

13. _____

14. _____

15. _____

4.3 LISTEN—STRESS

Mark the stressed syllable on each of these words with a (') before the stressed syllable.

or phan

cre ate

per fume

fra gile

safe ty

be lief

dis guise

pro fit

pre fer

ex clude

Module 5—Introducing More Vowels: /ɪ/, /ɛ/, /æ/, and /ʊ/

This module looks at the front vowels /ɪ/, /ɛ/, and /æ/ and one back vowel, /ʊ/. In addition, further practice with /a/, /ɑ/ and /ɔ/ will be presented.

The front vowel /ɪ/ is considered a (lower) high-front vowel, since the tongue's body is not as close to the palate as when saying /i/. It is the vowel that is typically heard in the pronunciations of "p<u>i</u>ck," "h<u>i</u>t," and "k<u>i</u>ss."

/ɛ/ is a (lower) mid-front vowel. In General American English, it is normally heard in words such as "n<u>e</u>ck," "h<u>ea</u>d," and "<u>e</u>gg." If you contrast the tongue position for the productions of /ɪ/ versus /ɛ/, you will find that the front bulge of the tongue is lower for /ɛ/ than for /ɪ/.

/æ/ is considered a low-front vowel. It is typically heard in the pronunciations of "h<u>a</u>t," "m<u>a</u>d," and "b<u>a</u>g." If contrasted to /ɛ/, /æ/ is produced with the bulge of the tongue in a lower position.

/ʊ/ is a (lower) high-back vowel typically heard in the pronunciation of "w<u>oo</u>d," "sh<u>ou</u>ld," and "b<u>oo</u>k." Comparing this vowel to /u/, one notices that the back hump of the tongue drops somewhat from /u/ to /ʊ/. Similar to /u/, /ʊ/ also requires lip rounding.

Words with /ɪ/: kid, ill, which, bit

Words with /ɛ/: ten, wet, red, sell

Words with /æ/: cat, ran, sack, patch

Words with /ʊ/: look, put, foot, could

Helpful Hints

1. /ɪ/ is transcribed like a capital "I," only it is smaller, the same size as lowercase letters. Orthographically, /ɪ/ is often spelled with the letter "i," as in "fish" or "pig." However, many different spellings, such as "ui" as in "built," "y" as in "gym," or "ie" as in "sieve," can be pronounced as /ɪ/.

2. /ɛ/ is not transcribed as a capital "E"; rather, its edges are rounded. Actually, it is the symbol for the Greek letter epsilon. The symbol /ɛ/ has the same size as lowercase letters. Most of the time, /ɛ/ is spelled with "e," as in "hen" or "bet." However, /ɛ/ can be spelled in a variety of ways such as "ai" ("said"), "ea" ("health"), or "ue" ("guess").

3. /æ/ is symbolized as a digraph; two letters form one symbol. In this case, an "a" letter is directly attached to the letter "e." The /æ/ symbol is the same size as lowercase letters. In most cases, /æ/ is spelled with "a," as in "mat" or "can." However, other spellings can infrequently be seen, such as "au" ("laugh") or "ai" ("plaid").

4. /ʊ/ is derived from the lowercase version of the Greek symbol upsilon. It looks somewhat like a "u," rounded at the bottom, and has two hor-

izontal wings that protrude on either side. It is the same size as lower-case letters. /ʊ/ is most often spelled with "u" ("put"), "oo" ("foot"), or "ou" ("could").

Exercises

5.1

Say the following words. Underline those words that contain /ɪ/, the vowel that is typically heard in "p<u>i</u>ck."

lead tin this white pill give ice in build seize

Underline the words that contain /ɛ/, the vowel that is typically heard in "hen."

edge desk leap these text fed reel she meant tent

Underline the words that contain /æ/, the vowel that is typically heard in "bat."

sack cane map great tax back bake weigh jade that

Underline the words that contain /ʊ/, the vowel that is typically heard in "wood."

bush loose good cook put room would boot luck bull

5.2

Underline the words that typically contain the vowels /ɪ/ ("pick"), /ɛ/ ("hen"), /æ/ ("bat"), or /ʊ/ ("wood").

beet–bid
meet–mitt
pill–peel
bed–bead
bait–bet
tack–take
mane–man
loop–look
pull–pool
cool–cook

5.3

Write the following words under the correct vowel symbol. At the end, all lists should contain the same number of words.

/ɪ/	/ɛ/	/æ/	/ʊ/

rat hood stem list should scratch bill bench chest nook
fit scrap ten ship clap full

5.4

How many words in the following list contain /ɪ/?

shin kit kite friend wrist write pin pine ❑ 3 ❑ 4 ❑ 5

How many words in the following list contain /ɛ/?

seal sell fence clean beet end eel breeze ❑ 3 ❑ 4 ❑ 5

How many words in the following list contain /æ/?

ash barn bath bathe half lamp lane past ❑ 3 ❑ 4 ❑ 5

How many words in the following list contain /ʊ/?

soot suit loot shook wool use huge cue ❑ 3 ❑ 4 ❑ 5

5.5

The following words are written in phonetic transcription. Write in the words they represent.

/tʊk/ _____

/pɪt/ _____

/kæt/ _____

/pɛt/ _____

/bæt/ _____

/pʊt/ _____

/bɪb/ _____

/bɛd/ _____

5.6

Say the following words, and look at the transcription of the vowel sounds. According to General American English pronunciation, which ones are correct ☺ and which ones are incorrect ☹?

foot	/ʊ/	☺	☹
full	/ɛ/	☺	☹
fill	/ɪ/	☺	☹
fell	/ɛ/	☺	☹
mad	/ɛ/	☺	☹
sent	/ɛ/	☺	☹
sack	/æ/	☺	☹
dress	/ɛ/	☺	☹
brook	/ʊ/	☺	☹

5.7

Underline the words that are typically produced with /ɪ/ in the stressed syllable.

igloo   chicken   license   filter   likely   injure   afflict   tiger

Underline the words that are typically produced with /ɛ/ in the stressed syllable.

beckon   weaving   ahead   ceiling   compete   condensed   heaven

settle

Underline the words that are typically produced with /æ/ in the stressed syllable.

bandage gather shampoo bagel rainbow aback complain attract

Underline the words that are typically produced with /ʊ/ in the stressed syllable.

bushel grumpy tunnel football pudding useful salute wooden

Listen to the Examples in Module 5.

5.1 LISTEN

The following words contain the stop-plosives /p/, /b/, /t/, /d/, /k/, and /g/ with the vowels /ɪ/, /ɛ/, and /æ/, and /ʊ/. Transcribe the entire word.

1. _____
2. _____
3. _____
4. _____
5. _____
6. _____
7. _____
8. _____

9. _____

10. _____

5.2 LISTEN

Transcribe the following words that contain the stop-plosives and the vowels /i/, /ɑ/, /u/, /ɪ/, /ɛ/, /æ/, or /ʊ/.

Melissa (age 6;4)   Gail (age 6;0)

1. _____   1. _____
2. _____   2. _____
3. _____   3. _____
4. _____   4. _____
5. _____   5. _____
6. _____   6. _____
7. _____   7. _____
8. _____   8. _____
9. _____   9. _____
10. _____   10. _____
11. _____   11. _____
12. _____   12. _____
13. _____   13. _____
14. _____   14. _____
15. _____   15. _____
16. _____   16. _____
17. _____   17. _____
18. _____   18. _____
19. _____   19. _____
20. _____   20. _____

5.3 LISTEN

Transcribe the following words that contain /p/, /b/, /t/, /d/, /k/, and /g/ with the vowels /ɪ/, /ɛ/, /æ/, or /ʊ/

1. /pɛt/
2. /tæg/
3. /pɪt/
4. /kæp/
5. /tæk/
6. /bɛt/
7. /bæk/
8. /gʊd/
9. /kæt/

10. /tʊk/
11. /kʊk/
12. /tæp/
13. /gæp/
14. /dɛd/
15. /tɪp/
16. /bæg/
17. /bʊg/
18. /dɔgi/ → /dagi/
19. /kʊki/
20. /pʊt/
21. _____
22. _____
23. _____
24. _____
25. _____
26. _____
27. _____
28. _____
29. _____
30. _____
31. _____
32. _____
33. _____
34. _____
35. _____
36. _____
37. _____
38. _____
39. _____
40. _____

5.4 LISTEN—STRESS

All of the following two-syllable words contain the stop-plosives /p/, /b/, /t/, /d/, /k/, or /g/ and the following vowels: /i/, /ɑ/, /u/, /ɪ/, /ɛ/, /æ/, or /ʊ/. Transcribe the word and put the stress marker (ˈ) in front of the stressed syllable.

1. /ˈtɪpi/
2. /ˈduti/
3. /ˈkuku/
4. /ˈkʌki/ → /ˈkʊki/

5. /ˈbɑbi/
6. /ˈkupɑn/
7. /ˈgʌdi/ → /ˈgʊri/
8. /ˈduwɛt/ → /duˈɛt/
9. /ˈɪglu/
10. /ˈkuti/

5.5 LISTEN

Each of the following words contains /a/ followed by /ɑ/, and the third word in the series contains /ɔ/. Listen and transcribe the last five words.

[dag]	[dɑg]	[dɔg]	_____
[bat]	[bɑt]	[bɔt]	_____
[pap]	[pɑp]	[pɔp]	_____
[tat]	[tɑt]	[tɔt]	_____
[bɔb]	[bɑb]	[bab]	_____

Module 6—The Fricatives /f/, /v/, /s/, /z/, /ʃ/, /ʒ/, /θ/, /ð/, and /h/

This module introduces the fricatives: /f/, /v/, /s/, /z/, /ʃ/, /ʒ/, /θ/, /ð/, and /h/.

Fricatives are those consonants in which the active and passive articulators come together so closely that an audible friction sound results when air is pushed through the constriction.

/f/ and /v/ are labio-dental fricatives. There is a narrow opening between the active articulator, the inner edge of the lower lip (*labio-*) and the passive articulator, the edges of the upper incisors (-*dental*). /f/ is voiceless, /v/ is voiced.

/s/ and /z/ are apico-alveolar fricatives. There is a narrow opening between the tip of the tongue (*apico-*) and the alveolar ridge (*alveolar*). Some individuals produce a predorsal-alveolar /s/ and /z/. The tongue tip is behind the lower incisors, and the tongue body arches upward, creating a narrow opening between the anterior third of the tongue body (*predorsal-*) and the alveolar ridge (*alveolar*). /s/ is voiceless, /z/ is voiced.

/ʃ/ and /ʒ/ are considered either coronal-prepalatal or coronal-postalveolar fricatives. For production of these consonants, a narrow opening occurs between the edges of the tongue (*coronal-*) and the most anterior portion of the palate (*prepalatal*). Another possible production is a slightly more anterior one. Here a narrow opening is created between the coronal portion of the tongue and a point posterior to the highest point of the alveolar ridge (*postalveolar*). /ʃ/ is voiceless, /ʒ/ is voiced.

/θ/ and /ð/ are apico-dental or interdental fricatives. The apico-dental articulation is created by a narrow opening between the apex of the tongue (*apico-*) and the posterior surface of the upper incisors (*dental*). A second possibility is that the tongue tip is slightly protruded between the upper and lower incisors (*interdental*). /θ/ is voiceless, /ð/ is voiced.

/h/ is considered to be a fricative according to the International Phonetic Alphabet notation; however, /h/ does not fit this given description as neatly as the other fricatives that were just introduced. For this discussion, /h/ is a voiceless glottal fricative. See Chapter 5 for more details about this production.

Helpful Hints

1. /f/ is often spelled with the letter "f," as in "five" or "fine." However, it can be spelled "ph" as in "phone," "gh" as in "rough," or "lf" as in "half." /v/ is usually orthographically represented by "v"; however, the letter "f" can also indicate /v/, as in "of."

2. /s/ can be spelled with "s" ("sun"), "ss" ("miss"), "c" ("city"), "sc" ("scene"), and "z" ("blitz"). On the other hand, /z/ is often orthographically represented by "s" ("has," "colors"). Other spellings for /z/ include "z" ("zoo"), "ss" ("scissors"), "zz" ("buzz"), and "es" ("washes").

3. The symbol /ʃ/ is an integral sign that is often used in mathematics. The symbol is as large as an uppercase letter and extends below the written line. /ʃ/ can be spelled with "sh" as in "sheep" but is also heard in words that contain "ti" ("election," "nation") or "ci" ("social," "special"). The symbol /ʒ/ is as large as a lowercase letter but extends below the written line. /ʒ/ is an infrequent sound heard in words that have been borrowed from other languages, such as "Jacque," "rouge," or "Peugeot." More common spellings of /ʒ/ include "si" ("occasion") and "su" ("pleasure").

4. The /θ/ symbol is the Greek theta, an uppercase "0" with a bar through it. The symbol /ð/ is a lowercase Greek delta with a line through the upper portion. Both symbols are as large as uppercase letters. /θ/ and /ð/ are represented orthographically by "th." For beginning transcribers, it is often difficult to distinguish between the voiceless and the voiced "th." One possibility might be to say the word first with voicing and then without. For example, say "the" first with voicing on the first sound and then without (whispered). This should help in determining if the sound is a voiceless /θ/ or a voiced /ð/.

5. The /h/ is typically represented orthographically with the letter "h"; however, it can be spelled "wh" as in "who." This sound can occur only at the beginning of a syllable in American English. The words "house," "helping," and "ahead" demonstrate this phonotactic constraint.

Exercises

6.1

Underline those words that have /f/ at the beginning, middle, or end of the word.

fun half have stuff elephant tough though of

Underline those words that have /v/ at the beginning, middle, or end of the word.

vote vacuum telephone laugh stove ever move shoving

Underline those words that have /s/ at the beginning, middle, or end of the word.

lasso sun shine loss whistle measure decent prison

Underline those words that have /z/ at the beginning, middle, or end of the word.

lousy zipper easy days squeeze vessel purpose icy

Underline those words that have /ʃ/ at the beginning, middle, or end of the word.

shop ration wish sugar guess cautious school pleasure

Underline those words that have /ʒ/ at the beginning, middle, or end of the word.

beige   stage   vision   wishful   leisure   music   business   treasure

Underline those words that have /θ/ at the beginning, middle, or end of the word.

thin   tooth   bath   bathe   thumb   the   that   think

Underline those words that have /ð/ at the beginning, middle, or end of the word.

this   mother   leather   thing   thirty   soothe   these   thorn

Underline those words that have /h/ at the beginning of a syllable.

hospital   where   ahoy   history   behind   behave   whoever

6.2

The following words are written in phonetic transcription. Write in orthographically the words they represent.

[sik] _____

[sɪk] _____

[hɪz] _____

[fit] _____

[fɪt] _____

[ʃip] _____

[ʃɪp] _____

[sut] _____

[sʊt] _____

[hu] _____

6.3

Voiceless and voiced th-sounds: /θ/ and /ð/. Beginning transcribers often have trouble distinguishing voiceless /θ/ from voiced /ð/. Say the following words and note whether the th-sounds are voiceless or voiced. Write in the appropriate symbol.

with _____

the _____

these _____

path _____

think _____

breathe _____

thick   _____

them   _____

weather   _____

bathe   _____

6.4

Say the following word pairs. Transcribe the fricatives in the order in which they occur.

Example: 1. "sip" 2. "zip" 1. [s] 2. [z]

1. vat	2. fat	1. [ ]	2. [ ]
1. half	2. have	1. [ ]	2. [ ]
1. said	2. shed	1. [ ]	2. [ ]
1. thin	2. fin	1. [ ]	2. [ ]
1. math	2. mash	1. [ ]	2. [ ]
1. cave	2. case	1. [ ]	2. [ ]
1. growth	2. grows	1. [ ]	2. [ ]
1. rouge	2. roof	1. [ ]	2. [ ]
1. beige	2. bathe	1. [ ]	2. [ ]
1. their	2. share	1. [ ]	2. [ ]

6.5

The following words contain either /θ/ or /ð/. Write the word under the correct phonetic symbol. At the end both lists should be equal in length.

/θ/	/ð/

clothing   thumb   Thursday   leather   sixth   thus   mouth   three

breathes   rhythm

6.6

Underline the words that are typically produced with /f/.

phase   photo   even   trophy   cough   leave   diver   gopher

Underline the words that are typically produced with /s/.

ration   excite   mission   hats   nest   cell   lesson   chosen

Underline the words that are typically produced with /ʃ/.

chandelier   action   erosion   matures   promotion   radish   marsh   seize

Underline the words that are typically produced with /θ/.

mother   toothbrush   booth   neither   further   fourteenth   worthless   together

Underline the words that are typically produced with /h/.

keyhole   whole   when   hockey   fought   sight   doghouse   uphill

6.7

Underline the words that are typically produced with /θ/ in the *stressed* syllable.

either   bathtub   fourteenth   thunder   feather
author   thrifty   although   northern   beneath

Underline the words that are typically produced with /f/ in the *stressed* syllable.

female   phonetics   vinegar   affair   facility
thankful   flower   butterfly   confirm   gopher

Underline the words that are typically produced with /s/ in the *stressed* syllable.

deceive   syrup   lobster   zebra   pansy
ladies   buckets   promotes   postage   distort

Underline the words that are typically produced with /ʃ/ in the *stressed* syllable.

shiny   machine   enclosure   vision   unsure
leisure   wishful   television   motion   afresh

Underline the words that are typically produced with /h/ in the *stressed* syllable.

forehead   inhale   Hawaii   happy   halibut
rehearse   ahoy   mohair   pothole   yahoo

Listen to the Examples in Module 6.

6.1 LISTEN

The following words contain /i/, /ɑ/, or /u/ with one of the fricatives /f/, /v/, /s/, /z/, /ʃ/, /ʒ/, /θ/, /ð/, or /h/ and/or the stop-plosives /p/, /b/, /t/, /d/, /k/, or /g/. Transcribe the word.

1. _____
2. _____
3. _____
4. _____
5. _____
6. _____
7. _____
8. _____
9. _____
10. _____
11. _____
12. _____

6.2 LISTEN

The following words contain /i/, /ɑ/, or /u/ with one of the fricatives /f/, /v/, /s/, /z/, /ʃ/, /ʒ/, /θ/, /ð/, or /h/ and/or the stop-plosives /p/, /b/, /t/, /d/, /k/, or /g/. Transcribe the word.

1. _____
2. _____
3. _____
4. _____
5. _____
6. _____
7. _____
8. _____
9. _____
10. _____
11. _____
12. _____

6.3 LISTEN

The following words contain the vowels /i/, /ɑ/, /u/, /ɪ/, /ɛ/, /æ/, or /ʊ/ and stop-plosives or fricatives. Transcribe the words.

1. _____
2. _____
3. _____

4. _____
5. _____
6. _____
7. _____
8. _____
9. _____
10. _____
11. _____
12. _____
13. _____

6.4 LISTEN

The following words contain the vowels /i/, /ɑ/, /u/, /ɪ/, /ɛ/, /æ/, or /ʊ/ and stop-plosives or fricatives. Transcribe the words.

1. _____
2. _____
3. _____
4. _____
5. _____
6. _____
7. _____
8. _____
9. _____
10. _____
11. _____
12. _____

6.5 LISTEN

The following words contain the vowels /i/, /ɑ/, /u/, /ɪ/, /ɛ/, /æ/, or /ʊ/ and stop-plosives or fricatives. Transcribe the words.

1. _____
2. _____
3. _____
4. _____
5. _____
6. _____
7. _____
8. _____
9. _____
10. _____
11. _____

6.6 LISTEN—STRESS

Place the stress marker (') in front of the stressed syllable.

a pplause

stam pede

e rase

cir cus

car go

ca ssette

com ply

tur quoise

dis grace

pro vide

Module 7—The Diphthongs /e͡ɪ/, /o͡ʊ/, /a͡ɪ/, /a͡ʊ/, and /ɔ͡ɪ/

This module introduces the diphthongs: /e͡ɪ/, /o͡ʊ/, /a͡ɪ/, /a͡ʊ/, and /ɔ͡ɪ/. Diphthongs are those vowels in which there is a change of quality during the production. This results in an onglide (the first part of the vowel) and an offglide portion (the last part of the vowel).

Please note that there are several different ways to transcribe the diphthongs. Please consult with your instructor and see which way he or she would like you to transcribe these vowel sounds. Use those transcriptions in the following exercises.

The diphthong /e͡ɪ/ is normally heard in words such as "c<u>a</u>ke," "r<u>ai</u>n," and "s<u>ay</u>."

The diphthong /o͡ʊ/ can typically be heard in words such as "t<u>oe</u>," "sn<u>ow</u>," and "b<u>oa</u>t."

The diphthong /a͡ɪ/ is a typical pronunciation in words such as "m<u>y</u>," "s<u>ig</u>n," and "l<u>i</u>me."

The diphthong /a͡ʊ/ is a common pronunciation in the words "n<u>ow</u>," "h<u>ou</u>se," and "<u>ou</u>t."

The diphthong /ɔ͡ɪ/ is normally heard in words such as "f<u>oi</u>l," "t<u>oy</u>," and "j<u>oi</u>n."

Helpful Hints

1. The most frequent spellings for /e͡ɪ/ include "a" as in "acorn" or "acre," "a-e" as in "bake" or "lane," and "ai" as in "pain" or "aid." However, there are several other spellings that can be seen for this diphthong. These include "ea" ("great"), "ei" ("weigh"), "ay" ("play"), "ey" ("they"), "et" ("ballet"), and "ee" ("matinee").
2. The diphthong /o͡ʊ/ has over twenty different spellings (Dewey, 1971). The most common ones include "o" as in "no" or "go," "o-e" as in "bone" or "stole," and "oa" as in "oak" or "boat." According to the lists compiled by Blockcolsky (1990) based on the second edition of the *Random House Unabridged Dictionary* and *Webster's Third New International Dictionary*, the following spellings are fairly common: "ow" ("owe") and "ou" ("doughnut").
3. The diphthong /a͡ɪ/ can also be spelled a number of ways. Common spellings are "i" ("ivy," "hi"), "i-e" ("bike," "mice"), "y" ("eye," "by"), "ui" ("guide"), "igh" ("high," "light"), "eigh" ("height"), and "ia" ("dial," "trial").
4. The most frequent spellings for the diphthong /a͡ʊ/ include "ou" ("bounce," "loud") and "ow" ("chowder," "cow"). According to Blockcolsky (1990), these spellings predominate common words of American English.
5. The diphthong /ɔ͡ɪ/ has two common spellings: "oi" as in "boil" or "choice" and "oy" as in "toy" or "royal."

7.1

Underline the words that have the /eɪ/ diphthong. This diphthong is heard in the word "sail."

<u>eight</u>   chamber   wagon   calf   <u>reindeer</u>   they   item   shade   lettuce   suede

Underline the words that have the /oʊ/ diphthong. This diphthong is heard in the word "goat."

tone   <u>both</u>   gone   bowl   cough   <u>whole</u>   noise   ounce   <u>coat</u>   yoga

Underline the words that have the /aɪ/ diphthong. This diphthong is heard in the word "bite."

<u>type</u>   sly   eyelash   air   trip   give   <u>light</u>   <u>write</u>   relieve   river

Underline the words that have the /aʊ/ diphthong. This diphthong is heard in the word "mouse."

bowl   <u>down</u>   <u>loud</u>   boost   cougar   <u>noun</u>   shower   rough   <u>mouth</u>   trout

Underline the words that have the /ɔɪ/ diphthong. This diphthong is heard in the word "joy."

<u>choice</u>   <u>coin</u>   powder   couch   <u>soil</u>   join   voice   hoof   door   <u>foil</u>

7.2

The following words are written in phonetic transcription. Write the word in orthography.

[keɪk]	"cake"
[taɪm]	"time"
[soʊp]	"soup"
[haʊs]	"house"
[tɔɪ]	"toy"
[boʊt]	"boat"
[kaɪt]	"kite"
[voʊt]	"vote"
[bɔɪz]	"boys"
[saɪt]	"site"

7.3

Transcribe the vowel in the following pairs of words

ice _"a͡ɪ s"_   ace _____

kite _"ka͡ɪt"_   coat _____

bike _"ba͡ɪk"_   bake _____

foil _"fɔ͡ɪl"_   foul _____

ties _____   toes _____

boy _____   bay _____

out _____   oat _____

voice _____   vase _____

now _____   no _____

void _____   vowed _____

7.4

Put the following words into the correct column under the diphthong that is in the word. At the end all the columns should be even.

/e͡ɪ/	/o͡ʊ/	/a͡ɪ/	/a͡ʊ/	/ɔ͡ɪ/

noise   clothes   hound   boast   paste   shout   rake   time

round   choice   rope   mine   join   clay   climb

7.5

The following words are written in transcription. Write the word in orthography.

[ʃa͡ɪn] _____

[ðe͡ɪ] _____

[ʃa͡ʊt] _____

[sa͡ɪnz] _____

[vɔ͡ɪd] _____

[be͡ɪð] _____

[ʃo͡ʊz] _____

[be͡ɪʒ] _____

[ða͡ʊ] _____

[ko͡ʊd] _____

7.6

Underline the words that have one of the diphthongs in the *stressed* syllable.

poison   outdo   voyage   highway   joyful   bouquet

fountain   lousy   dinette   daisy   eighteen   diaper

neighbor   broken   polka   outrage   poker   diamond

7.7

Put the stress marker (') before the stressed syllable of the following words.

pas tel	bu cket
De cem ber	ju ven ile
ro mance	pa rent
a gree ment	com pu ter
wa llet	par snip
con tain er	fa mil iar
tou pee	a chieve
mul ti ply	um bre lla
hu mane	or gan
clar i net	in tro duce

Listen to the Examples in Module 7.

7.1 LISTEN

The following words contain the diphthong /eɪ/ and stop-plosives or fricatives. Transcribe the words.

1. _____
2. _____
3. _____
4. _____
5. _____
6. _____
7. _____
8. _____
9. _____
10. _____

7.2 LISTEN

The following words contain the diphthong /o͡ʊ/ and either stop-plosives or fricatives. Transcribe the words.

1. _____
2. _____
3. _____
4. _____
5. _____
6. _____
7. _____
8. _____
9. _____
10. _____

7.3 LISTEN

The following words contain the diphthong /a͡ɪ/ and either stop-plosives or fricatives. Transcribe the words.

1. _____
2. _____
3. _____
4. _____
5. _____
6. _____
7. _____
8. _____
9. _____
10. _____

7.4 LISTEN

The following words contain the diphthong /a͡ʊ/ with either stop-plosives or fricatives. Transcribe the words.

1. _____
2. _____
3. _____
4. _____
5. _____
6. _____
7. _____
8. _____
9. _____
10. _____

7.5 LISTEN

The following words contain the diphthong /ɔɪ/ with either stop-plosives or fricatives. Transcribe the words.

1. _____
2. _____
3. _____
4. _____
5. _____
6. _____
7. _____
8. _____
9. _____
10. _____

7.6 LISTEN

The following words contain either diphthongs and/or the vowels /i/, /ɑ/, or /u/ plus stop-plosives or fricatives. Transcribe the words.

1. _____
2. _____
3. _____
4. _____
5. _____
6. _____
7. _____
8. _____
9. _____

7.7 LISTEN

The following words contain the diphthongs and/or the vowels /i, ɑ, u, ɪ, ɛ, æ, or ʊ/ plus the stop-plosives and fricatives. Transcribe the words.

1. _____
2. _____
3. _____
4. _____
5. _____
6. _____
7. _____
8. _____
9. _____
10. _____

7.8 LISTEN

The following words contain the diphthongs and/or the vowels /i, ɑ, u, ɪ, ɛ, æ, or ʊ/ plus the stop-plosives and fricatives. Transcribe the following words.

Vicky (age 3;0)   Cindy (age 6;0)

1. _____   1. _____
2. _____   2. _____
3. _____   3. _____
4. _____   4. _____
5. _____   5. _____
6. _____   6. _____
7. _____   7. _____
8. _____   8. _____
9. _____   9. _____
10. _____   10. _____

7.9 LISTEN—STRESS

The following two-syllable words contain the diphthongs and/or the vowels /i, ɑ, u, ɪ, ɛ, æ, or ʊ/ plus the stop-plosives and fricatives. Transcribe the words, and put the stress marker before the stressed syllable.

1. _____
2. _____
3. _____
4. _____
5. _____
6. _____
7. _____
8. _____
9. _____
10. _____

Module 8—The Nasals /m/, /n/, and /ŋ/, the Approximants (Consisting of the Glides /w/ and /j/ plus the Liquids /l/ and /r/) and the Affricates /tʃ/ and /dʒ/

This module introduces several different consonants: the nasals, the approximants, and the affricates. The nasals /m/, /n/, and /ŋ/ are the only consonants in American English that are produced with the velum lowered so that airflow is through the nasal passage. The approximants /w/, /j/, /l/, and /r/ are produced with the articulators coming close to one another, however, not nearly as close as the constriction that creates the fricatives. /w/ and /j/ are often categorized as glides, /l/ and /r/ as liquids. The third group of consonants, the affricates /tʃ/ and /dʒ/, consist of a stop-plosive portion releasing to a homorganic fricative portion of the sound.

The nasal /m/ is normally heard in words such as "<u>m</u>ake," "ha<u>mm</u>er," and "gu<u>m</u>."

The nasal /n/ can typically be heard in words such as "<u>n</u>o," "wi<u>nn</u>er," and "te<u>n</u>."

In American English, the nasal /ŋ/ is only noted at the end of a word or syllable. It is a typical pronunciation in words such as "si<u>ng</u>," "si<u>ng</u>ing," and "thi<u>n</u>k."

The approximant (glide) /w/ is restricted to the beginning of a word or syllable in American English. It is a common pronunciation in the words "<u>w</u>in," "a<u>w</u>ay," and "<u>wh</u>en."

The approximant (glide) /j/ is also restricted to the beginning of a word or syllable in American English. It is normally heard in words such as "<u>y</u>ou," "<u>y</u>ellow," and "<u>y</u>o<u>y</u>o."

The lateral approximant (liquid) /l/ is typically heard in words such as "<u>l</u>ike," "wi<u>ll</u>ing," and "tai<u>l</u>."

The central approximant (liquid) /r/ is restricted to the beginning of a word or syllable in American English. It is a common pronunciation in "<u>r</u>abbit," "<u>r</u>un," and "a<u>r</u>ound."

The affricate /tʃ/ is heard in the typical pronunciation of "<u>ch</u>ew," "<u>ch</u>ur<u>ch</u>," and "wat<u>ch</u>."

The affricate /dʒ/ is a common pronunciation in the words "<u>j</u>ump," "<u>j</u>u<u>dge</u>," and "lo<u>dge</u>."

 Helpful Hints

1. The most frequent spelling for /m/ is the letter "m," but other spellings can infrequently be seen. For example, "mm" is pronounced as /m/ in words such as "hammer" and "swimming." In addition, the letters "lm," "mb," and "mn" can be pronounced as /m/. For example, some

individuals may pronounce the "lm" as /m/ in "palm" or "calm," while others may pronounce those words with an /l/ + /m/ combination. Words such as "comb" or "thumb" exemplify the "mb" spelling, while "hymn" demonstrates the "mn" spelling for /m/.

2. /n/ is most frequently spelled as "n," but four other spellings can be noted: "gn," "kn," "nn," and "pn." The spelling "gn" is pronounced as /n/ in words such as "gnat" and "gnawing," while the spelling "kn" as /n/ is noted in words such as "knee" and "knock." The letters "nn" represent /n/ in "running" or "bunny," while "pn" is pronounced /n/ in "pneumonia."

3. The most common spelling for /ŋ/ is "ng" in words such as "ring," "wing," and "thing." When the letter "n" is followed by "k" or "g,"—even if the "n" is in one syllable and the "k" or "g" is in the following syllable—/ŋ/ is typically the pronunciation. Words such as "mongoose" (/mɑŋgus/), "think" (/θɪŋk/), and "tango" (/tæŋgoʊ]/) exemplify this.

4. The most common spelling for /w/ is the letter "w," which is demonstrated in words such as "word," "win," and "wed." However, /w/ can also be spelled "wh" as in "whip" or "when." Historically, "wh" words have been pronounced with the voiceless /ʍ/. This is considered an allophonic variation of /w/ and is very infrequently heard in the pronunciation of speakers of American English. Other spellings for /w/ include "u" when it follows the letter "q," as in "queen" or "quiet." On occasion the letter "o" may be pronounced as /w/ as in "one" or "once."

5. The sound /j/ is commonly spelled "y" as in "yellow" or "you," but is heard when "i" is combined with "o" in words such as "union" (here /j/ is at the beginning of the word and at the beginning of the second syllable) and "Junior" (at the beginning of the second syllable). /j/ can also be heard in words where consonants are followed by "u" as in "figure," "music," or "ambulance."

6. The sound /l/ is commonly spelled "l" or "ll" as in "lamp" or "telling."

7. The sound /r/ is most frequently spelled with the letters "r" or "rr" as in "rip" or "stirring." On occasion, /r/ can be spelled "wr," where the "w" is a silent letter. Words such as "write" and "wren" exemplify this.

8. The affricate /tʃ/ is often spelled as "ch," "t," and "tch." The letters "ch" are pronounced /tʃ/ in "chew" and "which," the spelling "t" is pronounced /tʃ/ in words such as "feature" and "lecture," and the letters "tch" are pronounced /tʃ/ as in "watch" and "ditch." Less frequent spellings include "c" as in "cello," and "t" may be pronounced as /tʃ/ in words such as "question" and "culture."

9. The affricate /dʒ/ is commonly spelled with "g" or "j." The words "germ" and "joy" exemplify these spellings. Less common spellings include "dg" ("ledge" or "dodge"), "gg" ("exaggerate"), and "gi" ("legion," "religion"). When "d" is followed by "j," it is pronounced /dʒ/ as in "adjust" and "adjourn." In addition, when a vowel follows "d," it can be occasionally pronounced as /dʒ/ as in "soldier" and "educate."

8.1

Underline the words that contain either the /m/, /n/, or /ŋ/ sounds.

album   robber   opener   nickel   strong   flying
rainbow   knight   signature   gnome   winter   famous

Underline the words that contain either /w/ or /j/ sounds.

once   show   write   you   wrist   yellow
wrinkle   unit   yodel   universal   wedding   now

Underline the words that contain either /l/ or /r/ sounds.

foolish   lounge   rocky   stall   wrote   carrot
garage   orange   station   ceiling   clock   whale

Underline the words that contain either the /tʃ/ or /dʒ/ sounds.

cheese   witch   June   germ   edge   wage
Peggy   magic   major   figure   dragon   pledge

8.2

The following words are written in phonetic transcription. Write the word orthographically.

/m/, /n/, /ŋ/

[min] _____

[nu] _____

[sɑŋ] _____

[mun] _____

[nɑt] _____

[mɪnt] _____

[θɪŋk] _____

[maɪk] _____

[noʊz] _____

[maʊs] _____

/w/, /j/

[wi] _____

[ju] _____

[wɪʃ] _____

[juzd] _____

[jɛs] _____

[wʊd] _____

[weɪt] _____

[wɑk] _____

[juθ] _____

[jist] _____

/l/, /r/

[lup] _____

[rid] _____

[lɑst] _____

[rɑɪd] _____

[ræft] _____

[leɪk] _____

[lik] _____

[lɑʊd] _____

[reɪk] _____

[roʊst] _____

/tʃ/, /dʒ/

[tʃu] _____

[dʒɑb] _____

[tʃɪp] _____

[bædʒ] _____

[dʒæk] _____

[dʒus] _____

[tʃiz] _____

[tʃeɪs] _____

[tʃuz] _____

[dʒɔɪ] _____

8.3

Transcribe the following pairs of words.

moon	_____	noon	_____
rake	_____	lake	_____
sin	_____	sing	_____
meat	_____	neat	_____
rich	_____	ridge	_____
room	_____	loom	_____
lock	_____	rock	_____
mope	_____	nope	_____
wrong	_____	long	_____
cheap	_____	jeep	_____
reed	_____	weed	_____
west	_____	rest	_____
mice	_____	nice	_____
lap	_____	wrap	_____
wedge	_____	ledge	_____
rich	_____	witch	_____
yes	_____	Les	_____
moan	_____	loan	_____
lick	_____	wick	_____
job	_____	rob	_____

8.4

Underline each of the words that has /m/, /n/, or /ŋ/ in the stressed syllable.

measure	canal	finish	mountain	prisoner	moustache
musical	command	humid	winner	honey	boating
segment	polishing	necklace	medal	human	jasmine

Underline each of the words that has /w/, /j/, /r/, or /l/ in the stressed syllable.

away	wagon	united	union	awake	someone
younger	latitude	limousine	delete	raisin	receipt
erase	await	kayak	Yahoo		

Underline each of the words that has /tʃ/ or /dʒ/ in the stressed syllable.

chestnut   Japan   jockey   chosen   coaches   agent

peachy   bewitch   suggest   ostrich   region

The following words are written in phonetic transcription. Write the word orthographically.

[blitʃ]   _____

[meɪlmæn]   _____

[nɔɪzi]   _____

[maɪgret]   _____

[pæŋkeɪk]   _____

[muvi]   _____

[roʊzi]   _____

[nɑkɪŋ]   _____

[niɑn]   _____

[rɪŋɪŋ]   _____

[dɑŋki]   _____

[reɪbiz]   _____

[kɑkrotʃ]   _____

[rɛdwʊd]   _____

[wɑʃklɑθ]   _____

[kiwi]   _____

[tʃɪli]   _____

[reɪlweɪ]   _____

[junaɪt]   _____

[dʒɛlifɪʃ]   _____

[juzɪŋ]   _____

[kaɪoʊti]   _____

[dʒɪpsi]   _____

[daɪdʒest]   _____

[ɛnreɪdʒ]   _____

8.6

There are many words with the sound /bj/, /pj/, /fj/, /vj/, /kj/, /mj/, or /kw/ spelled with "u." "Puny" and "fuel" exemplify this. Underline each of the following words if you hear /j/ or /w/ within the word.

fool   fuel   curve   beauty   cute   queen

quite   curl   quilt   choir   liquid   view

square   bootie   music   amuse   amend   cube

8.7

To note the boundary between syllables, a period "." is used. The following words are marked according to this principle. Mark the stressed syllable (ˈ) for the following words.

/toʊ.ki.oʊ/

/bæ.gɪdʒ/

/ɛn.geɪdʒ/

/sæn.wɪtʃ/

/maɪ.sɛlf/

/nɛf.ju/

/ræ.kun/

/i.vɛnt/

/reɪ.ʃoʊ/

/ri.lif/

Listen to the Examples in Module 8.

8.1 LISTEN

Transcribe the following words with /m/, /n/, or /ŋ/.

1. _____

2. _____

3. _____

4. _____

5. _____

6. _____

7. _____

8. _____

9. _____

10. _____

8.2 LISTEN

Transcribe the following words with /m/, /n/, or /ŋ/.

1. _____

2. _____

3. _____

4. _____

5. _____

6. _____

7. _____

8. _____

9. _____

10. _____

8.3 LISTEN

Transcribe the following words with /w/, /j/, /r/, or /l/.

1. _____

2. _____

3. _____

4. _____

5. _____

6. _____

7. _____

8. _____

9. _____

10. _____

8.4 LISTEN

breathy quality to voice

Transcribe the following words with /w/, /j/, /r/, or /l/.

1. /ˈlæso/ → /ˈlæsoʊ/   /motəb/

2. /ˈvækʌm/ → /ˈvækjʌm/

✱ 3. /ˈjɛlo/ → /ˈjɛloʊ/   "yellow"

4. /ˈwɪndo/ → /ˈwɪndoʊ/

5. /bʌtji/ → /byuti/

6. /ˈlaʊsi/ → /ˈlaʊzi/

7. /rɑki/

8. /lusɪŋ/ → /luzɪŋ/

9. /redio/

10. /wrɑʃɛd/

8.5 LISTEN

Transcribe the following words with /tʃ/ and /dʒ/.

1. _____

2. _____

3. _____

4. _____

5. _____

6. _____

7. _____

8. _____

9. _____

10. _____

11. _____

12. _____

13. _____

14. _____

15. _____

16. _____

17. _____

18. _____

19. _____

Module 9—The Central Vowels /ʌ/, /ə/, /ɝ/, and /ɚ/

This module introduces the four central vowels: /ʌ/, /ə/, /ɝ/, and /ɚ/. These vowels are characterized by a centralized positioning of the body of the tongue. Two of the central vowels, /ɝ/ and /ɚ/, have r-coloring. Thus, these vowels have perceptual and production qualities that are similar to the r-sound. Also, two of these vowels, /ʌ/ and /ɝ/, are stressed vowels. As such, their productions are marked by more intensity, typically a higher fundamental frequency and a longer duration when compared to their unstressed counterparts. The stressed vowel /ʌ/ has as its unstressed counterpart /ə/, while the stressed /ɝ/ has the corresponding unstressed vowel noted in /ɚ/. The /ʌ/ vowel can be heard in words such as "hut" or "stuck," while the /ə/ vowel is the vowel in the first syllable of "above" and "away." The central vowel with r-coloring /ɝ/ can be heard in "bird" or "word," while /ɚ/ is the vowel at the end of the second syllable in "father" and "mother."

Helpful Hints

1. The central vowel /ʌ/ can be spelled in a number of different ways. The most common spelling is "u" as in "shut" and "luck." However, it can also be spelled "o-e" as in "come" and "some," "oe" as in "does," and "ou" as in "rough" and "cousin."
2. The central vowel /ə/ can be spelled countless ways. This is due to the fact that vowel reduction occurs frequently. Vowel reduction, which was covered in Chapter 4, occurs as the rate of speaking increases or as the stress on a vowel is decreased. In these cases, the length of the vowel is reduced, and it is often produced as a schwa vowel, /ə/. Theoretically, most vowels could be reduced. Dewey (1971) notes a total of forty-three different spellings. Some common spellings are "a" and "o," when the stress is on the second syllable as in "amaze," "assign," "occur," and "object." The important thing to note with this vowel is that it represents the "uh" quality but in unstressed syllables. Several exercises will be directed to listening and transcribing this vowel.
3. The stressed central vowel with r-coloring /ɝ/ has four fairly common spellings: "er," "ir," "or," and "ur." The letters "er" represent this sound in words such as "herb" or "mermaid. The spelling "ir" is pronounced /ɝ/ in words such as "bird" and "first," while this sound can be heard in "word" or "world," spelled with "or." The letters "ur" represent this sound in words such as "purse" and "turn." The letters "ear" can also represent this sound in words such as "earth" and "pearl."
4. The unstressed central vowel with r-coloring /ɚ/ is commonly represented with the spellings "er," "or," and "ar." The spelling "er" as /ɚ/ can be noted at the end of words such as "player" or "danger." The "or" spelling as /ɚ/ is exemplified by the word endings in "pastor" and "tractor," while "ar" is noted as the last sound in words such as "pillar" and "burglar."

9.1

Underline the words that contain /ʌ/ or /ɝ/.

bird	cuff	dough	jump	fudge	bus
huge	word	clear	shirt	stir	east
church	fire	cup	nut	tune	cute

9.2

Underline the words that could contain /ə/ in typical pronunciations. Remember that this vowel will be in the unstressed syllable.

ago	ego	avoid	acre	balloon	cologne
copy	costume	canoe	afraid	petite	attack
agent	eighteen	buffet	salute	mesa	maybe

9.3

Underline the words that contain /ɚ/ in typical pronunciations. Remember that this vowel will be in the unstressed syllable.

father	mayor	major	freighter	antler	laser
percent	surprise	survey	bazaar	wonderful	longer
chowder	doctor	urgent	early	perspire	strainer

9.4

The following words are written in phonetic transcription. They contain either the stressed central vowel /ʌ/ or the stressed central vowel /ɝ/ with r-coloring. Write the words orthographically.

[tʃɝtʃ] _____

[dʒʌdʒ] _____

[sʌŋ] _____

[stɝ] _____

[ɝθ] _____

[ɝdʒ] _____

[bʌŋk] _____

[kʌm] _____

[lʌntʃ] _____

[tʌŋ] _____

9.5

The following words are written in phonetic transcription. They contain either the unstressed central vowel /ə/ or the unstressed central vowel with r-coloring /ɚ/. Write each of the words orthographically.

[sɪstɚ] _____

[teɪlɚ] _____

[əblum] _____

[əweɪ] _____

[bətɑn] _____

[pəlut] _____

[bæŋkɚ] _____

[hæmstɚ] _____

[səpoʊz] _____

[pəlis] _____

9.6

Look at the transcription of the central vowel sounds in the following words. According to the typical pronunciation, which ones are correct ☺ and which ones are incorrect ☹?

[ʌproʊtʃ]	☺	☹
[əvɔɪd]	☺	☹
[kəmpit]	☺	☹
[ɝli]	☺	☹
[bɚθdeɪ]	☺	☹
[fɑðɚ]	☺	☹
[məŋki]	☺	☹
[pɚhæps]	☺	☹
[beɪkɚ]	☺	☹
[mʌʃrum]	☺	☹

9.7

Stressing: Put the stress marker (') before the stressed syllable.

ca len dar   ca the dral

vol ca no   di a gram

re co mmend   de ter gent

pre ci sion   se cure ly

po pu lar   dis a ppear

Listen to the Examples in Module 9.

9.1 LISTEN

Transcribe the following one- and two-syllable words with /ʌ/.

1. _____
2. _____
3. _____
4. _____
5. _____
6. _____
7. _____
8. _____
9. _____
10. _____

9.2 LISTEN

Transcribe the following one- and two-syllable words with /ʌ/.

Matt (age 10;2)   Gail (age 6;0)

1. _____   1. _____
2. _____   2. _____
3. _____   3. _____
4. _____   4. _____
5. _____   5. _____
6. _____   6. _____
7. _____   7. _____
8. _____   8. _____
9. _____   9. _____
10. _____   10. _____

9.3 LISTEN

Transcribe the following one- and two-syllable words with /ɝ/.

1. _____
2. _____
3. _____
4. _____
5. _____
6. _____
7. _____
8. _____

9. _____
10. _____
11. _____
12. _____
13. _____
14. _____
15. _____
16. _____
17. _____
18. _____

9.4 LISTEN

Transcribe the following two-syllable words with /ə/.

1. _____
2. _____
3. _____
4. _____
5. _____
6. _____
7. _____
8. _____
9. _____
10. _____
11. _____
12. _____
13. _____
14. _____
15. _____
16. _____
17. _____
18. _____
19. _____
20. _____

9.5 LISTEN

Transcribe the following two-syllable words with /ɚ/.

1. _____
2. _____
3. _____
4. _____
5. _____

6. _____
7. _____
8. _____
9. _____
10. _____
11. _____
12. _____
13. _____
14. _____
15. _____
16. _____
17. _____

9.6 LISTEN

Transcribe the following two-syllable words with /ʌ/, /ɝ/, /ə/, and/or /ɚ/. Place the stress marker (') before the stressed syllable of each word.

1. ɝ _____
2. ɝ, ə _____
3. ɝ, ə _____
4. ɚ, ə _____
5. ʌ _____
6. ə, ʌ _____
7. ʌ, ʌ _____
8. ʌ, ə _____
9. ʌ, ə _____
10. ɚ _____

9.7 LISTEN

Transcribe the following two-syllable words with /ʌ/, /ɝ/, /ə/, and/or /ɚ/. Place the stress marker (') before the stressed syllable of each word.

1. _____
2. _____
3. _____
4. _____
5. _____
6. _____
7. _____
8. _____
9. _____
10. _____

MODULE 10—*The Centering or Rhotic Diphthongs* /ɑ͡ɚ/, /ɛ͡ɚ/, /ɪ͡ɚ/, *and* /o͡ɚ/

Centering diphthongs as those diphthongs that are produced with a central vowel as an offglide. In General American English, the central vowel with r-coloring /ɚ/ is commonly used as the offglide, thus the label *rhotic diphthong.*

Theoretically, any vowel could be combined with /ɚ/ to form a rhotic diphthong; however, in General American English the more common ones appear to be /ɑ͡ɚ/, /ɛ͡ɚ/, /ɪ͡ɚ/, and /o͡ɚ/. These rhotic diphthongs will be covered in this module.

It is important to note that there are typically at least two different ways to transcribe these diphthongs: as noted above, with the central vowel with r-coloring, or with the /r/ symbol. Thus, /ɑr/, /ɛr/, /ɪr/, and /or/ can be seen as possible transcriptions. A further complication is that /or/ is often transcribed as /ɔ͡ɚ/ or /ɔr/.

Please check with your instructor as to the way these transcriptions should be written. This workbook will use the central vowel with r-coloring /ɚ/ throughout the exercises.

Word examples include the following:

/ɑ͡ɚ/—"farm," "bar," "tar"

/ɛ͡ɚ/—"hair," "bear," "chair"

/ɪ͡ɚ/—"clear," "beer," "here"

/o͡ɚ/—"bore," "door," "store"

Please note that pronunciations may vary from speaker to speaker and depend upon dialectal variations. Check with your instructor to determine which pronunciations are more common in your area.

Helpful Hints

1. The centering diphthong /ɑ͡ɚ/ is most commonly spelled with "ar" as in "chart" and "harp." However, "ear" and "uar" can be noted, as in "heart" and "guard."
2. /ɛ͡ɚ/ can be spelled with "ear" as in "bear," "air" as in "chair," or "ar" as in "care." Other spellings include "arr" as in "carry" and "err" as in "ferry." Pronunciations can vary between /ɛ͡ɚ/ and /e͡ɚ/ with these words.
3. The centering diphthong /ɪ͡ɚ/ can be spelled several ways. For example, "ear" is noted in "hear," "ier" in "fierce," and "eer" in "cheer." Pronunciations can vary between /ɪ͡ɚ/ and /i͡ɚ/.
4. The centering diphthong /o͡ɚ/ is commonly spelled "oa" or "or." For example, the spelling "oa" is noted in "board," while /o͡ɚ/ is spelled as "or" in "born." The spelling "aur" is uncommon but is present in the word "aura," for example. Pronunciations can vary between /o͡ɚ/ and /ɔ͡ɚ/.

10.1

Underline the words that could be pronounced with the centering diphthong /ɑ͡ɚ/.

charm	barn	carry	farm	dare	pearl
darling	pair	wars	bargain	harbor	certain

Underline the words that could be pronounced with the centering diphthong /ɛ͡ɚ/.

very	cherry	fear	pierce	sheriff	errand
car	rare	there	hardy	parsley	absurd

Underline the words that could be pronounced with the centering diphthong /ɪ͡ɚ/.

clear	carrot	start	bird	cheer	deer
here	near	fire	birch	ear	sheer

Underline the words that could be pronounced with the centering diphthong /o͡ɚ/.

oar	board	world	worship	born	worm
door	force	ourself	horn	horse	court

10.2

The following words are written in phonetic transcription with the centering or rhotic diphthongs. Write the word orthographically.

[t͡ʃɑ͡ɚd͡ʒ] _____

[ho͡ɚs] _____

[ɪ͡ɚɪŋ] _____

[skwɛ͡ɚ] _____

[nɛ͡ɚo] _____

[bɑ͡ɚli] _____

[t͡ʃɛ͡ɚi] _____

[nĩ͡ɚɚ] _____

10.3

Underline the words with one of the centering diphthongs: /ɑ͡ɚ/, /ɛ͡ɚ/, /ɪ͡ɚ/, or /o͡ɚ/.

barn	burn
fare	fir

purr	pear
sore	sir
bird	board
curry	Kerry
furry	ferry
her	hair
sure	share
heart	her

10.4

The following words contain either the centering diphthong /ɑ˞/, /ɛ˞/, /ɪ˞/, or /o˞/ or the central vowel with r-coloring /ɝ/. Write the words orthographically.

[sɝˑdʒən] _____

[θɝˑti] _____

[wɛ͡ɚˑha͡ʊs] _____

[ɑ͡ɚˑmi] _____

[ho͡ɚˑsʃu] _____

[tɑ͡ɚˑ] _____

[mɝˑme͡ɪd] _____

[hɛ͡ɚˑɪŋ] _____

[hɪ͡ɚˑɪŋ] _____

10.5

The following words are written orthographically and in phonetic transcription. Put a stress marker before the primary stressed syllable. Fill in the blanks in the phonetic transcription with the appropriate vowel symbols.

strawberry	[strɑ.b_ _i]
carefully	[k_ _.fʊ.li]
murmuring	[m_ _.m_ _.ɪŋ]
ceramics	[s_ _.æ.mɪks]
embarass	[ɛm.b_ _.əs]
glorious	[gl_ _.i.əs]
pioneer	[pa͡ɪ.ə.n_ _]
dinosaur	[da͡ɪ.nə.s_ _]
turbulence	[t_ _.bju.ləns]
performance	[p_ _.f_ _.məns]

Listen to the Examples in Module 10.

10.1 LISTEN

Transcribe the following words that contain the centering diphthong /ɑɚ/, /ɛɚ/, /ɪɚ/, or /oɚ/.

1. _____
2. _____
3. _____
4. _____
5. _____
6. _____
7. _____
8. _____

10.2 LISTEN

Transcribe the following words that contain the centering diphthong /ɑɚ/, /ɛɚ/, /ɪɚ/, or /oɚ/.

1. _____
2. _____
3. _____
4. _____
5. _____
6. _____
7. _____
8. _____

10.3 LISTEN

The following words contain either the centering diphthong /ɑɚ/, /ɛɚ/, /ɪɚ/, or /oɚ/, or the central vowel with r-coloring /ɝ/. Transcribe the words.

Matt (age 10;0)

1. _____
2. _____
3. _____
4. _____
5. _____
6. _____
7. _____
8. _____
9. _____
10. _____

10.4 LISTEN

The following words contain three syllables. Transcribe the words: (1) Please put a period "." to mark the syllable boundaries. (2) Mark the primary stressed syllable by placing a (') before the stressed syllable. (3) Note the frequent use of the schwa vowel in unstressed syllables.

1. _____
2. _____
3. _____
4. _____
5. _____
6. _____
7. _____
8. _____
9. _____
10. _____
11. _____
12. _____
13. _____
14. _____
15. _____
16. _____
17. _____
18. _____
19. _____
20. _____

Module 11—Introducing the Diacritics

This module will introduce the diacritics. The first part of the exercises will consist of identifying the symbols that are used for the diacritics. The listening portion of the module will contrast the diacritics that are used more frequently when transcribing disordered speech.

Dentalized, Palatalized, Velarized, and Lateralized

Dentalized refers to an articulatory variation in which the tongue approaches the upper incisors. It is marked by a /ˌ/ placed under the IPA symbol. For the word "team" /tim/, a dentalized production of /t/ would be noted as /t̪im/.

Palatalization refers to an articulation in which the tongue approaches the palate. Only sounds that are not palatal sounds can be palatalized. For those sounds in which the alveolar ridge is the passive articulator (/n, t, d, s, z, l/ and the postalveolars /ʃ, ʒ, r/), this means that the tongue placement is more posterior. For velar consonants (/k, g, ŋ/), palatalization indicates that the articulation has moved somewhat more forward. The elevated /ʲ/ after the symbol in question is the diacritic used for palatalization. Thus, /sʲɑk/ for "sock" would indicate a palatalized /s/.

Velarization refers to the posterior movement of the tongue placement: for example, in the direction of the velum for palatal sounds. According to the IPA, the symbol for velarization is a /ˠ/ placed after the symbol in question. The exception to this is the velarized or dark l-sound. The dark l-sound (/ɫ/) is typically found in word-final position, before a consonant and following back vowels.

Lateralization refers to the airstream being released laterally during a sound production. In Standard American English, there is one lateral consonant, /l/. Note how the tongue tip is positioned on the alveolar ridge and the edges of the tongue are fairly flat, allowing the air to escape on both sides. Lateral releases are noted by the /ˡ/ (an elevated /l/) placed behind the sound in question. Thus, /dˡ/ would indicate a laterally released /d/. However, children can lateralize /s/ and /z/ sounds. When this occurs, the symbols used are /ɬ/ and /ɮ/, because this is seen as a primary, rather than a secondary articulation. The /ɬ/ is the voiceless lateral alveolar fricative, while /ɮ/ is the voiced lateral fricative.

Exercises

11.1

Look at the following transcriptions and note whether the diacritic indicates a sound is dentalized, palatalized, velarized, or lateralized. Write the correct term in the space provided.

[sʲup] _____

[t̪iθ] _____

[ʃʲɑp] _____

[ʃˠu] _____

[ɬɪp] _____

[ʒɪpɚ] _____

[fuɬ] _____

[d̪ɑk] _____

[pipəɬ] _____

[tˠuz] _____

[sʲun] _____

[s̪e͡ɪlɚ] _____

11.2

The following words are written orthographically. After each of the words, the term *dentalized, palatalized, velarized,* or *lateralized* is written. Transcribe the word using the correct diacritic.

sun	palatalized /s/	_____
toe	dentalized /t/	_____
sister	lateralized /s/	_____
shopping	velarized /ʃ/	_____
pulled	velarized /l/	_____
touch	palatalized /t/	_____
zebra	lateralized /z/	_____
stool	dentalized /s/	_____
singing	palatalized /s/	_____

Devoicing, Partial Devoicing, Voicing, and Partial Voicing

There are voiced and voiceless consonants of American English. However, on occasion, voiced consonants can be totally or partially devoiced. On the other hand, voiceless consonants can be produced with total or partial devoicing. If total voicing or devoicing occurs, the corresponding symbol is used. For example, if /s/ would become totally voiced, we would transcribe this as /z/. If /d/ would be produced with total devoicing, /t/ would be transcribed. For partial devoicing and voicing, specific diacritics are used. The diacritic for partial devoicing is a small circle placed under the sound symbol (if that placement interferes with the clarity of the basic symbol, it is acceptable to put the circle above the sound symbol). Partial voicing is noted by a diacritic mark like a lowercase "v" under the respective sound symbol. Therefore, /z̥/ would indicate a partially devoiced /z/, while /s̬/ would be the transcription for a partially voiced /s/.

11.3

The following words are written orthographically and in phonetic transcription. Indicate whether the transcription demonstrates (1) partial devoicing, (2) total devoicing, (3) partial voicing, or (4) total voicing.

tan	[dæn]	_____
big	[b̥ɪg]	_____
zoo	[su]	_____
get	[g̊ɛt]	_____
log	[lɑk]	_____
beige	[be͡ɪʒ̊]	_____
fan	[f̬æn]	_____
walk	[wɑk̬]	_____
visit	[vɪz̥ət]	_____
winner	[ʍɪnɚ]	_____

11.4

Transcribe the following words with the noted changes in production.

Sunday	partial voicing of /s/	_____
gopher	partial devoicing of /g/	_____
clever	partial voicing of /k/	_____
leisure	partial devoicing of /ʒ/	_____
shaking	partial voicing of /ʃ/	_____
bathe	partial devoicing of /ð/	_____
wearing	total devoicing of /w/	_____
baseballs	partial devoicing of /z/	_____
kissing	partial voicing of /s/	_____
tongues	partial devoicing of /z/	_____

Aspiration, Nonaspiration, and Unreleased Stop-Plosives

Stop-plosive consonants can be produced with a notable release of air which is labeled *aspiration*. Aspiration is that slight puff of air that you hear after the /p/ and /t/ if you pronounce the word "pie" or "toe." This is transcribed as /pʰ/ or /tʰ/, the small raised /ʰ/ representing the diacritic for aspiration. The voiceless stop-plosives /p/, /t/, and /k/ are typically aspirated at the beginning of a word. However, the voiceless stop-plosives are unaspirated following /s/, as in the word "speed." The symbol for unaspirated is /˭/ following the stop-plosive. In this case, "speed" could be transcribed /sp˭id/. Typically, the diacritics for aspiration and nonaspiration are not used to indicate normal pronunciations. The third diacritic in this group is the one for unreleased stop-plosives. Stop-plosives can be unreleased at the end of a word. *Unreleased* indicates that the articulators come together but there is no releasing movement, The diacritic for unreleased is /˺/, which is placed after the stop-plosive symbol in question. Therefore, an unreleased /t/ might be a possible pronunciation for "street," /strit˺/. It is a good idea to note unreleased stop-plosives. Unreleased stop-plosives at the end of words or utterances are considered a normal pronunciation; however, they may sound like a deletion of a final consonant when you are later listening to your tape recording.

11.5

The following words are written in phonetic transcription. Identify the word orthographically and write whether the diacritic used indicates an aspirated, an unaspirated, or an unreleased production.

Transcription	*Word Orthography*	*Diacritic Used*
/pʰɪloʊ/	_____	_____
/roʊbɑt˺/	_____	_____
/ɝˑnəst˭/	_____	_____
/ʃrʌb˺/	_____	_____
/ækrəbæt˭/	_____	_____
/tʰɑlɚ/	_____	_____
/rəgrɛt˭]	_____	_____
/sp˭iɚˑmɪnt/	_____	_____
/kʰætəlɑg/	_____	_____
/tʌgboʊt˺/	_____	_____

11.6

Write the following words in phonetic transcription. Use the diacritic that is indicated.

sparrow	unaspirated /p/	_____
report	unreleased /t/	_____
position	aspirated /p/	_____
skeleton	unaspirated /k/	_____
dialogue	unreleased /g/	_____
schedule	unaspirated /k/	_____
turpentine	aspirated initial /t/	_____
dynamite	unaspirated /t/	_____
Wichita	aspirated /t/	_____
expand	unreleased /d/	_____

Flap

The flap (also called a tap or one-tap trill) is an allophonic variation of /t/ and /d/. This variation often occurs when either /t/ or /d/ are produced between two vowels, such as in "matter" or "sadder." The flap articulation involves a single rapid contact between the active and passive articulators. The contact is very brief; there is no build-up of air pressure. Instead, it is a rapid movement toward the alveolar ridge. The tongue may approximate the alveolar ridge or touch it briefly. The diacritic symbol for the flap is /ɾ/.

11.7

Transcribe the following words, first noting a pronunciation with either a /t/ or /d/. Next transcribe the word with a flap. Say both words and listen to the differences.

Word	Transcription with /t/ or /d/	Transcription with Flap
ladder	_____	_____
butter	_____	_____
city	_____	_____
dirty	_____	_____
cloudy	_____	_____
stutter	_____	_____
charity	_____	_____
satisfy	_____	_____
guitar	_____	_____
variety	_____	_____

Syllabics

Unstressed syllables often become reduced syllables. If the vowel nucleus is reduced, a syllabic can result. In this case, the consonant becomes the nucleus of the syllable. Syllabics are marked by a small vertical line placed under the consonant that has become the syllable nucleus. Thus, "little" in which the final /əl/ is reduced to /l/ is transcribed as /l̩/, thus, /lɪtl̩/. Typically, only certain sounds become syllabics: /l/, /m/, and /n/ are the most common. The articulatory position of the syllabic relative to the final consonant of the preceding syllable is important. Some authors (e.g., Edwards, 2003) state that there needs to be a homorganic relationship between the final consonant of the preceding syllable and the syllabic. Thus, the active articulator must be the same (or approximately the same) for both consonants. In order for a syllabic to occur, the consonants /p/ and /b/ must precede /m/, while /t/, /d/, /s/, and /z/, must precede /n/ and /k/, and /g/ must precede /ŋ/. However, there are exceptions to this rule. Edwards (2003) notes that /t/ preceding the syllabic /l/ will typically cause the /t/ to be pronounced as [ɾ], while /t/ before the syllabic /n/ will result in [ʔ], the glottal stop.

11.8

Transcribe the following words, first without a syllabic, i.e., as an unreduced syllable, and second, with a syllabic consonant. Say the two pronunciations, noting the differences.

Word	Unreduced Syllable	With Syllabic
shuttle	[ʃʌtəl] or [ʃʌɾəl]	[ʃʌt̩] or [ʃʌɾ̩]
bottle	_____	_____
handle	_____	_____
button	_____	_____
flatten	_____	_____
rotten	_____	_____
cattle	_____	_____
widen	_____	_____
little	_____	_____
rattle	_____	_____

Labialization/Nonlabialization of Consonants

Most consonants are produced without lip rounding. The consonants /w/ and /ʃ/ are the exceptions: They do have lip rounding. The term *labialization* is used when normally unrounded consonants are now articulated with lip rounding. Nonlabialization denotes the unrounding of normally rounded consonants. The diacritic used for labialization is an elevated /ʷ/ placed after the symbol in question. The diacritic for nonlabialization is an arrow pointing in both directions. Therefore, /sʷ/ indicates a labialized /s/ production, while /ʃ↔/ is an /ʃ/ produced without the characteristic lip rounding.

11.9

Transcribe the following words, first without labialization and, second, with labialization of the underlined portion. Listen to the differences as you pronounce the two words.

Word	Transcription Without Labialization	Transcription with Labialization
<u>sh</u>op	_____	_____
<u>sh</u>eep	_____	_____
<u>sh</u>ed	_____	_____
<u>sh</u>ow	_____	_____
<u>sh</u>ower	_____	_____
wi<u>sh</u>	_____	_____
lea<u>sh</u>	_____	_____

shell   _____   _____

ru<u>sh</u>   _____   _____

Diacritics with Vowels

The diacritics that are used with vowels are categorized according to (1) the rounding or unrounding and (2) the changes in tongue placement for the vowels. Changes in tongue placement can reflect raising/lowering or advancing/retracting the tongue.

If a normally rounded vowel such as /u/ is produced with less rounding than normal, then a small "c" character is placed under the vowel in question. Thus /ṵ/ would indicate a production that clearly has less rounding than normal. If an unrounded vowel, such as /i/, is produced with lip rounding, then an inverted "c" ("ɔ") is placed under the vowel in question. /i̹/ would indicate lip rounding during the /i/ production.

Changes in tongue position are described in terms of (1) the extent to which the tongue is raised or lowered in the direction of the hard or soft palate (vertical dimensions), and (2) whether the highest point of the tongue for vowel production is more anteriorly (labeled "advanced") or more posteriorly located (labeled "retracted"). The diacritic for raised is /ˍ/, which is placed under the vowel symbol in question, while /ˌ/ is the symbol used for a more lowered tongue position. The diacritic for a more advanced tongue position is "+" placed under the vowel; for a more retracted position, "–" is placed under the vowel symbol.

Examples:

/æ̝/ The tongue is slightly elevated from the normal /æ/ position.

/ṵ/ The tongue is slightly lower than the normal /u/ position.

/u̟/ The tongue is more anteriorly positioned than for the normal /u/.

/i̠/ The tongue is more posteriorly positioned than for the normal /i/.

11.10

The following words are written in phonetic transcription with the diacritics for the vowel production. Write the word orthographically and then note what the diacritic represents.

Transcribe the following words with the noted diacritics.

Transcribed Word	Written Word	Meaning of Diacritic
/kɑ̝t/	cot	/ɑ/ is produced with a higher tongue position
/kli̹n/	_____	_____
/ʃʊ̜d/	_____	_____
/stri̠t/	_____	_____
/klæ̟s/	_____	_____

/θɪ̝ŋk/	________________	________________
/klæ̟səfa͡ɪ/	________________	________________
/θɪ̞sl̩/	________________	________________
/tʃɑ̞k/	________________	________________
/wɪ̝θ/	________________	________________

11.11

wealthy	elevated /ɛ/	________________
glamorous	retracted /æ/	________________
sympathy	lowered /ɪ/	________________
understood	advanced /ʊ/	________________
measuring	lowered /ɛ/	________________
cucumber	advanced /u/	________________
option	raised /ɑ/	________________
agreement	advanced /i/	________________
cassette	retracted /ɛ/	________________
thankful	raised /æ/	________________
pushing	advanced /ʊ/	________________
breathing	lowered /i/	________________

Nasality/Nonnasality

Nasality is marked with a diacritic if a nonnasal sound (all the vowels and consonants with the exception of /m/, /n/, and /ŋ/) become excessively nasal. The diacritic for this is the tiled (˜) placed over the sound symbol in question. Thus, /bẽˈbĩ/ would indicate that both vowels were perceived as having an excessive nasal quality. On the other hand, if one of the nasal consonants /m/, /n/, or /ŋ/ is produced without this nasal quality (which could be the case if the nasal cavity was congested or if a child has excessively large adenoids), then the tilde is used with two lines through it ͊ to indicate lack of nasality.

11.12

The following words are written in phonetic transcription. Write the word orthographically and identify the diacritic.

Word	*Written Word*	*Identify the Diacritic*
/rətr̃ĩt/	________________	________________
/tɛn͊tətɪv/	________________	________________
/skræ̃tʃi/	________________	________________

/fɪn͋əʃ/		
/dra͡ʊt/		
/m͋ɪn͋/		
/tɛn͋θ/		
/gre͡ɪps/		
/glʌ̃vz/		
/m͋ɝm͋ɚ/		

Listen to the Examples in Module 11.

11.1 LISTEN—DENTALIZED

The first word spoken is a typical pronunciation. Note the sound at the beginning of the word. The second of the pair is the same word but with a dentalized production. Transcribe each of the words.

Word	*Transcription of Typical Production*	*Transcription of Dentalized Production*
song	/saŋ/	[s̪aŋ]
saw	/sa/	[sʲa]
sad	/sæd/	[s̪æd]
sick		
zoo		

11.2 LISTEN—PALATALIZED

The first word spoken is a typical pronunciation. Note the sound at the beginning of the word. The second of the pair is the same word but with a palatalized production. Transcribe each of the words.

Word	*Transcription of Typical Production*	*Transcription of Palatalized Production*
sent	/sɪnt/	[sʲɪnt]
soak	/sok/	[sʲok]
sell		
sit		
zebra		

11.3 LISTEN—LATERALIZED

The first word spoken is a typical pronunciation. Note the sound at the beginning of the word. The second of the pair is the same word but with a lateralized /s/ or /z/ production. Transcribe each of the words.

Word	Transcription of Typical Production	Transcription of Lateralized Production
sack	/sæk/	[ɬæk]
Sam	/sem/	[ɬem]
seem	/sim/	[ɬim]
side		
zoo		

11.4 LISTEN—ASPIRATED/NONASPIRATED STOP-PLOSIVES

Listen to the following words and note whether they are aspirated at the beginning of the word or demonstrate nonaspiration. Transcribe the word using the appropriate diacritic.

pot _____

spot _____

paid _____

spade _____

top _____

11.5 LISTEN—UNRELEASED STOP-PLOSIVES

Listen to the following words and note that the sound at the end is unreleased. Transcribe the word using the appropriate diacritic.

note _____

lap _____

look _____

rope _____

hat _____

11.6 LISTEN—NONLABIALIZED [ʃ]

The first word spoken is a typical pronunciation. Note the sound at the beginning of the word. The second of the pair is the same word but with a nonlabialized /ʃ/ production. Transcribe each of the words.

Word	Transcription of Typical Production	Transcription of Nonlabialized Production
shack		
she		
ship		
shell		
shop		

11.7 LISTEN—SYLLABICS

The first word spoken is a typical pronunciation with an unreduced second syllable. The second of the pair is the same word but with a syllabic production. Transcribe each of the words.

Word	*Transcription of Unreduced Second Syllable*	*Transcription of Syllabic*
title	_____	_____
turtle	_____	_____
cattle	_____	_____
saddle	_____	_____
waddle	_____	_____

11.8 LISTEN—FLAPS

The first word spoken is a typical pronunciation with a slowly articulated /t/ or /d/. The second of the pair is the same word but with a flap production. Transcribe each of the words.

Word	*Transcription of Articulated /t/ or /d/*	*Transcription of Flap*
leader	_____	_____
letter	_____	_____
lady	_____	_____
glitter	_____	_____
soda	_____	_____
petal	_____	_____

Module 12—Dialect

 Listen to the Examples in Module 12.

12.1 LISTEN—THE VOWEL /ɑ/

The following words are spoken by a speaker from the North using /ɑ/.
Listen and transcribe the words.

Word	Transcription with /ɑ/
caught	_____
law	_____
chalk	_____
hawk	_____
taught	_____

12.2 LISTEN—CHANGES IN VOWELS /ɑ/ AND /a/

The following pairs of words are first spoken by a speaker from the North
using /ɑ/ and next by a speaker of Eastern New England pronouncing the
same word with either [a] or /a/. Listen to the differences and transcribe
the words.

Word	Transcription of Northern Speaker	Transcription of Eastern New England Speaker
shop	_____	_____
talk	_____	_____
lost	_____	_____
call	_____	_____
caught	_____	_____

12.3 LISTEN—CHANGES IN VOWELS NORTHERN VERSUS SOUTHERN DIALECT

The following pairs of words are spoken first by a speaker from the North
and next by a speaker of the South. Listen to the differences and transcribe
the words.

Word	Transcription of Northern Speaker	Transcription of Southern Speaker
I'll	_____	_____
shy	_____	_____
caught	_____	_____
cot	_____	_____
mine	_____	_____

12.4 LISTEN—R-LESSNESS

The following pairs of words are spoken first by a speaker from the North using central vowels with r-coloring and rhotic diphthongs and next by a speaker of Eastern New England pronouncing the same words often with the characteristic r-lessness. Listen to the differences and transcribe the words.

Word	Transcription of Northern Speaker	Transcription of Eastern New England Speaker
park	_____	_____
father	_____	_____
farm	_____	_____
car	_____	_____
charge	_____	_____

The following short phrases are spoken by individuals representing three regional dialects.

Transcribe the following:

Northern dialect

How are you today? _____

I am fine thank you. _____

It is wonderful weather. _____

There is sunshine and not rain. _____

It is simply marvelous. _____

Eastern dialect

How are you today? _____

I am fine thank you. _____

It is wonderful weather. _____

There is sunshine and not rain. _____

It is simply marvelous. _____

Southern dialect

How are you today? _____

I am fine thank you. _____

It is wonderful weather. _____

There is sunshine and not rain. _____

It is simply marvelous. _____

12.5 LISTEN—FOREIGN DIALECTS

Spanish American English   The following words are spoken by an adult speaker whose native language is Spanish. The word is first written orthographically. Transcribe what you hear the speaker saying.

Word	*Transcription*
have	_____
jeep	_____
think	_____
check	_____
teenager	_____

How are you today? _____

I am fine thank you. _____

It is wonderful weather. _____

There is sunshine and not rain. _____

It is simply marvelous. _____

Vietnamese American English   The following words are spoken by an adult speaker whose native language is Vietnamese. The word is first written orthographically. Transcribe what you hear the speaker saying.

Word	Transcription
cheese	_____
watch	_____
scratch	_____
father	_____
yellow	_____

How are you today?_____

I am fine thank you. _____

It is wonderful weather. _____

There is sunshine and not rain. _____

It is simply marvelous. _____

Cantonese American English The following words are spoken by an adult speaker whose native language is Cantonese. The word is first written orthographically. Transcribe what you hear the speaker saying.

Word	Transcription
ladder	_____
thin	_____
bad	_____
dog	_____
vase	_____

How are you today?_____

I am fine thank you. _____

It is wonderful weather. _____

There is sunshine and not rain. _____

It is simply marvelous. _____

Korean American English The following words are spoken by an adult speaker whose native language is Korean. The word is first written orthographically. Transcribe what you hear the speaker saying.

Word	Transcription
with	_____
thumb	_____
letter	_____
really	_____
first	_____

How are you today?_____

I am fine thank you. _____

It is wonderful weather. _____

There is sunshine and not rain. _____

It is simply marvelous. _____

Module 13—Spontaneous Speech and Articulation Testing

Exercises

13.1

The following is a portion of a language sample from Jeannette, age 4;6.

I want some jelly beans and some chocolate.	[aɪ wʌn sʌm ʒɛli bins æn sʌm sɑklət]
I don't know.	[aɪ doʊn noʊ]
I don't know who that is.	[aɪ doʊn noʊ hu dæt ɪs]
Ninja turtles fight the evil Ninjas.	[nɪnʒə tʊtəls faɪt də ivəl nɪnʒəs]
Then Shredder just comes.	[dɛn ʃrɛdə ʒʌst kʌms]
And all of these other things.	[æn ɑl əf dis ʌvə tɪŋs]

- **a.** Write down the inventory of Jeanette using both the vowels and consonants that are presented in this small sample.
- **b.** Note which vowels and consonants that are normally a portion of the American English inventory are not demonstrated in Jeanette's speech sample.
- **c.** Make a list of the words that Jeanette pronounces differently than would be expected when compared to the adult model of pronunciation.
- **d.** Note any consistent patterns of substitution of one sound for another.

13.2

The following transcription is from Matthew, age 4:6. Discuss what the diacritics/transcriptions indicate for each of the sounds. Which productions would be considered typical articulation, and which would be considered misarticulations?

[aɪ wʌnt tu goʊ ʈu s̪ʌ bitʃ]	I want to go to the beach.
[sʲæli ɫɛd wi kʊd˺ goʊ]	Sally said we could go.
[dærɪ wʌnts̪ tu sʷwɪm]	Daddy wants to swim.
[ɪt wɪɫ bi fʌn]	It will be fun.

Listen to the Examples in Module 13.

13.1 LISTEN—ARTICULATION TESTING

Transcribe the words of the following articulation test from John, age 4;6.

house	_____	carrot	_____
telephone	_____	orange	_____
cup	_____	thumb	_____
gun	_____	finger	_____
knife	_____	ring	_____
window	_____	jumping	_____
wagon	_____	pajamas	_____
wheel	_____	plane	_____
chicken	_____	blue	_____
zipper	_____	brush	_____
scissors	_____	drum	_____
duck	_____	flag	_____
matches	_____	santa	_____
lamp	_____	tree	_____
shovel	_____	yellow	_____
car	_____	vacuum	_____
rabbit	_____	bed	_____
fishing	_____	bathtub	_____
church	_____	bath	_____
feather	_____	stove	_____
pencils	_____	squirrel	_____
this	_____	sleeping	_____

ANSWERS TO TRANSCRIPTION WORKBOOK

Additional information, additions, and corrections can be found at www.phonologicaldisorders.com

Module 1

1.1 radio 2, purr 1, more 1, wax 2, watch 1, bought 1
1.2 did, goat, those; girls, find, books, lost; wants, Mindy, Nancy, shopping, Tuesday
1.3 2 sounds: her, up, the; 3 sounds: Gail, chain, tall; 4 sounds: broke, yellow, dunes; 5 sounds: pretty, running, sandy
1.4 not 3, fish 3, lift 4, thought 3, boat 3
1.5 yes, no, yes, no, no
1.6 stop, well, cactus
1.7 2, 3, 4, 4, 5
1.8 no, yes, yes, no, yes
1.9 she, watch, Peter
1.10 3, 2, 4, 3, 4
1.11 yes, no, yes, yes, yes
1.12 find, this, fries
1.1 **Listen** 3, 4, 3, 4, 5, 5, 4, 5, 3, 3, 2, 4, 4, 4, 4
1.2 **Listen** 3, 5, 4, 5, 5, 6, 5, 5, 5, 4, 4, 6, 6, 5, 4, 6, 5, 7, 8, 7, 7, 8, 7, 8, 6, 7, 5, 6, 7, 7, 7, 7, 5, 8, 7

Module 2

2.1 exam, college
2.2 <u>con</u>sole con<u>sole</u>, <u>con</u>tract con<u>tract</u>, <u>ob</u>ject ob<u>ject</u>, <u>con</u>tent con<u>tent</u>, <u>per</u>mit per<u>mit</u>
2.3 1st syllable: Christmas, campus, finger, listen, midnight, shower, letter; 2nd syllable: bamboo, routine, advice, discuss, baboon, return, roulette
2.4 1st syllable: concern, perhaps; 2nd syllable: forward, flower
2.5 alarm; illness; again, exist, bizarre, elope; winter, global, coffee, garden
2.6 'den tist, dis 'cuss, 'an gel, 'Mon day, co 'llect, la 'goon, en 'grave, 'bi gger, 'bin go, be 'lieve, in 'sure, 'in jure, 'mea sure, co 'llapse, a 'wake
2.7 1st syllable: logo, gossip, awesome, hamster; 2nd syllable: concoct, admire, antique, campaign
2.8 bacon, college, paper, severe
2.9 sue waits for bill but bill came late

2.10 1st, 1st, 1st, 2nd, 1st, 1st, 2nd, 2nd, 1st, 2nd, 1st, 1st, 2nd, 1st, 2nd, 1st, 2nd, 1st, 2nd, 2nd, 1st, 2nd, 1st, 2nd, 1st, 2nd, 2nd, 1st, 2nd, 1st

2.1 **Listen** 1st, 1st, 2nd, 1st, 2nd, 2nd, 2nd, 2nd, 1st, 2nd

2.2 **Listen** a 'quaint, gi 'raffe, 'gar den, un 'til, com 'pare, be 'lieve, 'com pact, con 'tract, per 'mit

2.3 **Listen**

1. 'ladder	15. 'under	29. a 'bove
2. 'scratching	16. be 'neath	30. 'liquid
3. a 'llow	17. 'pizza	31. a 'shamed
4. 'shadow	18. pre 'pare	32. 'survey
5. 'over	19. en 'dure	33. for 'get
6. 'insect	20. for 'give	34. e 'rupt
7. 'restful	21. 'peanut	35. com 'pete
8. 'challenge	22. 'either	36. a 'gain
9. re 'ceive	23. 'ocean	37. a 'round
10. 'running	24. re 'tire	38. 'detail
11. a 'cquaint	25. 'burger	39. chau 'ffeur
12. with 'draw	26. pa 'rade	40. 'cyclone
13. 'sugar	27. 'many	
14. 'locus	28. per 'spire	

Module 3

3.1 lip, lap, cut

3.2 /i/: league, beep, east, cheese; /ɑ/: top, blond, odd, chop; /u/: tune, hoop, juice, cool

3.3 [i], [i], [ɑ], [i], [ɑ], [u], [u], [i], [u], [ɑ], [ɑ], [u], [i], [u], [ɑ]

3.4 cooler [u], meatball [i], hockey [ɑ], peeking [i], season [i], lobby [ɑ], waffle [ɑ], losing [u], shopper [ɑ], tuba [u], recruit [u], ruin [u], retrieve [i], upon [ɑ], beater [i], aloof [u], Robert [ɑ], salute [u], meager [i], appeal [i], gooey [u], body [ɑ], locket [ɑ], season [i], along [ɑ], acute [u], topic [ɑ], untrue [u]

3.5 heat, keep, team, bean; hot, mop, lot, rock; soon, clue, shoe, flu

3.6 /i/: each, beak, east; /ɑ/: dock, boss, doll, fox; /u/: you, food, new, loose, tooth

3.7 4, 2, 4

3.8 peak, rot, wheel, fool, knock, eat, broom, sheep, pool, cop

3.9 correct, incorrect, correct, correct, incorrect, correct, incorrect, correct, incorrect, correct

3.10 /i/: easel, diesel, neon, appeal; /ɑ/: olive, body, hostage, comma, upon; /u/: doodle, losing, untrue, aloof

3.1 **Listen** [i], [u], [ɑ], [ɑ], [i], [u], [ɑ], [i], [u]

3.2 **Listen** [i], [u], [ɑ], [u], [u], [ɑ], [i], [ɑ], [u], [ɑ], [i], [ɑ], [i], [ɑ], [ɑ], [i], [u], [u], [u], [ɑ] (note the partial devoicing on final voiced plosives)

3.3 **Listen** [i], [ɑ], [u], [u], [ɑ], [ɑ], [u], [u], [ɑ], [i]

3.4 **Listen** [ɑ]–[ɔ], [ɔ]–[ɑ], [ɔ]–[ɑ]

3.5 **Listen** [ɑ]–[a], [a]–[ɑ], [a]–[ɑ]

3.6 **Listen** [i], [a], [i], [ɑ], [a], [ɑ] [a] (possibly [a̝]), [i], [i], [a], [ɑ], [ɔ], [ɔ], [u], [i], [i], [i], [u], [ɔ], [ɑ], [u], [i], [i], [u], [ɑ], [i], [ɑ], [u], [ɑ], [a]

Module 4

4.1 beginning, middle, not at all, end, end, middle, middle, not at all

4.2 beginning, end, end, beginning, end, not at all, beginning, middle

4.3 beginning, not at all, not at all, end, middle, middle, not at all, end

4.4 bean, dune, pill, read, seed, feet, gopher, collar, dollar, catch, baker, should, could

4.5 do, boot, keep, cop, peak, eat, coop, bought, talk, key

4.1 **Listen** [pi], [bi], [ti], [ki], [tu], [bɪt], [tɑp], [dɑg], [pɑt], [kip], [kɑt], [dɪd], [gɪk], [dɪp], [dʊd]

4.2 **Listen** [pɑp], [bik], [gɑt], [pu], [pɑ], [pip], [tut], [pɪt], [kɑp], [dɑt], [tɑp], [bab], [kab] (possibly [kab̥]), [it], [tɑk]

4.3 **Listen** 'or phan, cre 'ate, per 'fume, 'fra gile, 'safe ty, be 'lief, dis 'guise, 'pro fit, pre 'fer, ex 'clude

Module 5

5.1 /ɪ/: tin, this, pill, give, in, build; /ɛ/: edge, desk, text, fed, meant, tent; /æ/: sack, map, tax, back, that; /ʊ/: bush, good, cook, put, would, bull

5.2 bid, mitt, pill, bed, bet, tack, man, look, pull, cook

5.3 /ɪ/: list, bill, fit, ship; /ɛ/: stem, bench, chest, ten; /æ/: rat, scratch, scrap, clap; /ʊ/: hood, should, nook, full

5.4 4, 3, 5, 3

5.5 took, pit, cat, pet, bat, put, bib, bed

5.6 correct, incorrect, correct, correct, incorrect, correct, correct, correct, correct

5.7 /ɪ/: igloo, chicken, filter, injure, afflict; /ɛ/: beckon, ahead, condensed, heaven, settle; /æ/: bandage, gather, aback, attract; /ʊ/: bushel, football, pudding, wooden

5.1 **Listen** [gɛt], [pɪk], [tɪp], [kɛn], [tʊk], [bɪt], [tæp], [dɪg], [pæt], [pʊt]

5.2 **Listen** (Melissa): [dɑg], [tɪk], [kup], [gʊd], [kɛg], [dɪd], [dɪg], [kæp], [bɛd], [pæk] [gɛt], [pɪk], [tɪp], [kɛn], [tʊk], [bɪt], [tæp], [pɪg], [pæt], [pʊt]
(Gail): [dɑg], [tɪk] (t-dentalized), [kup], [gʊt], [kɛ͡ɪk], [dit], [dɪg] ([g] partially devoiced), [kæp], [bɛd] ([d] partially devoiced), [pæk] [gɛt], [pɪk], [tɪp] (ɪ lowered), [kɛn], [tʊk], [bɪt], [tæp], [pɪg] ([g] devoiced partially), [pæt], [pʊt] ([t] dentalized)

5.3 **Listen** [pɛt], [tæg], [pɪt], [kæp], [tæk], [bɛt], [bæk], [gʊd], [kæt], [tʊk], [kʊk], [tæp], [gæp], [dɛd], [tɪp], [bæg], [bʊgi], [dɑgi], [kʊki], [pʊt], [pɛk], [pɪk], [tʊk], [dɪp], [tɛd], [bʊk], [badi], [tæki], [dɛk], [pipt], [dæd], [gɛt], [dɪg], [dɑti], [bæt], [bægi], [tɑpt], [tɛdi], [kɪt], [pækt]

5.4 **Listen** ['tipi], ['duti], ['kuku], ['kʊki], ['babi], ['kupɑn], ['gʊdi], [du 'ɛt], ['ɪglu], ['kuti]

5.5 **Listen** [dɑg], [dɑg], [dɔg], [bɑt], [bat], [bɔt], [pap], [pɑp], [pɔp], [tɑt], [tat], [tɔt], [bɔb], [bɑb], [bab]

Module 6

6.1 /f/: fun, half, stuff, elephant, tough; /v/: vote, vacuum, stove, ever, move, shoving; /s/: lasso, sun, loss, whistle, decent; /z/: lousy, zipper, easy, days, squeeze; /ʃ/: shop, ration, wish, sugar, cautious; /ʒ/: beige, vision, leisure, treasure; /θ/: thin, tooth, bath, thumb, think; /ð/: this, mother, leather, soothe, these; /h/: hospital, ahoy, history, behind, behave, whoever

6.2 seek, sick, his, feet, fit, sheep, ship, suit, soot, who

6.3 [θ], [ð], [ð], [θ], [θ], [ð], [θ], [ð], [ð], [ð]

6.4 [v], [f]; [f], [v]; [s], [ʃ]; [θ], [f]; [θ], [ʃ]; [v], [s]; [θ], [z]; [ʒ], [f]; [ʒ], [ð]; [ð], [ʃ]

6.5 /θ/: thumb, Thursday, sixth, mouth, three; /ð/: clothing, leather, thus, breathes, rhythm

6.6 /f/: phase, photo, trophy, cough, gopher; /s/: excite, hats, nest, cell, lesson; /ʃ/: chandelier, action, promotion, radish, marsh; /θ/: tooth-brush, booth, fourteenth, worthless; /h/: keyhole, whole, hockey, doghouse, uphill

6.7 /θ/: bathtub, fourteenth, thunder, thrifty, beneath; /f/: female, affair, flower, confirm; /s/: deceive, syrup, promotes, postage; /ʃ/: shiny, machine, unsure, wishful, afresh; /h/: inhale, happy, halibut, rehearse, ahoy

6.1 **Listen** [fit], [tiθ], [ʃu], [sut], [hɑt], [tiz], [sɑs], [iv], [hup], [ʃuz], [θɑt], [ʃɑp]

6.2 **Listen** [piθ], [θɑk], [tɑθ], [zu], [hɑp], [af], [θup], [but], [hu], [ʃip], [θiθ], [bitθ]

6.3 **Listen** [ʃɪp], [stɑpt], [suð], [væn], [hæf], [fænz], [fʊt], [hɑk], [θɑts], [hʊf], [ðiz], [kɑfi], [suzi]

6.4 **Listen** [kɪs], [fæt], [sɪt], [hæt], [sæk], [zɪp], [ʃɛd], [ʃʊd], [ðɪs], [hʊk], [sɛd], [sun]

6.5 **Listen** [hɛdsɛt], [tispun], [buʃi], [tuθpɪk], [kætfud], [pɑpi], [ʃipdɑg], [siwid], [pɛgd], [hɑtdɑg], [tæbu]

6.6 **Listen** a 'pplause, stam 'pede, e 'rase, 'cir cus, 'car go, ca 'ssette, com 'ply, 'tur quoise, dis 'grace, pro 'vide

Module 7

7.1 /eɪ/: eight, chamber, reindeer, they, shade, suede; /oʊ/: tone, both, bowl, whole, coat, yoga; /aɪ/: type, sly, eyelash, light, write; /aʊ/: down, loud, noun, shower, mouth, trout; /ɔɪ/: choice, coin, soil, join, voice, foil

7.2 cake, time, soap, house, toy, boat, kite, vote, boys, sight

7.3 [aɪ]–[eɪ]; [aɪ]–[oʊ]; [aɪ]–[eɪ]; [ɔɪ]–[aʊ]; [aɪ]–[oʊ]; [ɔɪ]–[eɪ]; [aʊ]–[oʊ]; [ɔɪ]–[eɪ]; [aʊ]–[oʊ]; [ɔɪ]–[aʊ]

7.4 /eɪ/: paste, rake, clay; /oʊ/: clothes, boast, rope; /aɪ/: time, mine, climb; /aʊ/: hound, shout, round; /ɔɪ/: noise, choice, join

7.5 shine, they, shout, signs, void, bathe, shows, beige, thou, code

7.6 poison, voyage, highway, joyful, bouquet, fountain, lousy, daisy, diaper, neighbor, broken, polka, outrage, poker, diamond

7.7 pas 'tel, De 'cem ber, ro 'mance, a 'gree ment, 'wa llet, con 'tain er, tou 'pee 'mul ti ply, hu 'mane, clar i 'net, 'bu cket, 'ju ven ile, 'pa rent, com 'pu ter, 'par snip fa 'mil iar, a 'chieve, um 'bre lla, 'or gan, in tro 'duce

7.1 **Listen** [eɪp], [eɪt], [feɪk], [ʃeɪk], [peɪst], [ʃeɪd], [ðeɪ], [heɪ], [teɪst], [seɪf]

7.2 **Listen** [boʊt], [soʊk], [ʃoʊ], [foʊk], [ðoʊ], [doʊz], [ʃoʊd], [koʊt], [poʊk], [koʊk]

7.3 **Listen** [faɪt], [ʃaɪ], [taɪp], [daɪs], [baɪk], [gaɪd], [haɪt], [θaɪ], [paɪp], [skaɪz]

7.4 **Listen** [haʊs], [kaʊ], [ʃaʊt], [ðaʊ], [daʊt], [paʊt], [saʊθ], [vaʊ], [spaʊs], [skaʊt]

7.5 **Listen** [tɔɪ], [bɔɪ], [hɔɪst], [pɔɪz], [tɔɪz], [vɔɪs], [bɔɪz], [sɔɪ], [vɔɪst], [hɔɪsts]

7.6 **Listen** [toʊst], [blɑkt], [sɔɪbin], [bɔɪkat], [tɔɪʃap], [eɪdi], [haʊskoʊt], [deɪzi], [aʊtdu]

7.7 Listen [saɪdʃoʊ], [deɪtaɪm], [taɪdi], [heɪsti], [taɪkun], [keɪnaɪn], [haʊsgɛst], [baɪpæs], [aʊtbɪd], [oʊtkeɪk]

7.8 **Listen** (Vicky): [oʊbeɪ], [geɪtpoʊθt], [foʊtoʊ], [peɪθtæk], [hoʊboʊ], [aɪθaɪt], [taɪdi], [vɔɪθ], [ʃeɪdi], [ʃoʊdaʊn] (note the lack of lip round-ing on [ʃ])
(Cindy): [oʊbeɪ], [geɪtpoʊst], [foʊtoʊ], [heɪstæk], [hoʊboʊ], [aɪsaɪt], [taɪdi], [vɔɪs], [ʃeɪdi], [ʃoʊdaʊn]

7.9 **Listen** ['ʃuʃaɪn], ['kætfɪʃ], [ɑl'ðoʊ], ['bæθhaʊs], ['veɪkeɪt], ['aɪvi], [ri'vaɪv], [taɪ'fun], [tu'deɪ], ['bifsteɪk]

Module 8

8.1 /m, n, ŋ/: album, opener, nickel, strong, flying, rainbow, knight, sig-nature, gnome, winter, famous; /w, j/: once, you, yellow, unit, yodel, universal, wedding; /l, r/: foolish, lounge, rocky, stall, wrote, carrot, garage, orange, ceiling, clock, whale; /tʃ, dʒ/: cheese, witch, June, germ, edge, wage, magic, major, pledge

8.2 mean, new, song, moon, not, mint, think, Mike, nose, mouse: we, you, wish, used, yes, wood, wait, walk, youth, yeast; loop, reed, lost, ride, raft, lake, leak, loud, rake, roast; chew, job, cheap, badge, jack, juice, cheese, chase, choose, joy

8.3 [mun–nun], [reɪk–leɪk], [sɪn–sɪŋ], [mit–nit], [rɪtʃ–rɪdʒ], [rum–lum], [lɑk–rɑk], [moʊp–noʊp], [rɑŋ–lɑŋ], [tʃip–dʒip], [rid–wid], [wɛst–rɛst], [maɪs–naɪs], [læp–ræp], [wɛdʒ–lɛdʒ], [rɪtʃ–wɪtʃ], [jɛs–lɛs], [moʊn–loʊn], [lɪk–wɪk], [dʒɑb–rɑb]

8.4 measure, canal, mountain, musical, command, necklace, medal; away, wagon, union, awake, younger, latitude, delete, raisin, erase, await, Yahoo; chestnut, jockey, chosen, bewitch, suggest

8.5 bleach, mailman, noisy, migrate, pancake, movie, rosey, knocking, neon, ringing, donkey, rabies, cockroach, redwood, washcloth kiwi, chilly, railway, unite, jellyfish, using, coyote, gypsy, digest, enrage

8.6 fuel, beauty, cute, queen, quite, quilt, choir, liquid, view, square, music, amuse, cube

8.7 /ˈtoʊ.ki.oʊ/ /ˈbæ.gɪdʒ/ /ɛn.ˈgeɪdʒ/, /ˈsæn.wɪtʃ/ /maɪ.ˈsɛlf/ /ˈnɛf.ju/ /ræ.ˈkun/ /i.ˈvɛnt/ /ˈreɪ.ʃoʊ/ /ri.ˈlif/

8.1 **Listen** [mɛnju], [meɪbi], [wɪnɪŋ], [hɪmsɛlf], [saɪgan], [naɪtli], [flaɪɪŋ], [dɛdlaɪn], [klæsmeɪt], [klaɪmɪŋ]

8.2 **Listen** [mɪlk], [mæskat], [daŋki], [nikæp], [nɛktaɪ], [poʊnis], [bæbun], [suzi], [rɪŋɪn], [pɪkpɛn]

8.3 **Listen** [wɪloʊ], [reɪni], [rilaɪ], [waʃrum], [kabwɛb], [juzɪŋ], [hæfweɪ], [rijuz], [hjumeɪn], [hjugoʊ]

8.4 **Listen** [læsoʊ], [vækjum], [jɛloʊ], [wɪndoʊ], [bjuti], [laʊzi], [raki], [lusɪŋ], [reɪdioʊ], [wʊtʃɛd]

8.5 **Listen** [tʃɛloʊ], [dʒini], [tʃapsui], [foʊlɪdʒ], [astrɪtʃ], [idʒɪpt], [biwɪtʃ], [beɪsbalkoʊtʃ], [tʃeɪndʒɪŋ], [dʒɛlibinz], [tʃɪmni], [watʃdag], [dʒɪfi], [paɪprɛntʃ], [dʒeɪni], [tʃuɪŋ], [rɪtʃi], [aʊtstrɛtʃ], [hakikoʊtʃ]

Module 9

9.1 bird, cuff, jump, fudge, bus, word, shirt, stir, church, cup, nut

9.2 ago, avoid, balloon, cologne, canoe, afraid, petite, attack, buffet, salute, mesa

9.3 father, mayor, major, freighter, antler, lasar, percent, surprise, wonderful, longer, chowder, doctor, perspire, strainer

9.4 church, judge, sung, stir, earth, urge, bunk, come, lunch, tongue

9.5 sister, tailor, abloom, away, baton, polute, banker, hamster, suppose, police

9.6 incorrect, correct, correct, correct, incorrect, incorrect, incorrect, correct, correct, correct

9.7 'ca.len.dar, vol.'ca.no, re.co.'mmend, pre.'ci.sion, 'po.pu.lar, ca.'the.dral, 'di.a.gram, de.'ter.gent, se.'cure.ly, dis.a.'ppear

9.1 **Listen** [bʌg], [hʌŋ], [θʌmtæk], [brʌʃ], [dʌstɪŋ], [bʌbli], [fʌdʒ], [kʌps], [sʌnbeɪð], [ʃrʌb]

9.2 **Listen** (Cindy): [jʌŋ], [bʌni], [hʌŋgri], [pʌpi], [bʌɾi], [rʌŋ], [sʌdzi], [sʌndaʊn], [tʌtʃ], [krʌtʃ]
(Gail): [jʌŋ], [bʌni], [hʌŋgwi], [pʌpi], [bʌdi], [wʌŋ], [sʌdsi], [sʌndaʊn], [tʌtʃ], [kwʌtʃ]

9.3 **Listen** [bɝst], [ɝθi], [gɝlfrɛnd], [kɝfju], [nɝsmeɪd], [tɝnɪŋ], [tɝkɔɪz], [sɝveɪ], [wɝldli], [twɝld], [bɝdsid], [bɝθdeɪ], [nɝd], [θɝdi], [wɝkbʊk], [ɝdʒ], [vɝtʃu], [lɝnɪŋ]

9.4 **Listen** [ədapt], [kəmænd], [tənaɪt], [ləkras], [ʃəlæk], [leɪbəl], [əpoʊz], [əlaʊd], [əlaɪv], [əbdʒɛkt], [əbaʊt], [səksɛs], [məʃin], [ləgun], [kənɛkt], [kəmplit], [bəlun], [əgɪn], [kəkun], [kəsɛt]

9.5 **Listen** [sɚvaɪv], [reɪzɚ], [skiɚ], [litɚ], [pɚsu], [lizɚ], [fɚgat], [streɪndʒɚ], [lagɚ], [krækɚ], [hæmɚ], [neɪbɚ], [fɚgɪv], [wɛðɚ], [sɚpraɪz], [titʃɚ], [brɔɪlɚ]

9.6 **Listen** [ˈɝθkweɪk], [ˈɝbən], [ˈdʒɝnəl], [ˈkɝnəl], [ənˈliʃ], [ənˈtʌtʃt], [ˈdʌndʒən], [ˈpʌblək], [ˈpʌmkən], [ˈʃoʊldɚ]

9.7 **Listen** [ˈsʌnbɚn], [ˈsʌpɚ] [ˈsʌðɚn], [ˈtʌtʃdaʊn], [əˈmjus], [kənˈsɝn], [səbˈtrækt], [ənˈplʌg], [əpˈtaɪt], [ˈfɝnəs]

Module 10

10.1 charm, barn, farm, darling, bargain, harbor; very, cherry, sheriff, errand, rare, there; clear, cheer, deer, here, near, ear, sheer; oar, board, born, door, force, horn, horse court

10.2 charge, horse, earring, square, narrow, barley, cherry, nearer

10.3 barn, fare, pear, sore, board, Kerry, ferry, hair, share, heart

10.4 surgeon, thirty, wearhouse, army, horseshoe, tar, mermaid, herring, hearing

10.5 [ˈstrɑ.bɛɚ.i], [ˈkɛɚ.fʊ.li], [ˈmɝ.mə.ɪŋ], [sɚ.ˈæ.mɪks], [ɛm.ˈbɛɚ.əs], [ˈgloɚ.i.əs], [paɪ.ə.ˈniɚ], [ˈdaɪ.nə.sɑɚ] or [ˈdaɪ.nə.soɚ], [ˈtɝ.bju.ləns], [pɚ.ˈfoɚ.məns]

10.1 Listen [koɚs], [jiɚbʊk], [hɑɚʃ], [mɛɚid], [ɛɚmeɪl], [ɑɚtʃ], [hɛɚbrəʃ], [piɚst]

10.2 Listen [bɑɚn], [biɚd], [hɛɚɪŋ], [poɚtreɪt], [fiɚsli], [koɚni], [wiɚd], [hoɚsbæk]

10.3 Listen [kaɚpɪt], [paɚsli], [dʒɝzi], [vɛɚi], [ɑɚtʃɚ], [fɑɚðɚ], [bɛθdeɑ], [θɝtiz̥], [iɚplag), [hɑɚpun]

10.4 Listen [pɚ.ˈfɛk.ʃən], [ˈwɑ.tɚ.fɑl], [ˈdrʌ.dʒɚ.i], [ˈræz.bɛɚ.i], [ˈvɝ.bə.li], [ˈhaɪ.drə.dʒən], [kwɑ.ˈdru.plət], [ˈfri.kwən.si], [ˈtʃiz.bɚ.gɚ], [ˈgræs.hɑ.pɚ], [ˈoɚ.kə.strə], [ˈpaɚ.kɪŋ.lɑt], [ˈpoɚ.kju.paɪn], [ˈkra.kə.daɪl], [ˈmaɪ.krə.foʊn], [kɑm.prə.ˈhɛnd], [æd.ˈvɛn.tʃɚ], [di.ˈpaɚ.tʃɚ], [dʒɝm.bɚ.ˈi], [ɛn.ˈgeɪdʒ.mənt]

Module 11

11.1 palatalized, dentalized, palatalized, velarized, lateralized, lateralized, velarized, dentalized, velarized, velarized, palatalized, dentalized

11.2 [sʲʌn], [t̪oʊ], [l̟ɪɫtɚ], [ʃˤapɪŋ], [pʊɫd], [tʲʌtʃ], [ꞣibrə], [s̪tul], [sʲɪŋɪŋ]

11.3 total voicing, partial devoicing, total devoicing, partial devoicing, total devoicing, partial devoicing, partial voicing, partial voicing, partial devoicing, total devoicing

11.4 [s̬ʌndeɪ], [g̊oʊfɚ], [ꞣlevɚ], [liʒ̊ɚ], [ʃeɪkɪŋ], [beɪd̥], [ʍɛɚɪŋ], [beɪsbalz̥], [kɪs̬ɪŋ], [tʌŋz̥]

11.5 pillow, aspirated [p]; robot, unreleased [t]; earnest, unaspirated [t]; shrub, unreleased [b]; acrobat, unaspirated [t]; taller, aspirated [t]; regret, unaspirated [t]; spearmint, unaspirated [p]; catalog, aspirated [k]; tugboat, unreleased [t]

11.6 [spˀɛɚoʊ], [ripoɚtˀ], [pʰəzɪʃən], [skˀɛlətən], [daɪəlagˀ], [skˀɛdʒəl], [tʰɝpəntaɪn], [daɪnəmaɪtˀ], [wɪtʃətʰa], [ɛkspændˀ]—There are several possibilities for the transcription of these words. Variations will occur when you say them somewhat differently.

11.7 [lædɚ–lærɚ], [bʌtɚ–bʌrɚ], [sɪti–sɪri], [dɝti–dɝri], [klaʊdi–klaʊri], [stʌtɚ–stʌrɚ], [tʃɛɚti–tʃɛɚri], [sætəsfaɪ–særəsfaɪ], [gɪtɑɚ–gɪrɑɚ], [vɝaɪəti–vɝaɪəri]

11.8 [batəl, barəl—batl̩, barl̩], [hændəl, hænrəl—hændl̩, hænrl̩], [bʌtən, bʌrən—bʌtn̩, bʌʔn̩], [flætən, flærən—flætn̩, flæʔn̩], [ratən, rarən—ratn̩, raʔn̩], [kætəl, kærəl—kætl̩, kærl̩], [waɪdən, waɪrən—waɪdn̩, waɪʔn̩], [lɪtəl, lɪrəl—lɪtl̩, lɪrl̩], [rætəl, rærəl—rætl̩, rærl̩]

11.9 [ʃap–ʃap̅], [ʃip–ʃip̅], [ʃɛd–ʃɛd̅], [ʃoʊ–ʃoʊ̅], [ʃaʊə–ʃaʊə̅], [wɪʃ–wɪ ʃ̅], [liʃ–li ʃ̅], [ʃɛl–ʃɛl̅], [rʌʃ–rʌ ʃ̅]

11.10 clean, lowered; should, lowered; street, retracted; class, more anterior; think, lowered; classify, more anterior; thistle, raised; chalk, raised; with, lowered

11.11 [wɛl̩θi], [glæmə˞əs], [sɪmpəθi], [əndə˞stʊd], [mɛʒə˞ɪŋ], [kjʊkəmbə˞], [ɑpʃən], [əgrɪmənt], [kəsɛt], [θæŋkfʊl], [pʊʃɪŋ], [brɪdɪŋ]

11.12 retreat, nasalized; tentative, denasalized; scratchy, nasalized; finish, denasalized; drought, nasalized; mean, denasalized; tenth, denasalized; grapes, nasalized; gloves, nasalized; murmer, denasalized

11.1 **Listen** [saŋ–s̬aŋ], [sa–s̬a], [sæd–s̬æd], [sɪk–s̬ɪk], [zu–z̬u]

11.2 **Listen** [sɛnt–sʲɛnt], [soʊk–sʲoʊk], [sɛl–sʲɛl], [sɪt–sʲɪt], [zibrə–zʲibrə]

11.3 **Listen** [sæk–ɬæk], [sæm–ɬæm], [sim–ɬim], [saɪd–ɬaɪd], [zu–ʒu]

11.4 **Listen** [pʰat], [spʰat], [p˭eɪd], [spʰeɪd], [t˭ap]

11.5 **Listen** [noʊt], [læp̚], [lʊk̚], [roʊp̚], [hæt̚]

11.6 **Listen** [ʃæk], [ʃæk̅], [ʃi], [ʃi̅], [ʃɪp], [ʃɪp̅], [ʃɛl], [ʃɛl̅], [ʃap], [ʃap̅]

11.7 **Listen** [taɪtəl taɪrl̩], [tɝtəl tɝrl̩], [kætəl kærl̩], [sædəl særl̩], [wadəl warl̩]

11.8 **Listen** [lidə˞–lirə˞], [lɛtə˞–lɛrə˞], [leɪdi–leɪri], [glɪtə˞–glɪrə˞], [soʊdə–soʊrə], [pɛtəl–pɛrəl]

Module 12

12.1 **Listen** [kat], [la], [tʃak], [hak], [tat]

12.2 **Listen Northern:** [ʃap], [tak], [last], [kal], [kat]
   New England: [ʃap], [tak], [last], [kal], [kat]

12.3 **Listen Northern:** [aɪl], [ʃaɪ], [kat], [kat], [maɪn]
   Southern: [al], [ʃaə], [kat], [kat], [maən]

12.4 **Listen Northern:** [paɚk], [faðɚ], [faɚm], [kaɚ], [tʃaɚdʒ]
   Eastern: [pak], [faða], [fam], [ka], [tʃaɚtʃ]

Northern speaker
How are you today? [haʊ aɚ ju tədeɪ]
I am fine thank you. [aɪm faɪn θæŋk ju]
It's wonderful weather. [ɪts wʌndə˞fəl wɛðə˞]
There is sunshine and not rain. [ðɛɚ ɪs sʌnʃaɪn nat reɪn]
It is simply marvelous. [ɪt ɪs sɪmpli maɚvələs]

Eastern speaker
How are you today? [haʊ jə duən]
I am fine thank you. [am faɪn θæŋk ju]
It is wonderful weather. [ɪts wʌndəfʊl wɛðə]
There is sunshine and not rain. [ðɛɚz sʌnʃaɪ n̩ nat reɪn]
It is simply marvelous. [ɪts sɪmpli mavələs]

Southern speaker

How are you today? [haʊ ɑ͡ ju͡ tədeɪ]

I am fine thank you. [ɑm fɑn θæŋk ju]

It is wonderful weather. [ɪts wɑndəfəl wɛða]

There is sunshine and not rain. [ðɛɚs sʌnʃɑɪn ən noʊ͡ reɪn]

It is simply marvelous. [ɪts sɪmpli mɑvələs]

12.5 Listen Spanish American: [hæf], [dʒip], [θɪŋk], [tʃɛkʰ], [tinetʃɚ]

How are you today? [haʊ ɑ͡ɚ ju tade̥]

I am fine thank you. [ɑ͡ɪm fɑ͡ɪn tæŋk ju]

It is wonderful weather. [ɪz wʌndafʊl wɛðɛɚ]

There is sunshine and not rain. [ðɛ͡ɚ ɪs sʌ̃ʃɑɪn ənoʊ͡ reɪn]

It is simply marvelous. [ɪt ɪs sɪmpəl mɑ͡ɚvaləs]

Vietnamese American: [tis̟], [watʰ], [skræs], [fadə], [jɛloʊ]

How are you today? [ha͡ʊa ju tade]

I am fine thank you. [ɑ͡ɪəm fɑ͡ɪ tæŋk ju]

It is wonderful weather. [ɪd ə wʌndafəl wɛdɑ]

There is sunshine and not rain. [dɛ͡ɚ ɪs sʌnsɑɑn nat rɛn]

It is simply marvelous. [ɪt ə sʌnli mavələ]

Cantonese American: [læɾɚ], [θɪn], [bædʰ], [daga], [ve͡ɪs]

How are you today? [haʊ͡ ɑ͡ɚ ju təde]

I am fine thank you. [ɑəm fɑ͡ɪ θeŋk ju]

It is wonderful weather. [ɪt ɪs wʌndafal rɛðɚ]

There is sunshine and not rain. [ðɚsə sʌnʃe͡ɪn natə re͡ɪn]

It is simply marvelous. [ɪt ɪs sɪmple mabələs]

Korean American: [rɪθ], [tʌm], [lɛɾɚ] [rili], [faɚst]

How are you today? [haʊ͡ ɑ͡ɚ jutade]

I am fine thank you. [ɑəm fɑ͡ɪn tæŋk ju]

It is wonderful weather. [ɪt ɪs wʌndafəl rɛðɚ]

There is sunshine and not rain. [ðɛ͡əsə s̟ʌn ʃɑɪn natə re͡ɪn]

It is simply marvelous. [ɪt ɪs sɪmpli mɑ͡ɚbᵊləs]

Module 13

13.1

a) Vowels: [i, ɪ, ɛ, æ, u, ʊ, ɑ, ʌ, ə, a͡ɪ, o͡ʊ]; Consonants: [b, t, d, k, m, n, ŋ, f, v, s, ʃ, ʒ, h, w, l, r]

Syllable initiating: [b, t, d, k, n, f, v, s, ʃ, ʒ, h, w, l, r]

Syllable terminating: [t, m, n, ŋ, s, l]

Jeannette uses far more consonants in the syllable-initiating position when compared to the syllable-terminating one. [m] is the only consonant that is used syllable-terminating but not syllable-initiating. This could be due to the nature of the topic of the language sample.

b) Vowels that Jeannette does not display: [ɝ, ɚ, e͡ɪ, a͡ʊ, ɔ͡ɪ]. She does not use the [a] or the [ɔ] vowels but this could be dialect related.

Consonants that Jeannette does not display: [p, g, θ, ð, z, tʃ, dʒ, j]

c) words that are pronounced differently: jelly, chocolate, that, turtles, the, then, Shredder, just, these, other, things

d) Consistent patterns: [dʒ] is replaced with [ʒ], [ð] is replaced by [d] and [θ] by [t], however, there is one instance of [v] replacing [ð] in the word *other*. She has one instance of a correct [r] in *Shredder* but lacks any vowels with r-coloring.

13.2

[aɪ wʌnt tu goʊ t̪u s̪ʌ bitʃ]
I want to go to the beach.
The dentalized [t] and [s] could be considered misarticulations. The dentalized [t] will probably not be very noticeable but the dentalized [s] is produced as a substitution for [ð].

[sʲæli ɬɛd wi kʊdˀ goʊ]
Sally said we could go.
The palatalized [s] would be considered a misarticulation as well as the lateralized [s] in said. It is interesting that she uses two very different variations of s-productions. The unreleased [d] in *could* would be considered normal

[dærɪ wʌnts̪ tu sʷwim]
Daddy wants to swim.
The flap in the middle of *daddy* would be considered normal. The dentalized [s] at the end of *wants* is probably not due to assimilation effects; however, the rounded [s] on *swim* would be caused by the [w], which has lip rounding.

[ɪt wɪɬ bi fʌn]
It will be fun.
The dark-l would be considered a normal variation.

13.1 LISTEN

house	[haʊs]	rabbit	[wæbɪt]
telephone	[tɛləfoʊn]	fishing	[fɪʃin]
cup	[kʌp]	church	[tʃɔtʃ]
gun	[gʌn]	feather	[feðə]
knife	[naɪf]	pencils	[pɛnsals]
window	[wɪndoʊ]	this	[ðɪs]
wagon	[wægɪn]	carrot	[kewət]
wheel	[wil]	orange	[ɔwɪntʃ]
chicken	[tʃɪkɪn]	thumb	[θʌm]
zipper	[zɪpə]	finger	[θɪŋgʊ]
scissors	[sɪzɔs]	ring	[wɪŋ]
duck	[dʌk]	jumping	[dʒʌmpin]
matches	[mæʃtəs]	pajamas	[pədʒæməs]
lamp	[læmp]	plane	[pleɪn]
shovel	[ʃʌval]	blue	[blu]
car	[kaə]	brush	[bwʌʃ]

drum	[dwʌm]	bed	[bɛd̥]
flag	[flæg]	bathtub	[bæθtʌb]
Santa	[sæntə]	bath	[bæθ]
tree	[twi]	stove	[stoᵘf]
yellow	[jɛlo͡ʊ]	squirrel	[skwʌl]
vacuum	[vækjum]	sleeping	[slipin]

abduct Opening the vocal folds, thus moving the vocal folds away from the midline of the glottis.

acoustic phonetics Branch of phonetics that documents the transmission properties of speech sounds. Professionals specializing in acoustic phonetics study speech sounds in the form of sound waves that travel through the air from a speaker to a listener.

acoustic resonator A container filled with air that is set into vibration.

active articulator The anatomical structure that actually moves during the generation of speech sounds.

adduct Closing the vocal folds, thus moving the vocal folds toward the midline of the glottis.

affricate A manner of articulation defined by a stop-plosive portion releasing to a homorganic (*hom* = same, *organic* = active articulator) fricative portion. The stop-plosive and fricative are articulated in one movement and are functionally (phonemically) considered one unit.

affrication The replacement of fricatives by homorganic affricates.

allophones Variations in phoneme realizations that do not change the meaning of a word when they are produced in various contexts.

allophonic similitude The number of features affected in an assimilation process is such that the altered segment is perceived to be an allophonic variation of the speech sound, i.e., it does not change the phoneme value.

alphabetic systems Based on the same principles that govern ordinary alphabetic writing consisting of the use of a single symbol to represent a speech sound; there exists a one-to-one relationship between the symbol and the sound.

alveolar The alveolar ridge as passive articulator.

alveolar pressure The pressure within the lungs.

alveolar ridge A protuberance formed by the alveolar process, which is the thickened portion of the maxilla (upper jaw) housing the teeth.

alveolarization: The change of nonalveolar sounds, mostly interdental and labio-dental sounds, into alveolar ones.

analphabetic systems Each sound segment is represented by a composite notation made up of a number of symbols. These symbols are abbreviated descriptive labels for the sound segment.

anticipatory assimilation See *regressive assimilation*.

apical The tip of the tongue, or apex of the tongue, as active articulator.

approach phase The first phase in the production of stop-plosives, characterized by the articulators moving from a previous open state to a closed state; the velum is raised, blocking off air flow to the nasal cavity. Also called *shutting phase*.

approximant A manner of articulation in which the articulators come close to one another (approximate), but not nearly as close as the constriction that creates the fricative speech sounds. The distance between active and passive articulators is wider; there is a much broader passage of air. The consonants /r/, /l/, /w/, and /j/ are approximants.

articulation disorder Difficulties with the motor production aspects of speech, or an inability to produce certain speech sounds.

articulators Those anatomical structures directly involved in the generation of speech sounds, including the lips, tongue, mandible (lower jaw), teeth, hard palate, and velum.

articulatory phonetics Branch of phonetics that examines production features of speech sounds. Professionals specializing in articulatory phonetics are primarily concerned with how the different speech sounds are generated; they describe and classify speech sounds according to parameters of their actual production.

articulatory system Contains the mandible, tongue, lips, teeth, alveolar ridge, hard palate, and velum and is important in forming the individual speech sounds.

aspiration The puff of air that is created when increased air pressure is released. Aspiration occurs due to a greater build-up of pressure within the oral cavity during certain voiceless stop-plosive productions.

assimilation The adaptive articulatory change that results in neighboring sound segments becoming similar in their production. Also called *harmony processes*.

atmospheric pressure The pressure equal to the outside air.

auditory phonetics Branch of phonetics that studies how speech sound waves are identified and perceived by the listener.

back vowels On a horizontal, front-to-back plane, those vowels in which the hump of the tongue is farther back, creating a narrowing in the upper pharynx.

broad transcription See *phonemic transcription*.

canonical babbling Stage 4 of prelinguistic development, which extends from approximately 6 months on.

cavity features Reference active and passive articulators as distinctive features.

centering diphthongs Those diphthongs in which the offglide consists of a central vowel.

central approximant /r/; produced with a central airflow in which the articulators come close to one another but not close enough to create turbulent airflow or friction. Also referred to as a liquid or rhotic consonant.

central vowels On a horizontal, front-to-back plane, those vowels in which the hump of the tongue is in a centralized position. When contrasted to the front or the back vowels, the central vowels have a more neutral tongue position.

chain shifts Systematic changes in vowel systems in which the vowels shift in respect to their articulatory features. The articulatory features may change according to tongue height, tongue position (fronting or backing of the tongue), or rounding of the lips.

checked syllables See *closed syllables.*

citation form The spoken form of a word produced in isolation, as distinguished from the form it would have when produced in conversational speech.

close vowels Vowels that are produced with the tongue closer to the palate.

closed syllables Syllables that do contain a coda. Also called *checked syllables.*

close-mid vowel Vowel in which the tongue is halfway between a close and an open-mid vowel. Examples are /e/ and /o/.

closure phase See *stop phase.*

cluster reduction Articulatory simplification of consonant clusters by omitting one consonant (in two-consonant clusters) and one or two consonants (in three-consonant clusters).

coalescence When during an assimilation process two neighboring speech sounds are merged and form a new and different segment.

coarticulation Changes in the production features of consonants and vowels as they are influenced by surrounding sounds.

coda All the sound segments of a syllable following the peak.

code switching Changing back and forth between two or more languages or dialects. In this context it is used to indicate the changing back and forth from African American Vernacular English and Standard American English.

cognates Pairs of similar sounds.

complementary distribution Two allophones of a phoneme that cannot normally replace one another, as they occur in mutually exclusive contexts.

complex wave A wave that consists of more than just one frequency.

consonant cluster variations In reference to dialects, those phonological differences that affect strings of consonants.

consonants Speech sounds produced with a relatively closed vocal tract, typically with significant articulatory constriction.

contact assimilation When one segment affects a sound that directly precedes or follows it. Also called *contiguous assimilation.*

contiguous assimilation See *contact assimilation.*

continuant A type of consonant in which the vocal tract is not completely blocked, but rather a continuous flow of air is achieved. Vowels, fricatives, nasals, and approximants are continuants.

contrastive analysis See *relational analysis*.

contrastive stress When one syllable within a two-word utterance becomes prominent.

cooing and laughter Stage 2 of prelinguistic development, from approximately 2 to 4 months of age.

coronal As active articulator, the front and lateral edges of the tongue (including the apex).

creole A pidgin language that has become the mother tongue of a community.

culture A way of life developed by a group of individuals to meet psychosocial needs; consists of values, norms, beliefs, attitudes, behavioral styles, and tradition.

deaffrication The production of affricates as homorganic fricatives.

denasalization The replacement of nasals by homorganic stops.

dental The upper teeth as passive articulators.

derhotacization The loss of r-coloring in central vowels with r-coloring [ɝ] and [ɚ].

devoicing The replacement of a voiceless for a normally voiced sound.

diacritics Small letter-shaped symbols or marks that can be added to a vowel or consonant symbol to modify or refine its phonetic value.

dialect A neutral label that refers to any variety of a language that is shared by a group of speakers.

dialectology The study of sociolects, dialects correlated to social differences.

digraph A combination of two letters representing one sound.

diphthongization An allophonic variation of a vowel in which vowels that are typically produced as monophthongs are articulated as diphthongs.

diphthongs *(di* = two, *phthong* = sound) Vowels that undergo a change in quality during their production.

distinctive features The smallest indivisible sound properties that establish phonemes.

distribution of phonemes See *distribution requirement*.

distribution requirement The rule-governed patterns of sounds and syllables within a particular language; the restrictions on word and syllable shapes relative to which types of phonemes can occur in which word positions. Also called *distribution of phonemes*.

dorsum Body of the tongue. Also defined as the broad superior surface of the tongue, the body of the tongue comprised of the front and back, or simply as the back of the tongue.

dysarthria A disorder characterized by weakness, paralysis, a lack of coordination, and changes in the muscle tone of the entire speech mechanism. It may be caused by a neuromuscular disorder, a stroke (cerebrovascular accidents), infectious processes, tumors, degenerative diseases, and traumatic insults as a result of head injuries.

dysphagia A swallowing disorder characterized by difficulty in preparing for the swallow or in moving material from the mouth to the stomach.

epenthesis Refers to the insertion of a sound segment into a word, thereby changing its syllable structure. The intrusive sound can be a vowel as well as a consonant, but most often it is restricted to a schwa insertion between two consonants.

ethnic dialects Those dialects that are in general related to ethnic background.

ethnicity Commonalities such as religion, nationality, and region that may evolve into a specific way of living as a subculture.

extrinsic muscles Those muscles having at least one attachment to structures outside the referenced structure.

falling diphthong A diphthong in which the gliding movement of the tongue moves from a higher to a lower articulatory position.

final-consonant deletion The omission of a syllable-arresting consonant.

first word An entity of relatively stable phonetic form that is produced consistently by the child in a particular context. This form must be recognizably related to the adultlike word form of a particular language.

forced vibration When one object sets another object into vibration.

formal Standard English The most formal spoken language based on the written language, is exemplified in guides of usage and in grammar texts. When there is a question as to whether a form is considered Standard English, then these grammar texts are consulted.

formants Vocal tract resonances.

fortis consonants Those plosives that have clearly more intraoral pressure, which translates into a stronger puff of air (aspirated stop-plosives); from the Latin word meaning "strong."

free variation Two allophones of one phoneme that could be exchanged for one another in similar contexts. Therefore, it is optional and unpredictable whether one or the other is produced in that context for that particular phoneme.

free vibration The natural vibratory response of an object, which is dependent upon the mass, tension, and stiffness of that object.

fricatives A manner of articulation that results when the active and passive articulators approximate each other so closely that the air is forced with considerable pressure through the constriction that is formed. As the air is pressed through this narrow passageway, its flow creates an audible noise, a frictionlike quality, labeled frication, which gives these consonants their name.

fronting Sound substitutions in which the active and/or passive articulators are more anteriorly located for the production than the target sound.

front vowels On a horizontal, front-to-back plane, those vowels which have a more forward location of the bulge or hump of the tongue.

fundamental frequency Average number of glottal openings per second.

General American English Norm or typical pronunciation. Also called *Standard American English*.

glides See *semi-vowel approximants*.

gliding of liquids/fricatives The replacement of liquids or fricatives by glides.

glottal As passive articulator there is narrowing of the glottis, the space between the vocal folds.

glottis The space between the vocal folds.

grapheme A letter or combination of letters that supposedly represents a speech sound.

grooved channel fricative A fricative in which the channel for the airflow is extremely narrow. Both /s/ and /z/ are considered grooved channel fricatives, as the air flows through a narrow opening that is created by a sagittal (front-to-back), v-shaped furrow of the tongue.

harmonics Whole-numbered multiples of the fundamental frequency.

harmony processes See *assimilation*.

high vowels On a vertical, up-and-down plane, those vowels that have the greatest degree of tongue elevation relative to the palate.

hyperadduction Excessive adduction of the vocal folds.

hypernasality An excessive amount of perceived nasal cavity resonance due to lack of necessary velopharyngeal port closure.

hyperpharynx See *nasopharynx*.

hypertension Too much muscular action and tension.

hypopharynx See *laryngopharynx*.

hypotension Lack of muscular tension.

independent analysis Evaluates the child's phonological system independently of the adult target form.

informal Standard English A form of English that takes into account the assessment of the members of the American English speaking community as they judge the "standardness" of other speakers. This notion exists on a continuum ranging from standard to nonstandard speakers of American English. It relies far more heavily on grammatical structure than pronunciation patterns.

International Phonetic Alphabet The most widely used phonetic notation system.

intonation The feature of pitch when it functions linguistically at the sentence level.

intrinsic muscles Those muscles having both attachments within the referenced structure.

jargon stage Stage 5 of prelinguistic development, which is from approximately 10 months on.

labial Phonetic descriptor used when the bottom lip is used as an active articulator or the top lip is used as a passive articulator.

labialization The replacement of a nonlabial sound by a labial one.

laryngopharynx That portion of the pharynx that extends from the oropharynx to the entrance of the esophagus. Also called *hypopharynx*.

lateral approximant /l/; a type of consonant in which the air passes laterally over the sides of the tongue while the tongue blocks the center of the oral cavity.

lax vowels Those that are produced with less muscular tenseness, thus laxness, of the tongue and of the entire articulatory mechanism.

lenis consonants Those stop-plosives that have clearly less intraoral pressure (unaspirated stop-plosives), which translates into less air pressure during their production; derived from the Latin word meaning "weak."

limited English proficient student Any individual between the ages of 3 and 21 who is enrolled or preparing to enroll in an elementary or secondary school and who was not born in the United States or whose native language is a language other than English. Also individuals who are Native Americans or Alaska Natives and come from an environment where a language other than English has had a significant impact on them are included in this definition. The difficulties in speaking, writing, or understanding the English language compromise these individuals' abilities to successfully achieve in classrooms, where the language of instruction is English, or to participate fully in society.

linear phonologies A theoretical model in which all meaning-distinguishing sound segments are serially arranged.

linguistics Field of study that is concerned with the nature of language and communication.

lip retraction of vowels See *unrounded vowels*.

lip spreading of vowels See *unrounded vowels*.

long vowels Those vowels that are longer in duration.

low vowels On a vertical, up-and-down plane, those vowels that have the least degree of tongue elevation relative to the palate.

major class features Features established to characterize and distinguish between production possibilities that result in three sound classes that are essentially quite different, such as distinguishing vowels from consonants.

malocclusion Any abnormality in the alignment of the upper and the lower teeth, the alignment of the upper and lower jaws, the relationship of the upper and lower teeth to one another, or the positioning of individual teeth.

manner of articulation Refers to the type of constriction the active and passive articulators produce for the realization of a particular consonant; the way in which the airstream is modified as a result of the interaction of the articulators.

mechanical resonator The actual object itself is set into motion.

mediodorsal The middle one-third of the tongue as active articulator.

mediopalatal The second third of the hard palate as passive articulator.

mediopharynx See *oropharyx*.

mergers A variable that impacts dialects, consisting of the neutralization of features; phonemic distinctions are lost. Thus, two sounds tend to become more like each other. The phonemic boundary between the two becomes indistinct, and one sound may emerge as the prevalent pronunciation.

mid vowels On a vertical, up-and-down plane, those vowels that have the tongue approximately midway between the highest and the lowest vowel articulation.

minimal pairs Words that differ in only one phoneme value, such as "bee" and "beet" or "hit" and "him."

monophthongization An allophonic variation of a vowel in which vowels that are typically produced as diphthongs are articulated as monophthongs.

monophthongs (*mono* = one, *phthong* = sound) Vowels that remain qualitatively the same throughout their entire production.

multilinear phonologies See *nonlinear phonologies*.

narrow slit channel fricative A fricative produced with the channel for the airflow that is wider and flatter than that for a grooved fricative. The sh-productions, /ʃ/ and /ʒ/, are examples.

narrow transcription See *phonetic transcription*.

nasal cavities Two narrow chambers that begin at the soft palate and end at the exterior portion of the nostrils.

nasal emission Consonants produced with a great deal of nasal noise. Occurs on specific consonants that have a high degree of pressure in the oral cavity during their production.

nasal sounds (nasals) A manner of articulation defined by a complete blockage of the oral cavity; the articulators come together, creating a closure in the oral cavity, and the velum is lowered so that the airstream is directed through the nasal cavity. In American English, "m," "n," and "ng" are nasals.

nasalization An allophonic variation of a vowel in which vowels produced in the context of a nasal consonant ([m], [n], or [ŋ]) become nasalized.

nasopharynx That portion of the pharynx that extends from the upper portion of the nasal cavity to the soft palate. Also called *hyperpharynx*.

natural frequency The frequency at which an object vibrates. Also called its *resonant frequency*.

natural processes Those processes that are common in the speech development of children across languages.

noncontiguous assimilation See *remote assimilation*.

noncontinuants Those sounds in which there is complete obstruction of the flow of air. In American English, the stop-plosives and affricates are noncontinuants.

nonlinear phonologies A theoretical model in which there is a hierarchical interaction between segments and other linguistic units.

nonnasal sounds Those sounds produced with the velopharyngeal port closed; airflow passes through the oral cavity only.

nonphonemic diphthongs Those diphthongs that do not have phonemic value; the production of these sounds as diphthongs (as opposed to their articulation as monophthongs) does not change the meaning of a word.

nonpulmonic Referring to those sounds that are produced using "other airstream mechanisms" (IPA, 1999, p. 9).

nonreduplicated babbling One type of canonical babbling, which is marked by variation of both consonants and vowels from syllable to syllable. Also called *variegated babbling*.

nonresonant consonants A type of consonant based on the resonant qualities of the sound. Stop-plosives, fricatives, and affricates are nonresonant consonants.

nonsegmental phonologies See *nonlinear phonologies*.

nucleus The most prominent portion of a syllable, occupied by a vowel or syllabic consonant; syllable nuclei are louder than the other components of the syllable, thus, they are more intense than the surrounding consonants.

obstruents Those sounds that are produced with a complete or narrow constriction at some point in the vocal tract. The stop-plosives, fricatives, and affricates are obstruents.

occlusion The alignment of the upper and the lower teeth, the alignment of the upper and lower jaws, the relationship of the upper and lower teeth to one another, thus, the positioning of individual teeth.

offglide The second or final vowel portion of the diphthong.

onglide The first vowel portion of the diphthong.

onset All the segments prior to the peak of the syllable.

open syllables Syllables that do not contain a coda. Also called *unchecked syllables*.

open vowels Vowels that are articulated with the tongue farther away from the palate.

open-mid vowel A vowel in which the tongue is halfway between a close-mid and open vowel. Examples are /ɛ/ and /ɔ/.

oral cavity Mouth area that extends from the lips to the soft palate.

oropharynx That portion of the pharynx that extends from the soft palate to the hyoid bone. Also called the mediopharynx.

overbite Upper jaw is too far advanced relative to the lower jaw.

overlaid function See *secondary function*.

partial assimilation When the changed segment during an assimilation process is closer to but not identical to the sound that was the source of the change.

passive articulator The immovable portion of the vocal tract that is paired with the active articulator; consists of those structures that do not or cannot move during the production of speech sounds.

peak The most prominent, acoustically most intense part of the syllable.

perceptual phonetics Branch of phonetics that studies how speech sound waves are identified and perceived by the listener.

perseverative assimilation See *progressive assimilation.*

pharyngeal cavity A muscular and membranous tube-like structure, extending from the epiglottis to the soft palate.

phonation The production of tones resulting from vibration of the vocal folds.

phonatory system Consists of the larynx and is responsible for phonation.

phone Any particular occurrence of a sound segment that is used by a speaker when saying a word, regardless of whether the target language uses it.

phoneme The smallest linguistic unit that is able, when combined with other such units, to establish word meanings and distinguish between them; the central unit of phonology.

phonemic assimilation When the number of features affected during an assimilation process is such that the altered segment is perceived to be a different speech sound altogether, i.e., a different phoneme.

phonemic contrasts The ability of an individual to use phonemes contrastively within a language.

phonemic diphthongs Diphthongs that have phoneme value; the production of these sounds as diphthongs (as opposed to their articulation as monophthongs) can change the meaning of a word.

phonemic inventory All the vowels and consonants an individual uses as contrastive phonemes.

phonemic transcription Based on the phoneme system of that particular language; each symbol represents a phoneme. Also called *broad transcription.*

phonetic notation A set of symbols that stand for sound segments; a specific type of symbol system to describe each speech sound within a given language.

phonetic transcription (as one of two types of transcription) The use of a phonetic categorization that includes as much production detail as possible. Also called *narrow transcription.*

phonetic transcription (used in a general sense) The use of phonetic notation to record utterances or parts of utterances.

phonetic variability The rather unstable pronunciations of the child's first fifty words.

phonetically consistent forms Vocalizations used consistently but without a recognizable adult model (Dore, Franklin, Miller, & Ramer, 1976).

phonetics The science and study of speech emphasizing the description of speech sounds according to their production, transmission, and perceptual features.

phonological disorder An impaired system of phonemes and phoneme patterns.

phonological idioms As the child attempts to master other complexities of language, accurate sound productions are later replaced by inaccurate ones.

phonology Studies the structure and systematic patterning of sounds in a particular language; includes the description of the sounds a language uses and the rules governing how these sounds are organized.

phonotactic constraints The rule-governed patterns of sounds and syllables within a particular language; the restrictions on word and syllable shapes relative to which types of phonemes can occur in which word positions.

phonotactic processes In reference to dialects, those variations in which phonemes are added or deleted when compared to informal Standard English.

phonotactics The specific branch of phonology that deals with restrictions in a language on the permissible combinations of phonemes. Phonotactics identifies permissible syllable structure, consonant clusters, and vowel sequences within a particular language.

physiological phonetics Branch of phonetics that examines the anatomical-physiological prerequisites for speech and hearing, in particular the functional adequacy of all structures that are a portion of the speech process.

pidgin A system of communication that has grown up among people who do not share a common language but who want to talk to each other.

pitch The perceptual correlate of frequency.

postdorsal The posterior one-third of the tongue as active articulator.

postpalatal The posterior one-third of the hard palate as passive articulator.

predorsal The anterior one-third of the tongue as active articulator.

prelinguistic behavior Vocalizations prior to the first true words.

prepalatal The first third of the hard palate as passive articulator.

primary cardinal vowels (*cardinal* = chief, fundamental) Refers to those vowels that are considered to be the vowel points on which the system hinges.

primary function The life-supporting tasks of the speech mechanism. Also called *vital function*.

progressive assimilation A sound segment modifies a following sound. Also called *perseverative assimilation*.

prosodic features See *suprasegmental features*.

prosodic variability In reference to dialects, noted differences in intonational contours of sentences, the timing of sounds and syllables, and stress patterns of words which may distinguish a particular dialect.

protowords Vocalizations used consistently but without a recognizable adult model (Menn, 1978).

pulmonic sounds Those sounds that use air from the lungs for sound production.

quasi-words Vocalizations used consistently but without a recognizable adult model (Stoel-Gammon & Cooper, 1984).

r-coloring When a vowel has perceptual qualities that are similar to the r-sound.

race A biological label that is defined in terms of observable physical features (such as skin color, hair type and color, head shape and size), and biological characteristics (such as genetic composition).

received pronunciation Was considered to be the most "official" version of English spoken in the British Isles and was commonly used by most announcers on radio and television.

reduction An allophonic variation of vowels that occurs as the rate of speaking increases or as the stress on a vowel is decreased; the length is reduced, and the vowel becomes centralized; the vowels typically are reduced to a schwa vowel.

reduplicated babbling One type of canonical babbling, which is marked by similar strings of consonant-vowel productions; the consonants stay the same from syllable to syllable.

reduplication The replacement of a syllable or part of a syllable by a repetition of the preceding syllable.

reflexive crying and vegetative sounds Stage 1 of prelinguistic development, from birth to approximately 2 months of age.

reflexive vocalizations Those vocalizations in Stage 1 of the prelinguistic development, which include cries, coughs, grunts, and burps that seem to be automatic responses reflecting the physical state of the infant.

regional dialects Those dialects corresponding to various geographical locations.

regression As the child attempts to master other complexities of language, accurate sound productions are later replaced by inaccurate ones.

regressive assimilation A sound segment modifies a preceding sound. Also called *anticipatory assimilation*.

relational analysis The expected adult inventory is used as a basis for comparison of phonological abilities.

release phase The third phase of stop-plosive production, which consists of a sudden separation of the articulators that then allows for the burst of air that gives these sounds their characteristic quality.

remote assimilation A type of assimilation in which at least one other segment separates the assimilated sounds in question, especially when the sounds are in two different syllables. Also called *noncontiguous assimilation*.

resonance The selective absorption and reinforcement of sound energies, which create the characteristic quality of certain speech sounds.

resonant consonants A type of consonant based on the resonant quality of the sound. Nasals and approximants are considered to be resonant consonants.

resonant frequency See *natural frequency*.

resonatory system A series of cavities, the oral, nasal, and pharyngeal cavities, that play a vital role in resonance.

respiratory system Consists primarily of the lungs and airways, including the trachea, rib cage, abdomen, and diaphragm. These structures are directly related to respiration, the exchange of gases necessary for sustaining life, and are necessary to generate the airflow that makes voice and speech possible.

rhotic diphthong A centering diphthong in which the offglide represents a central vowel with r-coloring.

rhyme The nucleus plus the coda of a syllable.

rhythm The manner in which stressed and unstressed syllables succeed each other.

rising diphthong A diphthong in which the gliding movement of the tongue moves from a lower to a higher articulatory position.

rounded vowels Those vowels that are produced when the mouth opening is reduced by contraction of the muscles of the lips.

sagittal midline The median plane that divides the body, or in this case the vocal tract, into right and left halves.

secondary cardinal vowels Those vowels that differ only in the lip rounding/unrounding when compared to their primary cardinal vowel counterparts.

secondary function A function that is merely placed onto the original function. Also called *overlaid function*.

semivowel A type of consonant that denotes the similarity between the articulation of these consonants and other vowels. /w/ and /j/ (also called glides) are considered semivowels.

semivowel approximants Consonants that have a gliding movement of the active articulator from a partly constricted position into a more open position. Also called *glides*.

sense-group An organizational unit imposed upon prosodic data.

short vowels Those vowels that are shorter in duration.

shutting phase See *approach phase*.

sibilant A fricative with greater acoustic energy and more high-frequency components than other fricatives. Sibilants include /s/, /z/, /ʃ/, and /ʒ/.

slit fricatives Fricatives with a wider and flatter channel shape. Also divided into wide and narrow slit channel fricatives.

social dialect A dialect correlated to social differences.

sonorants Speech sounds that are produced with a relatively open vocal tract, creating a resonant quality of the sounds. Those sounds that have more acoustic energy, that are louder. In American English vowels, nasals, and approximants are considered sonorants.

sonority A sound's loudness relative to that of other sounds with the same length, stress, and pitch.

sound spectrogram The visual display of an acoustic analysis; frequency is displayed on the vertical axis, duration on the horizontal axis, and intensity is noted by the darkness of the tracings.

source features Specific laryngeal features as distinctive features.

speech mechanism Cumulative label for the structures that are involved in producing speech.

speech melody A general term used to reference pitch fluctuations relative to their linguistic function.

speech sounds Individual units of speech.

speech Referring to oral, verbal communication; as a communication mode, speech is the exchange of information through speaking or talking.

Standard American English See *General American English.*

stimulability testing A type of testing that probes the client's ability to produce the correct articulation of a misarticulated sound when some kind of "stimulation" is provided by the clinician. Many variations in this procedure exist, but commonly the clinician asks the client to "watch and listen to me, and then you try to say it exactly like I did."

stop phase The second phase of stop-plosive production in which the articulators are held closed for a period of time (40–150 ms), during which there is a build-up of air pressure behind the closure. Also called *closure phase.*

stop-plosives Consonants defined by complete blockage of the oral cavity; the articulators come together creating a closure in the oral cavity to block off the airflow, which results in a build-up of air pressure behind this occlusion; the velum is raised. This pressure is released suddenly, which creates the characteristic "explosive" sound of these consonants.

stopping The replacement of fricatives and affricates by stops.

stress The degree of force of an utterance or the prominence produced by means of respiratory effort.

subglottal That area below the vocal folds.

substitution processes In reference to a dialect, a sound in one dialect corresponds to a different sound in another dialect.

suprasegmental features Those modifications that occur that are related to intonation, stress, and timing. Also called *prosodic features.*

syllabic sound A speech sound that can function as the nucleus of a syllable. Vowels are syllabic sounds, but also nasals and the lateral approximant /l/ can, under certain circumstances, be syllabic sounds.

syllable initiating Segments that are the onset of a syllable.

syllable terminating Segments that are the coda of a syllable.

tempo The speed of speaking.

tense vowels Vowels that are produced with more muscular tenseness of the tongue and of the entire articulatory mechanism.

timbre Refers to the tonal quality that differentiates two sounds of the same pitch, loudness, and duration.

tone-unit An organizational unit imposed upon prosodic data.

tone The changes in fundamental frequency, perceived as pitch, when they function linguistically at the word (morpheme) level.

total assimilation The label given during an assimilation process when the changed segment and the source of the change become identical.

transfer The incorporation of language features into a non-native language, based on the occurrence of similar features in the native language.

unchecked syllables See *open syllables*.

underbite Lower jaw protrusion is excessive relative to the upper jaw.

unrounded vowels Those vowels that are produced with the muscles of the lips either quite inactive or neutral, or with the contraction of specific muscles that draw back the corners of the lips; also labeled vowels with lip spreading or lip retraction.

unstressed syllable deletion The omission of an unstressed syllable. Also called *weak syllable deletion*.

variegated babbling See *nonreduplicated babbling*.

vegetative sounds Those vocalizations in Stage 1 of the prelinguistic development that include grunts and sighs associated with activity and clicks and other noises that are associated with feeding.

velar Referring to the velum as passive articulator of speech sounds.

velopharyngeal mechanism The structures and muscles of the velum (soft palate) and those of the pharyngeal walls.

velopharyngeal port The passage that connects the oropharynx and the nasopharynx.

vernacular dialects Those varieties of spoken American English that are considered to be outside the continuum of informal Standard English.

vital function See *primary function*.

vocables Vocalizations used consistently but without a recognizable adult model (Ferguson, 1976).

vocal play Stage 3 of prelinguistic development, from approximately 4 to 6 months of age.

vocal tract All speech-related systems above the vocal folds.

voicing Term used to denote the presence or absence of simultaneous vocal fold vibration resulting in voiced or voiceless consonants; in phonological processes the replacement of a voiced for a voiceless sound.

vowelization (vocalization) The replacement of syllabic liquids and nasals, foremost [l], [r], and [n], by vowels.

vowels Speech sounds produced with a relatively open vocal tract, without articulatory constriction.

weak syllable deletion See *unstressed syllable deletion*

wide slit channel fricative A fricative produced with a widening and flattening of the channel produced by the tongue. /θ/ and /ð/ are examples.

Abercrombie, D. (1967). *Elements of general phonetics.* Chicago: Aldine.

Akmajian, A. Demers, R., Farmer, A., & Harnish, R. (2001). *Linguistics: An introduction to language and communication* (5th ed.). Cambridge, MA: MIT Press.

Altaha, F. (1995). Pronunciation errors made by Saudi University students learning English: Analysis and remedy. *I.T.L. Review of Applied Linguistics,* 109–123.

American Speech-Language-Hearing Association. (1987). Ad hoc committee on dysphagia report. *ASHA, 29,* 57–58.

American Speech-Language-Hearing Association. (2002). *Incidence and prevalence of speech, voice, and language disorders in the United States—2002 edition: Factsheet.* Rockville, MD: Author.

American Speech-Language-Hearing Association. (2003). *American English dialects* [Technical Report]. Retrieved March 12, 2007, from www.asha.org/policy.

Andrews, N., & Fey, M. (1986). Analysis of the speech of phonologically impaired children in two sampling conditions. *Language, Speech, and Hearing Services in Schools, 17,* 187–198.

Angelocci, A., Kopp, G., & Holbrook, A. (1964). The vowel formants of deaf and normal-hearing eleven- to fourteen-year-old boys. *Journal of Speech and Hearing Disorders, 29,* 156–170.

Arlt, P., & Goodban, M. (1976). A comparative study of articulatory acquisition as based on a study of 240 normals, aged three to six. *Language, Speech, and Hearing Services in Schools, 7,* 173–180.

Atkinson-King, K. (1973). Children's acquisition of phonological stress contrasts. *UCLA Working Papers in Phonetics, 25,* 184–191.

Bailey, G., Maynor, N., & Cukor-Avila, P. (1991). *The emergence of Black English: Text and commentary.* Philadelphia/Amsterdam: John Benjamin.

Bailey, G., & Ross, G. (1992). The evolution of a vernacular. In M. Rissanen et al., *History of Englishes: New methods and interpretations in historical linguistics* (pp. 519–531). Berlin: Mouton de Gruyter.

Ball, M., & Kent, R. (1997). *The new phonologies: Developments in clinical linguistics.* San Diego: Singular.

Ball, M., & Rahilly, J. (1999). *Phonetics: The science of speech.* London: Arnold.

Bankson, N., & Byrne, M. (1962). The relationship between missing teeth and selected consonant sounds. *Journal of Speech and Hearing Disorders, 24,* 341–348.

Battle, D. (1993). *Communication disorders in multicultural populations.* Boston: Andover Medical Publishers.

Bauman-Waengler, J. (2008). *Articulatory and phonological impairments: A clinical focus.* (3rd ed.). Boston: Allyn and Bacon.

Benguerel, A.-P., & Cowan, H. (1974). Coarticulation of upper lip protrusion in French. *Phonetica, 30,* 41–55.

Bernhardt, B., & Stemberger, J. (1998). Handbook of phonological development from the perspective of constraint-based nonlinear phonology. San Diego: Academic Press.

Blache, S. (1978). *The acquisition of distinctive features.* Baltimore: University Park Press.

Blache, S. (1989). A distinctive-feature approach. In N. Creaghead, P. Newman, & W. Secord, *Assessment and remediation of articulatory and phonological disorders* (2nd ed., pp. 361–382). New York: Macmillan.

Black, J. (1949). Natural frequency, duration, and intensity of vowels in reading. *Journal of Speech and Hearing Disorders, 14*, 216–221.

Bleile, K. (2002). Evaluating articulation and phonological disorders when the clock is running. *American Journal of Speech-Language Pathology, 11*, 243–249.

Blockcolsky, V. (1990). *Book of words: 17,000 words selected by vowels and diphthongs.* Tucson: Communication Skill Builders.

Blockcolsky, V., Frazer, J., & Frazer, D. (1987). *40,000 selected words.* Tucson, AZ: Communication Skill Builders.

Blosser, J. L., & Neidecker, E. A. (2002). *School programs in speech-language pathology: Organization and service delivery* (4th ed.). Boston: Allyn and Bacon.

Bok Lee, H. (1999). Korean. In International Phonetic Association, *Handbook of the International Phonetic Association* (pp. 120–123). Cambridge, UK: Cambridge University Press.

Boone, D., McFarlane, S., & Von Berg, S. (2004). The voice and voice therapy. Boston: Pearson/Allyn and Bacon.

Borden, G., Harris, K., & Raphael, L. (2003). *Speech science primer: Physiology, acoustics, and perception of speech* (4th ed.). Baltimore: Lippincott Williams & Wilkins.

Bosma, J. F. (1975). Anatomic and physiologic development of the speech apparatus. In E. L. Eagles (Ed.), *Human communication and its disorders: Volume 3.* New York: Raven Press.

Boysson-Bardies, B., de, & Vihman, M. (1991). Adaptation to language. *Language, 67*, 297–339.

Bronstein, A. (1960). *The pronunciation of American English. An introduction to phonetics.* New York: Appleton-Century-Crofts.

Browman, C., & Goldstein, L. (1986). Towards an articulatory phonology. *Phonology Yearbook, 3*, 219–252.

Brown, R. (1973). *A first language: The early stages.* Cambridge, MA: Harvard University Press.

Brown, V. (1990). *The social and linguistic history of a merger: /i/ and /e/ before nasals in Southern American English.* Unpublished doctoral dissertation, Texas A & M University, College Station.

Bruner, J. (1975). The ontogenesis of speech acts. *Journal of Child Language, 2*, 1–19.

Canning, B., & Rose, M. (1974). Clinical measurements of the speech, tongue and lip movements in British children with normal speech. *British Journal of Disorders of Communication, 9*, 45–50.

Carpenter, L. (2003). Dialect: Language variations across cultures. In L. Shriberg & R. Kent, *Clinical phonetics* (3rd ed., pp. 389–408). Boston: Pearson Education.

Carrell, J., & Tiffany, W. R. (1960). *Phonetics: Theory and application to speech improvement.* New York: McGraw-Hill.

Carver, C. (1987). *American regional dialects: A word geography.* Ann Arbor: University of Michigan Press.

Chan, A., & Li, D. (2000). English and Cantonese phonology in contrast: Explaining Cantonese ESL learners' English pronunciation problems. *Language, Culture, and Curriculum, 13*, 67–85.

Chen, H. P., & Irwin, O. C. (1946). Infant speech: Vowel and consonant types. *Journal of Speech Disorders, 11*, 27–29.

Cheng, L. L. (1994). Asian/Pacific students and the learning of English. In J. Bernthal & N. Bankson (Eds.), *Child phonology: Characteristics, assessment, and intervention with special populations* (pp. 255–274). New York: Thieme.

Cherney, L. R. (1994). Dysphagia in adults with neurologic disorders: An overview. In L. R. Cherney (Ed.), *Clinical management of dysphagia in adults and children* (2nd ed., pp. 1–33). Gaithersburg, MD: Aspen.

Cho, B.-E. (2004). Issues concerning Korean learners of English: English education in Korea and some common difficulties of Korean students. *The East Asian Learner, 1*, 31–36.

Chomsky, C. (1971). *Linguistic development in children from 6 to 10.* Office of Education (DHEW): Final Report. Washington, DC: Bureau of Research.

Chomsky, N. (1957). *Syntactic structures*. The Hague: Mouton.

Chomsky, N., & Halle, M. (1968). *The sound pattern of English*. New York: Harper and Row.

Colton, R. H., & Casper, J. K. (1990). *Understanding voice problems: A physiological perspective for diagnosis and treatment*. Baltimore: William & Wilkins.

Creaghead, N. A., & Newman, P. W. (1989). Articulatory phonetics and phonology. In N. A. Creaghead, P. W. Newman, & W. A. Secord (Eds.), *Assessment and remediation of articulatory and phonological disorders* (2nd ed., pp. 9–33). New York: Macmillan.

Cruttenden, A. (1985). Intonation comprehension in 10-year-olds. *Journal of Child Language, 12*, 643–661.

Crystal, D. (1986). Prosodic development. In P. Fletcher & M. Garman (Eds.), *Language acquisition* (2nd ed., pp. 174–197). Cambridge, UK: Cambridge University Press.

Crystal, D. (1987). *The Cambridge encyclopedia of language*. Cambridge, UK: Cambridge University Press.

Darley, F. L., Aronson, A. E., & Brown, J. R. (1975). *Motor speech disorders*. Philadelphia: W. B. Saunders.

Davis, B. L., & MacNeilage, P. F. (1990). Acquisition of correct vowel production: A quantitative case study. *Journal of Speech and Hearing Research, 33*, 16–27.

Demuth, K., & Fee, E. (1995). *Minimal words in early phonological development*. Unpublished master's thesis, Brown University, Providence, RI & Dalhousie University, Halifax, Nova Scotia.

Dewey, G. (1971). *English spelling: Roadblock to reading*. New York: Teachers College Press.

Diedrich, W. (1983). Stimulability and articulation disorders. In J. Locke (Ed.), *Assessing and treating phonological disorders: Current approaches. Seminars in Speech and Language, 4*. New York: Thieme-Stratton.

Dore, J., Franklin, M. B., Miller, R. T., & Ramer, A. L. (1976). Transitional phenomena in early language acquisition. *Journal of Child Language, 3*, 13–29.

Duckworth, M., Allen, G., Hardcastle, W., & Ball, M. J. (1990). Extensions to the International Phonetic Alphabet for the transcription of atypical speech. *Clinical Linguistics and Phonetics, 4*, 273–280.

Dworkin, J. P. (1991). *Motor speech disorders: A treatment guide*. St. Louis: Mosby-Year Book.

Eckert, P. (1988). Adolescent social structure and the spread of linguistic change. *Language in Society, 17*, 183–208.

Edwards, H. T. (2003). *Applied phonetics: The sounds of American English* (3rd ed.). Clifton Park, NY: Thomson Delmar Learning.

Elbers, L. (1982). Operating principles in repetitive babbling: A cognitive approach. *Cognition, 12*, 45–63.

Elbert, M., & Gierut, J. (1986). *Handbook of clinical phonology: Approaches to assessment and treatment*. San Diego: College-Hill Press.

Fairbanks, G., House, A., & Stevens, E. (1950). An experimental study in vowel intensities. *Journal of the Acoustical Society of America, 22*, 457–459.

Fairbanks, G., & Lintner, M. (1951). A study of minor organic deviations in functional disorders of articulation. *Journal of Speech and Hearing Disorders, 16*, 273–279.

Faircloth, S., & Faircloth, M. (1973). *Phonetic science: A program of instruction*. Englewood Cliffs, NJ: Prentice-Hall.

Fee, E. (1996). Syllable structure and minimal words. In B. Bernhardt, J. Gilbert, & D. Ingram (Eds), *Proceedings of the UBC International Conference on Phonological Acquisition* (pp. 85–98). Somerville, MA: Cascadilla Press.

Ferguson, C. (1976). Learning to pronounce: The earliest stages of phonological development in the child. In F. Minifie & L. Floyd (Eds.), *Communicative and cognitive abilities: Early behavioral assessment* (pp. 273–297). Baltimore: University Park Press.

Ferguson, C. A., & Farwell, C. (1975). Words and sounds in early language acquisition: English initial consonants in the first fifty words. *Language, 51*, 419–439.

Ferrand, C. T. (2007). *Speech science: An integrated approach to theory and clinical practice* (2nd ed.). Boston: Allyn and Bacon.

Fisicelli, R. M. (1950). *An experimental study of the prelinguistic speech development of institutionalized infants.* Unpublished doctoral dissertation, Fordham University, New York, NY.

Flexner, S. (Ed.). (1987). *The Random House dictionary of the English language* (2nd ed.). New York: Random House.

Flexner, S. B., & Hauck, L. C. (Eds.). (1987). *The Random House dictionary* (2nd ed.). New York: Random House.

Forchhammer, J. (1940). Vokal und Konsonant. *Archiv fuer vergleichende Phonetik, IV*, 51–66.

French, A. (1988). What shall we do with "medial" sounds? *British Journal of Disorders of Communication, 23*, 41–50.

French, A. (1989). The systematic acquisition of word forms by a child during the first-fifty-word stage. *Journal of Child Language, 16*, 69–90.

Froeschels, E. (1931). *Lehrbuch der Sprachheilkunde* (3rd ed.). Vienna: Deuticke.

Fudala, J., & Reynolds, W. (1994). *Arizona articulation proficiency scale* (2nd ed.). Los Angeles: Western Psychological Services.

Fudala, J., & Reynolds, W. (2000). *Arizona 3: Arizona articulation proficiency scale* (3rd ed.). Los Angeles: Western Psychological Services.

Garn-Nunn, P., & Lynn, J. (2004). *Calvert's descriptive phonetics* (3rd ed.). New York: Thieme Medical Publishers.

Gesell, A., & Thompson, H. (1934). *Infant behavior: Its genesis and growth.* New York: McGraw-Hill.

Gierut, J. (1998). Treatment efficacy: Functional phonological disorders in children. *Journal of Speech, Language, and Hearing Research, 41*, 85–100.

Gilbert, J. H., & Purves, B. A. (1977). Temporal constraints on consonant clusters in child speech production. *Journal of Child Language, 4*, 417–432.

Gladwell, M. (2001). *The tipping point: How little things can make a big difference.* New York: Back Bay Books/Little, Brown and Company.

Goldstein, B., & Washington, P. (2001). An initial investigation of phonological patterns in 4-year-old typically developing Spanish-English bilingual children. *Language, Speech, & Hearing Services in the Schools, 32*, 153–164.

González, G. (1988). Chicano English. In D. Bixler-Marquez & J. Ornstein-Galicia (Eds.), *Chicano speech in the bilingual classroom. Series VI, Vol. 6* (p. 71–89). New York: Lang.

Gorecka, A. (1989). *The phonology of articulation.* Unpublished doctoral dissertation. Massachusetts Institute of Technology, Cambridge, MA.

Grunwell, P. (1981). The development of phonology: A descriptive profile. *First Language, 2*, 161–191.

Grunwell, P. (1986). Aspects of phonological development in later childhood. In K. Durkin (Ed.), *Language development in the school years* (pp. 34–56). London: Croom Helm.

Grunwell, P. (1987). *Clinical phonology* (2nd ed.). Baltimore: Williams & Wilkins.

Hadding-Koch, K. (1961). *Acoustico-phonetic studies in the intonation of southern Swedish.* Travaux de l'Institut de phonetique de Lund, Vol. 3. Lund, Sweden: CWK Gleerups.

Haelsig, P., & Madison, C. (1986). A study of phonological processes exhibited by 3-, 4-, and 5- year-old children. *Language, Speech, and Hearing Services in Schools, 17*, 107–114.

Halle, M. (1983). On distinctive features and their articulatory implementation. *Natural Language and Linguistic Theory, 1*(1), 91–105.

Hallé, P., de Boysson-Bardies, B., & Vihman, M. (1991). Beginnings of prosodic organization: Intonation and duration patterns of disyllables produced by Japanese and French infants. *Language and Speech, 34*, 299–318.

Hane, A. (2003). A dyadic approach to the interactional context of language acquisition: The direct and indirect effects of early mother-infant vocal coordination in predicting language outcomes at 24 months. *Dissertation Abstracts International, 63,* 39–58.

Hanson, M. L. (1983). *Articulation.* Philadelphia: W. B. Saunders.

Hargrove, P. (1982). Misarticulated vowels: A case study. *Language, Speech, and Hearing Services in Schools, 13,* 86–95.

Hartman, J. (1985). Guide to pronunciation. In F. Cassidy (Ed.), *Dictionary of American regional English: Volume I, Introduction and A–C* (pp. xli–lx). Cambridge, MA: The Belknap Press of Harvard University Press.

Hawkins, S. (1979). Temporal coordination of consonants in the speech of children: Further data. *Journal of Phonetics, 13,* 235–267.

Haynes, W., & Moran, M. (1989). A cross-sectional developmental study of final consonant production in Southern Black children from preschool through third grade. *Language, Speech, and Hearing Services in Schools, 20,* 400–406.

Heffner, R.-M.S. (1975). *General phonetics.* Madison: University of Wisconsin Press.

Hellwag, C. F. (1781). *Dissertatio inauguralis physicomedica de formatione loquelae* (Unpublished dissertation), University of Tübingen, Tübingen, Germany.

Hidalgo, M. (1987). On the question of "standard" versus "dialect": Implications for teaching Hispanic college students. *Hispanic Journal of Behavioral Sciences, 9*(4), 375–395.

Hixon, T., Goldman, M., & Mead, J. (1973). Kinematics of the chest wall during speech production. *Journal of Speech and Hearing Research, 16,* 78–115.

Hodson, B., Scherz, J., & Strattman, K. (2002). Evaluating communicative abilities of a highly unintelligible preschooler. *American Journal of Speech-Language Pathology, 11,* 236–242.

Hoffman, P., Schuckers, G., & Daniloff, R. (1989). *Children's phonetic disorders: Theory and treatment.* Boston: Little, Brown.

Holmgren, K., Lindblom, B., Aurelius, G., Jalling, B., & Zetterstrom, R. (1986). On the phonetics of infant vocalization. In B. Lindblom & R. Zetterstrom (Eds.), *Precursors of early speech* (pp. 51–63). New York: Stockton Press.

Hornby, P. A., & Hass, W. A. (1970). Use of contrastive stress by preschool children. *Journal of Speech and Hearing Research, 13,* 395–399.

Hsu, H., & Fogel, A. (2001). Infant vocal development in a dynamic mother-infant communication system. *Infancy, 2,* 87–109.

Hsu, H., Fogel, A., & Cooper, R. (2000). Infant vocal development during the first 6 months: Speech quality and melodic complexity. *Infant and Child Development, 9,* 1–17.

Huthaily, K. (2003). *Phonological analysis of Arabic and English.* Master's thesis. University of Montana, Helena.

Ianucci, D., & Dodd, D. (1980). The development of some aspects of quantifier negation. *Papers & Reports on Child Language Development, 19,* 88–94.

Iglesias, A., & Goldstein, B. (1998). Language and dialectal variations. In J. Bernthal & N. Bankson (Eds.) *Articulation and phonological disorders* (pp. 147–161). Englewood Cliffs, NJ: Prentice-Hall.

Ingram, D. (1974). Phonological rules in young children. *Journal of Child Language, 1,* 49–64.

Ingram, D. (1981). *Procedures for the phonological analysis of children's language.* Baltimore: University Park Press.

Ingram, D. (1989a). *First language acquisition: Method, description, and explanation.* Cambridge, UK: Cambridge University Press.

Ingram, D. (1989b). *Phonological disability in children* (2nd ed.). London: Whurr.

International Phonetic Alphabet (IPA). (2005). The International Phonetic Alphabet (revised from 1993). *Journal of the International Phonetic Association, 23,* center pages.

International Phonetic Association. (1999). *Handbook of the International Phonetic Association.* Cambridge, UK: Cambridge University Press.

Irwin, J. V., & Wong, S. P. (1983). *Phonological development in children 18 to 72 months.* Carbondale: Southern Illinois University Press.

Irwin, O. C. (1945). Reliability of infant speech sound data. *Journal of Speech Disorders, 10,* 227–235.

Irwin, O. C. (1946). Infant speech: Equations for consonant–vowel ratios. *Journal of Speech Disorders, 11,* 177–180.

Irwin, O. C. (1947a). Infant speech: Consonantal sounds according to place of articulation. *Journal of Speech and Hearing Disorders, 12,* 397–401.

Irwin, O. C. (1947b). Infant speech: Consonant sounds according to manner of articulation. *Journal of Speech and Hearing Disorders, 12,* 402–404.

Irwin, O. C. (1948). Infant speech: Development of vowel sounds. *Journal of Speech and Hearing Disorders, 13,* 31–34.

Irwin, O. C. (1951). Infant speech: Consonantal position. *Journal of Speech and Hearing Disorders, 16,* 159–161.

Irwin, O. C., & Chen, H. P. (1946). Infant speech: Vowel and consonant frequency. *Journal of Speech and Hearing Disorders, 11,* 123–125.

Jakobson, R. (1941/1968). *Kindersprache, Aphasie und allgemeine Lautgesetze.* Uppsala, Sweden: Almquist and Wiksell.

Jakobson, R. (1949). On the identification of phonemic entities. *Travaux du Cercle Linguistique de Prague, 5,* 205–213.

Jakobson, R. (1971). Why "mama" and "papa"? In A. Bar-Adon & W. Leopold (Eds.), *Child language: A book of readings* (pp. 213–217). Englewood Cliffs, NJ: Prentice Hall.

Jakobson, R., & Halle, M. (1956). *Fundamentals of language.* The Hague: Mouton.

Jakobson, R., Fant, G., & Halle, M. (1952). *Preliminaries to speech analysis: The distinctive features and their correlates.* Cambridge, MA: MIT Press.

Jespersen, O. (1889). *The articulation of speech sounds.* Marburg: Elwert Verlag.

Jones, D. (1932). *An outline of English phonetics.* Leipzig: B.G. Teubner.

Kantner, C. E., & West, R. (1960). *Phonetics* (Rev. ed.). New York: Harper & Brothers.

Kent, R. D. (1997). *The speech sciences.* San Diego: Singular.

Kent, R. D., & Bauer, H. R. (1985). Vocalizations of one-year-olds. *Journal of Child Language, 13,* 491–526.

Kent, R. D., & Forner, L. (1980). Speech segment durations in sentence recitations by children and adults. *Journal of Phonetics, 8,* 157–168.

Kent, R. D., & Murray, A. D. (1982). Acoustic features of infant vocalic utterances at 3, 6, and 9 months. *Journal of the Acoustical Society of America, 72,* 353–365.

Khan, L. (1988, November). *Vowel remediation: A case study.* Paper presented at the American Speech-Language-Hearing Association Convention, Boston, MA.

Khan, L. (2002). The sixth view: Assessing preschoolers' articulation and phonology from the trenches. *American Journal of Speech-Language Pathology, 11,* 250–254.

Khan, L., & Lewis, N. (2002). *Khan-Lewis phonological analysis* (2nd ed.). Circle Pines, MN: American Guidance Service.

Kharma, N., & Hajjaj, A. (1989). *Errors in English among Arabic speakers: Analysis and remedy.* London: Longman International Education.

Kiesling, S. (1998). Men's identities and sociolinguistic variation: The case of fraternity men. *Journal of Sociolinguistics, 2,* 69–99.

Klein, H. (1984). Procedure for maximizing phonological information from single-word responses. *Language, Speech, and Hearing Services in Schools, 15,* 267–274.

Klein, H., Lederer, S., & Cortese, E. (1991). Children's knowledge of auditory/articulatory correspondences: Phonologic and metaphonologic. *Journal of Speech and Hearing Research, 34,* 559–564.

Kühnert, B., & Nolan, F. (2000). The origin of coarticulation. In W. Hardcastle and N. Hewlett (Eds.), *Coarticulation: Theory, data, and techniques.* (pp. 7–30). Cambridge, UK: Cambridge University Press.

Kuhl, P., & Meltzoff, A. (1996). Infant vocalizations in response to speech: Vocal imitation and developmental change. *Journal of the Acoustical Society of America, 4,* 2424–2438.

Labov, W. (1985). *The increasing divergence of black and white vernaculars: Introduction to the research reports.* Unpublished manuscript.

Labov, W. (1991). The three dialects of English. In P. Eckert (Ed.), *New ways of analyzing sound change* (pp. 1–44). New York: Academic Press.

Labov, W. (1994). *Principles of linguistic change. Volume 1: Internal factors.* Oxford, UK: Blackwell.

Labov, W. (1996, November). *The organization of dialect diversity.* Paper presented at 4th International Conference on Spoken Language Processing, Philadelphia.

Labov, W., Ash, S., & Boberg, C. (1997). *A national map of the regional dialects of American English.* Retrieved February 1, 2005, from the University of Pennsylvania Telsur Project website: http://www.ling.upenn.edu/phono_atlas/NationalMap/NationalMap.html

Labov, W., Ash, S., & Boberg, C. (2005). *Atlas of North American English.* Berlin: Mouton de Gruyter.

Labov, W., Yaeger, M., & Steiner, R. (1972). *A quantitative study of sound change in progress.* Philadelphia: U.S. Regional Survey.

Ladefoged, P. (1971). *Preliminaries to linguistic phonetics.* Chicago: University of Chicago Press.

Ladefoged, P. (1993). *A course in phonetics* (3rd ed.). New York: Harcourt Brace Jovanovich.

Ladefoged, P. (1997). Linguistic phonetic description. In W. Hardcastle & J. Laver (Eds.), *The handbook of phonetic sciences* (pp. 589–618). Oxford, UK: Blackwell.

Ladefoged, P. (1999). American English. In International Phonetic Association, *Handbook of the International Phonetic Association* (pp. 41–44). Cambridge, UK: Cambridge University Press.

Ladefoged, P. (2001). *A course in phonetics* (4th ed.). Fort Worth, TX: Harcourt Brace.

Ladefoged, P. (2005). *Vowels and consonants: An introduction to the sounds of languages* (2nd ed.). Malden, MA: Blackwell.

Ladefoged, P. (2006). *A course in phonetics* (5th ed.). Boston: Thomson Wadsworth.

Ladefoged, P., DeClerk, J., Lindau, M., & Papcun, G. (1972). An auditory-motor theory of speech production. *UCLA Working Papers in Phonetics, 22,* 48–75.

Ladefoged, P., & Maddieson, I. (1996). *The sounds of the world's languages.* Oxford, UK: Blackwell.

Lane, H., Perkell, J., Svirsky, M., & Webster, J. (1991). Changes in speech breathing following cochlear implant in postlingually deafened adults. *Journal of Speech and Hearing Research, 34,* 526–533.

Laver, J. (1994). *Principles of phonetics.* Cambridge, UK: Cambridge University Press.

Lee, H. B. (1999). Korean. In *Handbook of the International Phonetic Association* (pp. 120–122) Cambridge, UK: Cambridge University Press.

Lehiste, I. (1977). *Suprasegmentals* (2nd ed.). Cambridge, MA: MIT Press.

Lehiste, I., & Peterson, G. (1959). Vowel amplitude and phonemic stress in American English. *Journal of the Acoustical Society of America, 31,* 428–435.

Leonard, L., & Leonard, J. (1985). The contribution of phonetic context to an unusual phonological pattern: A case study. *Language, Speech, and Hearing Services in Schools, 16,* 110–118.

Leonard, L., Newhoff, M., & Mesalam, L. (1980). Individual differences in early child phonology. *Applied Psycholinguistics, 1,* 7–30.

Leopold, W. F. (1947). *Speech development of a bilingual child: A linguist's record.* Evanston, IL: Northwestern University Press.

Li, C., & Thompson, S. (1987). Chinese. In B. Comrie (Ed.), *The world's major languages* (pp. 811–833). New York: Oxford University Press.

Liberman, A., Cooper, F., Harris, K., & MacNeilage, P. (1963). Motor theory of speech perception. In *Stockholm Speech Communication Seminar, Vol. II, Paper D 3.* Stockholm, Sweden: Speech Transmission Laboratory, Royal Institute of Technology.

Lieberman, P. (1998). *Eve spoke: Human language and evolution.* New York: W.W. Norton.

Lipsitt, L. (1966). Learning processes of human newborns. *Merrill-Palmer Quarterly, 12*, 45–71.

Lipski, J. (2000). The linguistic situation of Central Americans. In S. McKay and S. Wong (Ed.), *New immigrants in the United States* (pp. 189–215). Cambridge, UK: Cambridge University Press.

Locke, J. L. (1983). *Phonological acquisition and change.* New York: Academic Press.

Locke, J. L. (1990). Structure and stimulation in the ontogeny of spoken language. *Developmental Psychobiology, 23*, 621–643.

Lof, G. (2002). Two comments on this assessment series. *American Journal of Speech-Language Pathology, 11*, 255–256.

Lowe, R. (1994). *Phonology: Assessment and intervention applications in speech pathology.* Baltimore: Williams & Wilkins.

Lowe, R. (1996). Assessment link between phonology and articulation: ALPHA (Rev. ed.). Mifflinville, PA: Speech and Language Resources.

Lowe, R., Knutson, P., & Monson, M. (1985). Incidence of fronting in preschool children. *Language, Speech, and Hearing Services in Schools, 16*, 119–123.

Lyons, J. (1981). *Language and linguistics.* Cambridge, UK: Cambridge University Press.

MacKay, I. (1987). *Phonetics: The science of speech production* (2nd ed.). Boston: Allyn and Bacon.

Malikouti-Drachman, A., & Drachman, G. (1975). The acquisition of stress in Modern Greek. *Salzburger Beiträge zur Linguistik, 2*, 277–289.

Mallinson, C. (2004). A good guide to African American English: A linguistic guide. *American Speech, 79*, 219–223.

Masataka, N. (1993). Effects of contingent and non-contingent maternal stimulation on the vocal behavior of three- and four-month-old Japanese infants. *Journal of Child Language, 20*, 303–312.

Masataka, N. (2001). Why early linguistic milestones are delayed in children with Williams syndrome: Late onset of hand banging as a possible rate-limiting constraint on the emergence of canonical babbling, *Developmental Science, 4*, 158–164.

McDonald, E. (1964). *A deep test of articulation—a picture form.* Pittsburgh: Stanwix.

Mehrabian, A. (1970). Measures of vocabulary and grammatical skills for children up to age six. *Developmental Psychology, 2*, 439–446.

Menn, L. (1971). Phonotactic rules in beginning speech. *Lingua, 26*, 225–251.

Menn, L. (1978). *Pattern, control and contrast in beginning speech: A case study in the development of word form and word function.* Bloomington: Indiana University Linguistics Club.

Menyuk, P. (1980). The role of context in misarticulations. In G. Yeni-Komshian, J. Kavanagh, & C. Ferguson (Eds.), *Child phonology: Vol. 1. Production* (pp. 211–226). New York: Academic Press.

Menzerath, P., & De Lacerda, A. (1933). *Koartikulation, Steuerung und Lautabgrenzung.* Berlin und Bonn: Fred. Dümmlers.

Meyer, E. A. (1910). Plastographic analysis. Untersuchung über Lautbildung. *Viëtor Festschrift.* Marburg, Germany: Elwert.

Miccio, A. (2002). Clinical problem solving: Assessment of phonological disorders. *American Journal of Speech-Language Pathology, 11*, 221–229.

Miccio, A., Elbert, M., & Forrest, K. (1999). The relationship between stimulability and phonological acquisition in children with normally developing and disordered phonologies. *American Journal of Speech-Language Pathology, 8*, 347–363.

Miller, G., & Nicely, P. (1955). An analysis of perceptual confusions among some English consonants. *Journal of the Acoustical Society of America, 27*, 338–352.

Mitchell, P. R., & Kent, R. (1990). Phonetic variation in multisyllable babbling. *Journal of Child Language, 17*, 247–265.

Morgan, M. (1998). More than a mood or an attitude: Discourse and verbal genres in African-American culture. In S. Mufwene, J. Rickford, G. Bailey, & J. Baugh

(Eds.), *African-American English: Structure, history, and use* (pp. 251–281). London: Routledge.

Mortensen, D. (2004). *Preliminaries to Mong Leng (Hmong Njua) phonology*. Retrieved September 25, 2006, from ist-socrates.berkeley.edu/~dmort/mong_leng_phonology.pdf

Moses, E. (1964). *Phonetics: History and interpretation*. Englewood Cliffs, NJ: Prentice-Hall.

Moskowitz, A. (1971). *Acquisition of phonology*. Unpublished doctoral dissertation, University of California, Berkeley.

Myers, F. L., & Myers, R. W. (1983). Perception of stress contrasts in semantic and non-semantic contexts by children. *Journal of Psycholinguistic Research, 12,* 327–338.

Nakazima, S. A. (1962). A comparative study of the speech developments of Japanese and American English in childhood (1): A comparison of the developments of voices at the prelinguistic period. *Studia Phonologica, 2,* 27–46.

National Institute on Deafness and Other Communication Disorders. *Strategic plan: Plain language version*. Retrieved April 23, 2001, from http://www.nidcd.nih.gov/about/director/nsrp.htm

Neary, T. (1978). *Phonetic feature systems for vowels*. Doctoral dissertation, University of Connecticut, Storrs. Reproduced by Indiana University Linguistic Club.

Nelson, K. (1973). Structure and strategy in learning to talk. *Monographs of the Society of Research in Child Development, 38* (149). Chicago: University of Chicago Press.

New Webster's dictionary of the English language. (1986). Chicago: Delair Publishing.

Newman, D. (2002). The phonetic status of Arabic within the world's languages: The uniqueness of the lu at al-d aad. *Antwerp Papers in Linguistics* (pp. 446–452). Antwerp, Belgium: University of Antwerp.

Nittrouer, S., Studdert-Kennedy, M., & McGowan, R. (1989). The emergence of phonetic segments: Evidence from the spectral structure of fricative-vowel syllables spoken by children and adults. *Journal of Speech and Hearing Research, 32,* 120–132.

Nittrouer, S., & Whalen, D. (1989). The perceptual effects of child–adult differences in fricative vowel coarticulation. *Journal of the Acoustical Society of America, 86,* 1266–1276.

No Child Left Behind Act of 2001, Public Law No. 107–110 (May 23, 2001).

Nordmark, J. O. (1968). Mechanisms of frequency discrimination. *Journal of the Acoustical Society of America, 44,* p. 1533.

Office of English Language Acquisition. (2002). *Survey of the states' limited English proficient students and available educational programs and services 2000–2001 summary report.* Washington, DC: National Clearinghouse for English Language Acquisition and Language Instruction Educational Programs.

Ohala, J. J. (1991, August). The integration of phonetics and phonology. *Proceedings of the XIIth International Congress of Phonetic Sciences*, Aix-en-Provence, *1,* 1–16.

Ohala, J. J. (2004). Phonetics and phonology then, and then, and now. In H. Quene & V. van Heuven (Eds.), *On speech and language: Studies for Sieb G. Nooteboom* (LOT Occasional Series 2, pp. 133–140). Netherlands Graduate School of Linguistics, Utrecht, Netherlands.

Ohala, M. (1999). Hindi. In *Handbook of the International Phonetic Association*. International Phonetic Association (pp. 100–103). Cambridge, UK: Cambridge University Press.

Ohde, R. N., & Sharf, D. J. (1992). *Phonetic analysis of normal and abnormal speech.* New York: Merrill.

Okada, H. (1999). Japanese. In *The handbook of the International Phonetic Association* (pp. 117–119). Cambridge, UK: Cambridge University Press.

Oller, D. K. (1980). The emergence of the sounds of speech in infancy. In G. Yeni-Komshian, J. Kavanagh, & C. A. Ferguson (Eds.), *Child phonology, Vol. I: Production* (pp. 93–112). New York: Academic Press.

Oller, D. K., Wieman, L. A., Doyle, W. J., & Ross, C. (1976). Infant babbling and speech. *Journal of Child Language, 3*, 1–11.

Olmsted, D. (1971). *Out of the mouth of babes: Earliest stages in language learning.* The Hague: Mouton.

Osberger, M., Levitt, H., & Slosberg, R. (1979). Acoustic characteristics of correctly produced vowels. [Abstract]. *Journal of the Acoustical Society of America, 66*, 13.

Otheguy, R., Garcia, O., & Roca, A. (2000). Speaking in Cuban: The language of Cuban Americans. In S. McKay & S. Wong (Ed.), *New immigrants in the United States* (pp. 165–188). Cambridge, UK: Cambridge University Press.

Owens, R. E. (2008). *Language development: An introduction* (7th ed.). Boston: Allyn and Bacon.

Panagos, J., & Prelock, P. (1982). Phonological constraints on the sentence production of language disordered children. *Journal of Speech and Hearing Research, 25*, 171–177.

Panconcelli-Calzia, G. (1957). Earlier history of phonetics. In L. Kaiser (Ed.), *Manual of phonetics* (pp. 17–33). Amsterdam: North-Holland Publishing.

Papaeliou, C., Minadakis, G., & Cavouras, D. (2002). Acoustic patterns of infant vocalizations expressing emotions and communicative functions. *Journal of Speech, Language and Hearing Research, 45*, 311–318.

Paul, H. (1898). *Prinzipien der Sprachgeschichte* (3rd ed.). Halle: Niemeyer.

Penfield, J., & Ornstein-Galacia, J. (1985). *Chicano English: An ethnic dialect.* Philadelphia: John Benjamin.

Perez, E. (1994). Phonological differences among speakers of Spanish-influenced English. In J. Bernthal & N. Bankson (Eds.), *Child phonology: Characteristics, assessment, and intervention with special populations* (pp. 245–254). New York: Thieme.

Perlman, A. L. (2000). Disordered swallowing. In J. B. Tomblin, H. L. Morris, & D. C. Spriestersbach (Eds.), *Diagnosis in speech-language pathology* (2nd ed., pp. 403–426). San Diego: Singular.

Pierce, J. E., & Hanna, I. V. (1974). *The development of a phonological system in English-speaking American children.* Portland, OR: HaPi Press.

Pike, K. L. (1943). *Phonetics.* Ann Arbor: University of Michigan Press.

Pollock, K., & Swanson, L. (1986, November). *Analysis of vowel errors in a disordered child during training.* Paper presented at the annual convention of the American Speech-Language-Hearing Association, Detroit, MI.

Poole, I. (1934). Genetic development of articulation of consonant sounds in speech. *Elementary English Review, 11*, 159–161.

Poole, S. C. (1999). *An introduction to linguistics.* New York: St. Martin's Press.

Powell, T., Elbert, M., & Dinnsen, D. (1991). Stimulability as a factor in the phonologic generalization of misarticulating preschool children. *Journal of Speech and Hearing Research, 34*, 1318–1328.

Power, T. (2003). *Practice for Arabic language backgrounds.* Retrieved September 15, 2007, from http://www.btinternet.com/~ted.power/l1arabic.html

Prather, E. M., Hedrick, D., & Kern, C. (1975). Articulation development in children aged two to four years. *Journal of Speech and Hearing Disorders, 40*, 179–191.

Preisser, D., Hodson, B., & Paden, E. (1988). Developmental phonology: 18–29 months. *Journal of Speech and Hearing Disorders, 53*, 125–130.

Raphael, L., & Bell-Berti, F. (1975). Tongue musculature and the feature of tension in English vowels. *Phonetica, 32*, 61–63.

Ratliff, M. (1992). *Meaningful tone: A study of tonal morphology in compounds, form classes, and expressive phrases in White Hmong.* Monograph Number 27, Southeast Asia. De Kalb: Northern Illinois University Center for Southeast Asian Studies.

Rickford, J. (1999). *African American Vernacular English: Features, evolution, and educational implications.* Oxford, UK: Blackwell.

Riesz, R. R. (1928). Differential intensity sensitivity of the ear of pure tones. *Physiological Review, 31*, p. 867.

Roach, P. (2004). British English: Received pronunciation. *Journal of the International Phonetic Association, 34*, 239–245.

Robb, M. P., & Saxman, J. H. (1990). Syllable durations of preword and early word vocalizations. *Journal of Speech and Hearing Research, 33*, 583–593.

Roberts, J., Burchinal, M., & Footo, M. (1990). Phonological process decline from 2½ to 8 years. *Journal of Communication Disorders, 23*, 205–217.

Rosenfeld-Johnson, S. (2001). *Oral-motor exercises for speech clarity.* Tucson, AZ: Innovative Therapists International.

Rousselot, P.-J. (1897–1901). *Principes de phonétique experimentale*, I–II. Paris: H. Welter.

Ruhlen, M. (1976). *Guide to the languages of the world.* San Diego: Los Amigos Research Associates.

Russell, G. (1928). *The vowel.* Columbus: Ohio State University Press.

Rvachew, S., & Nowak, M. (2001). The effect of target-selection strategy on phonological learning. *Journal of Speech, Language, and Hearing Research, 44*, 610–623.

Rvachew, S., Rafaat, S., & Martin, M. (1999). Stimulability, speech perception skills, and the treatment of phonological disorders. *American Journal of Speech-Language Pathology, 8*, 33–43.

Sagey, E. (1986*). The representation of features and relations in non-linear phonology.* Unpublished doctoral dissertation, Massachusetts Institute of Technology: Cambridge, MA.

Sankoff, D., & Laberge, S. (1978). The linguistic market and the statistical explanation of variability. In D. Sankoff (Ed.), *Linguistic variation: Models and methods* (pp. 239–250). New York: Academic Press.

Schneider, E. (1996). *Focus on the USA.* Philadelphia/Amsterdam: John Benjamins.

Schultze, F. (1880/1971). The speech of the child. In A. Bar-Adon & W. Leopold (Eds. & trans.), *Child language: A book of readings.* Englewood Cliffs, NJ: Prentice-Hall.

Schwartz, R. (1992). Clinical applications of recent advances in phonological theory. *Language, Speech, and Hearing Services in Schools, 23*, 269–276.

Sharkey, S., & Folkins, J. (1985). Variability of lip and jaw movements in children and adults: Implications for the development of speech motor control. *Journal of Speech and Hearing Research, 28*, 3–15.

Shibamoto, J., & Olmstead, D. (1978). Lexical and syllabic patterns in phonological acquisition. *Journal of Child Language, 5*, 417–456.

Shower, E. G., & Biddulph, R. (1931). Differential pitch sensitivity of the ear. *Journal of the Acoustical Society of America, 3*, p. 275.

Shprintzen, R. J. (1995). *Cleft palate speech management: A multidisciplinary approach.* St. Louis: Mosby Year-Book.

Shriberg, L., & Kent, R. (2003). *Clinical phonetics* (3rd ed.). Boston: Allyn and Bacon.

Shriberg, L., & Kwiatkowski, J. (1982). Phonological disorders III: A procedure for assessing severity of involvement. *Journal of Speech and Hearing Disorders, 47*, 242–256.

Shvachkin, N. K. (1973). The development of phonemic speech perception in early childhood. In C. A. Ferguson, & D. I. Slobin (Eds.), *Studies of child language development.* New York: Holt, Rinehart & Winston.

Sievers, E. (1876). *Grundzüge der Lautphysiologie zur Einführung in das Studium der Lautlehre der indogermanischen Sprachen.* Leipzig: Breitkopf und Hartel.

Sievers, E. (1901). *Grundzüge der Phonetik: Zur Einführung in das Studium der indogermanischen Sprachen.* Leipzig: Breitkopf und Hartel.

Singh, S., & Polen, S. (1972). Use of distinctive feature model in speech pathology. *Acta Symbolica, 3*, 17–25.

Sloat, C., Taylor, S., & Hoard, J. (1978*). Introduction to phonology.* Englewood Cliffs, NJ: Prentice-Hall.

Small, L. (2005). *Fundamentals of phonetics: A practical guide for students* (2nd ed.). Boston: Allyn and Bacon.

Smit, A. (1986). Ages of speech sound acquisition: Comparisons and critiques of several normative studies. *Language, Speech, and Hearing Services in Schools, 17,* 175–186.

Smit, A. (1993a). Phonologic error distributions in the Iowa-Nebraska Articulation Norms Project: Consonant singletons. *Journal of Speech and Hearing Research, 36,* 533–547.

Smit, A. (1993b). Phonologic error distributions in the Iowa-Nebraska Articulation Norms Project: Word-initial consonant clusters. *Journal of Speech and Hearing Research, 36,* 931–947.

Smit, A., Hand, L., Freilinger, J., Bernthal, J., & Bird, A. (1990). The Iowa Articulation Norms Project and its Nebraska replication. *Journal of Speech and Hearing Disorders, 55,* 779–798.

Smith, B., Brown-Sweeney, S., & Stoel-Gammon, C. (1989). A quantitative analysis of reduplicated and variegated babbling. *First Language, 9,* 175–189.

Smith, N. (1973). *The acquisition of phonology: A case study.* Cambridge, UK: Cambridge University Press.

Smitherman, G. (1996). *African-American English: From the hood to the amen corner.* Center for Interdisciplinary Studies of Writing, Speaker Series No. 5. Minneapolis: University of Minnesota.

Snow, D. (1998a). Children's imitations of intonation countours: Are rising tones more difficult than falling tones? *Journal of Speech, Language, and Hearing Research, 41,* 576–587.

Snow, D. (1998b). A prominence account of syllable reduction in early speech development: The child's prosodic phonology of tiger and giraffe. *Journal of Speech, Language, and Hearing Research, 41,* 1171–1184.

Snow, D. (2000). The emotional basis of linguistic and nonlinguistic intonation: Implications for hemispheric specialization. *Developmental Neuropsychology, 17,* 1–27.

Snow, D., & Balog, H. (2002). Do children produce the melody before the words? A review of developmental intonation research. *Lingua, 112,* 1025–1058.

Snow, K. (1961). Articulation proficiency in relation to certain dental abnormalities. *Journal of Speech and Hearing Disorders, 26,* 209–212.

Spencer, P., & Marschark, M. (2003). Cochlear implants: Issues and implications. In M. Marschark & P. Spencer (Eds.), *Oxford handbook of deaf studies, language and education* (pp. 434–450). Oxford, UK: Oxford University Press.

Stampe, D. (1979). *A dissertation on natural phonology.* New York: Garland.

Stark, R. (1980). Stages of speech development in the first year of life. In G. Yeni-Komshian, J. Kavanagh, & C. A. Ferguson (Eds.), *Child phonology, Vol. I: Production* (pp. 73–92). New York: Academic Press.

Stark, R. (1986). Prespeech segmental feature development. In P. Fletcher & M. Garman (Eds.), *Language acquisition: Studies in first language development* (pp. 149–173). Cambridge, UK: Cambridge University Press.

Starr, C. (1972). Dental and occlusal hazards to normal speech production. In K. Bzoch (Ed.), *Communicative disorders related to cleft lip and palate* (pp. 337–356). Boston: Little, Brown.

Steven, S. S., & Volkmann, J. (1940). The relation of pitch to frequency. *American Journal of Psychology, 53,* p. 329.

Stevens, S. S. (1935). The relation of pitch to intensity. *Journal of the Acoustical Society of America, 6,* p. 150.

Stockman, I. (1996). The promises and pitfalls of language sample analysis as an assessment tool for linguistic minority children. *Language, Speech, and hearing Services in Schools, 27,* 355–366.

Stoel-Gammon, C. (1985). Phonetic inventories, 15–24 months: A longitudinal study. *Journal of Speech and Hearing Research, 28,* 505–512.

Stoel-Gammon, C. (1987). Phonological skills in 2-year-olds. *Language, Speech, and Hearing Services in Schools, 18*, 323–329.

Stoel-Gammon, C., & Cooper, J. A. (1984). Patterns of early lexical and phonological development. *Journal of Child Language, 11*, 247–271.

Stoel-Gammon, C., & Herrington, P. (1990). Vowel systems of normally developing and phonologically disordered children. *Clinical Linguistics and Phonetics, 4*, 145–160.

Stoel-Gammon, C., & Menn, L. (1997). Phonological development: Learning sounds and sound patterns. In J. Berko Gleason (Ed.), *The development of language* (4th ed., pp. 69–121). Boston: Allyn and Bacon.

Subtelny, J., Mestre, J., & Subtelny, J. (1964). Comparative study of normal and defective articulation of /s/ as related to malocclusion and deglutition. *Journal of Speech and Hearing Disorders, 29*, 269–285.

Sussman, H., & Westbury, J. (1981). The effects of antagonistic gestures on temporal and amplitude parameters of anticipatory labial coarticulation. *Journal of Speech and Hearing Research, 24*, 16–24.

Sweet, H. (1877). *A handbook of phonetics*. Oxford, UK: Clarendon Press.

Sweet, H. (1890). *Primer of phonetics*. Oxford, UK: Oxford University Press.

Techmer, F. (1885). *Zur Veranschaulichung der Lautbildung*. Leipzig: Heilbronn.

Templin, M. (1957). *Certain language skills in children: Their development and interrelationships* (Institute of Child Welfare Monograph 26). Minneapolis: The University of Minnesota Press.

Terrell, S., & Terrell, F. (1993). African American cultures. In D. Battle (Ed.), *Communication disorders in multicultural populations* (pp. 3–37). Boston: Andover Medical.

Thelwal, R., & Akram Sa'Adeddin, M. (1999). Arabic. In International Phonetic Association, *Handbook of the International Phonetic Association* (pp. 51–54). Cambridge, UK: Cambridge University Press.

Thiele, G. (1980). *Handlexikon der Medizin*. München, Germany: Urban & Schwarzenberg.

Thomas, C. K. (1958). *Phonetics of American English*. New York: Ronald Press.

Trubetzkoy, N. S. (1939). *Grundzüge der Phonologie*. Prague: Travaux du Cercle, 4. Linguistique de Prague.

Turk, A., Jusczyk, P., & Gerken, L. (1995). Do English-learning infants use syllable weight to determine stress? *Language and Speech, 38*, 143–158.

Tyler, A., & Tolbert, L. (2002). Speech-language assessment in the clinical setting. *American Journal of Speech-Language Pathology, 11*, 215–220.

Uldall, E. (1960). Attitudinal meanings conveyed by intonation contours. *Language and Speech, 13*, 123–130.

U.S. Census Bureau. (2000). *Census 2000*. Retrieved April 27, 2007, from http://factfinder.census.gov.

U.S. Department of Commerce. (2003). *Yearbook of immigration statistics*. Springfield, VA: National Technical Information Service.

Val Barros, A.-M. (2003). *Pronunciation difficulties in the consonant system experienced by Arabic speakers when learning English after the age of puberty*. Master's thesis. University of West Virginia, Wheeling.

Van Riper, C. (1978). *Speech correction: Principles and methods* (6th ed.). Englewood Cliffs, NJ: Prentice-Hall.

Van Riper, C., & Irwin, J. (1958). *Voice and articulation*. Englewood Cliffs, NJ: Prentice-Hall.

Vandeputte, O., Vincent, P., & Hermans, T. (1986). *Dutch, the language of twenty million Dutch and Flemish people* (2nd ed.). Rekkem, Flanders, Belgium: Stichting Ons Erfdeel.

Vaux, B. (2005). English dialect survey. Retrieved January 12, 2005, from http://www.hcs.harvard.edu/~golder/dialect/

Velleman, S. (1998). *Making phonology functional: What do I do first?* Boston: Butterworth-Heinemann.

Velleman, S., & Strand, K. (1994). Developmental verbal dyspraxia. In J. Bernthal & N. Bankson (Eds.), *Child phonology: Characteristics, assessment and intervention with special populations* (pp. 110–139). New York: Thieme.

Velten, H. (1943). The growth of phonemic and lexical patterns in infant language. *Language, 19,* 281–292.

Vihman, M. (1984). *Individual differences in phonological development: Age one and age three.* Unpublished manuscript.

Vihman, M. (1992). Early syllables and the construction of phonology. In C. Ferguson, L. Menn, & C. Stoel-Gammon (Eds.), *Phonological development: Models, research, implications* (pp. 393–422). Timonium, MD: York Press.

Vihman, M. M. (1998). Early phonological development. In J. E. Bernthal & N. W. Bankson (Eds.), *Articulation and phonological disorders* (2nd ed., pp. 38–53). Boston: Allyn and Bacon.

Vihman, M. M., Ferguson, C. A., & Elbert, M. (1986). Phonological development from babbling to speech: Common tendencies and individual differences. *Applied Psycholinguistics, 7,* 3–40.

Vihman, M., & Greenlee, M. (1987). Individual differences in phonological development: Ages one and three years. *Journal of Speech and Hearing Research, 30,* 503–521.

Vihman, M. M., Macken, M. A., Miller, R., Simmons, H., & Miller, J. (1985). From babbling to speech: A reassessment of the continuity issue, *Language, 61,* 397–445.

von Essen, O. (1979). *Allgemeine und angewandte Phonetik* (5th ed.) Berlin: Akademie Verlag.

Waengler, H.-H. (1983). *Grundriss einer Phonetik des Deutschen* (4th ed.). Berlin: Akademie Verlag.

Washington, J. (1998). *African American English research: A review and future directions.* Retrieved January 21, 2006, from http://www.rcgd.isr.umich.edu/prba/perspectives/spring1998/jwashington.pdf

Watson, J. (2002). *The phonology and morphology of Arabic.* Oxford, UK: Oxford University Press.

Weiss, C. (1980). *Weiss comprehensive articulation test.* Allen, TX: DLM Teaching Resources.

Weiss, C. E., & Lillywhite, H. E. (1981). *Communication disorders* (2nd ed.). St. Louis: C.V. Mosby.

Weiss, C., Gordon, M., & Lillywhite, H. (1987). *Clinical management of articulatory and phonologic disorders* (2nd ed.). Boston: Williams & Wilkins.

Wellman, B. L., Case, I. M., Mengert, I. G., & Bradbury, D. E. (1931). Speech sounds of young children. In *University of Iowa Studies in Child Welfare, 5.* Iowa City: University of Iowa Press.

Wells, J. (1982). *Accents of English, Volume 2, British Isles.* Cambridge, UK: Cambridge University Press.

Wells, J. (1997). What happened to Received Pronunciation? *II Jornadas de Estudios Ingleses, 8,* p. 19–28.

Whalen, D., Levitt, A., & Wang, Q. (1991). Intonational differences between reduplicative babbling of French- and English-learning infants. *Journal of Child Language 18,* 501–516.

Wilkins, J. (1668). *An essay towards a real character and a philosophical language.* London: S. Gellibrand.

Winitz, H., & Irwin, O. C. (1958). Syllabic and phonetic structure of infants' early words. *Journal of Speech and Hearing Research, 1,* 250–256.

Wise, C. M. (1957). *Introduction to phonetics.* Englewood Cliffs, NJ: Prentice-Hall.

Wolfram, W. (1986). Language variations in the United States. In O. Taylor (Ed.), *Treatment of communication disorders in culturally and linguistically diverse populations* (pp. 73–116). San Diego: College-Hill Press.

Wolfram, W. (1991). *Dialects and American English*. Englewood Cliffs, NJ: Prentice-Hall.

Wolfram, W. (1994). The phonology of a sociocultural variety: The case of African American vernacular English. In J. Bernthal & N. Bankson (Eds.), *Child phonology: Characteristics, assessment and intervention with special populations* (pp. 227–244). New York: Thieme.

Wolfram, W., & Schilling-Estes, N. (2006). *American English: Dialects and variations* (2nd ed.). Malden, MA: Blackwell.

Yavaş, M. (1998). *Phonology: development and disorders*. San Diego: Singular.

Yeni-Komshian, G., Flege, J., Liu, S. (2000). Pronunciation proficiency in the first and second languages of Korean-English bilinguals. *Bilingualism: Language and Cognition, 3*, 131–150.

Yorkston, K., Beukelman, D., & Bell, K. (1988). *Clinical management of dysarthric speakers*. Boston: College-Hill Press.

Zemlin, W. R. (1986). Anatomy and physiology of speech. In G. Shames & E. Wiig (Eds.), *Human communication disorders: An introduction* (2nd ed., pp. 81–133). Columbus, OH: Merrill.

Zemlin, W. R. (1998). *Speech and hearing science: Anatomy and physiology* (3rd ed.). Englewood Cliffs, NJ: Prentice-Hall.

Zentella, A. (2000). Puerto Ricans in the United States: Confronting the linguistic repercussions of colonialism. In S. McKay & S. Wong (Ed.), *New immigrants in the United States* (pp. 137–164). Cambridge, UK: Cambridge University Press.

Lane, H., 35
Laver, J., 140
Lederer, S., 288
Lee, H.B., 185, 187, 188
Lehiste, I., 209, 211
Leonard, J., 93
Leonard, L., 93, 244
Leopold, W.F., 243, 250, 251
Levitt, A., 241
Levitt, H., 44
Lewis, N., 267
Li, C., 184
Li, D., 186
Liberman, A., 211
Lieberman, P., 24
Lillywhite, H.E., 215, 245, 255
Lindau, M., 80
Lindblom, B., 239
Lintner, M., 40
Lipsitt, L., 245
Lipski, J., 180
Liu, S., 174
Locke, J.L., 240, 242
Lof, G., 288
Lowe, R., 99, 265, 266, 267, 283
Lynn, J., 75, 79, 85
Lyons, J., 4

M

MacKay, I., 52, 61, 62, 113, 116, 121, 136, 207, 209
Macken, M.A., 240, 250
MacNeilage, P.F., 90, 211, 240
Maddieson, I., 187, 188, 190
Madison, C., 264
Malikouti-Drachman, A., 251
Mallinson, C., 172
Marschark, M., 109
Martin, M., 289
Masataka, N., 237, 241
Maynor, N., 172
McDonald, E., 119
McFarlane, S., 35
McGowan, R., 202
Mehrabian, A., 245
Meltzoff, A., 240
Mengert, I.G., 246, 247
Menn, L., 240, 242, 243, 250
Menyuk, P., 290
Menzerath, P., 201
Mesalam, L., 244
Mestre, J., 40
Meyer, E.A., 80
Miccio, A., 288
Miller, G., 120
Miller, J., 240, 250
Miller, R.T., 240, 241, 242, 250
Minadakis, G., 240
Mitchell, P.R., 237, 239, 242
Monson, M., 265

Morgan, M., 152
Mortensen, D., 182
Moses, E., 8
Moskowitz, A., 251
Murray, A.D., 241
Myers, F.L., 256
Myers, R.W., 256

N

Nakazima, S.A., 238
Neary, T., 80
Neidecker, E.A., 52
Nelson, K., 242
New Webster's Dictionary of English Language, 61
Newhoff, M., 244
Newman, D., 189
Newman, P.W., 22
Nicely, P., 120
Nittrouer, S., 202
Nolan, F., 201
Nordmark, J.O., 4
Nowak, M., 288

O

Office of English Language Acquisition, 150, 173
Ohala, J.J., 8
Ohde, R.N., 4, 5, 43
Okada, H., 109
Oller, D.K., 237, 238, 239, 243
Olmstead, D., 244
Olmsted, D., 246
Ornstein-Galacia, J., 177, 178, 179
Osberger, M., 44
Otheguy, R., 178
Owens, R.E., 241

P

Paden, E., 263, 264
Panagos, J., 290
Panconcelli-Calzia, G., 8
Papaeliou, C., 240
Papcun, G., 80
Paul, H., 201
Penfield, J., 177, 178, 179
Perez, E., 177, 179
Perkell, J., 35
Perlman, A.L., 29
Peterson, G., 211
Pierce, J.E., 240
Polen, S., 257
Pollock, K., 93
Poole, I., 247, 248, 250, 275
Poole, S.C., 6
Powell, T., 288
Power, T., 190, 191
Prather, E.M., 247, 248, 250, 275
Preisser, D., 263, 264
Prelock, P., 290
Purves, B.A., 253

preschool, 245–51
school-age, 252–56
vowel production in, 93
Citation form, 65
articulation test, spontaneous speech *versus,* 66
testing, 282
Click, 56
Clinical Assessment of Articulation & Phonology, 284
Closed syllables, 303
open syllables *versus,* 303
Close vowels, 80, 82
Cluster reduction, 264
Coalescence, 206
Coarticulation, 201, 230
anticipatory, 202
defined, 201
Cochlear implant, 109
Coda, 302
Code switching, 169
Cognates, 74
Communication, 68
defined, 2
disorders, 6
notation system and, 52
Communicative disorders, case study on, 15
Complementary distribution, 12–13, 17
Complex wave, 42
Consonant clusters, case study on, 274
Consonant-like sounds, 240
Consonants, 4, 56
active articulators, 111–13
age of acquisition of, 254
case study on, 108–9, 117, 143
cluster variations, 154
continuant, 124
diacritics used with, 214–23
fortis, 116
individual, 126–27
labialization of, 221–22, 389–90
lenis, 116
manner of articulation, 115–24
nasal, 128–29
noncontinuant, 124
nonlabialization of, 221–22, 389–90
non-pulmonic, 57
nonresonant, 125
obstruent, 125
passive articulators, 113–15
production features of, 108–45
pulmonic, 57
resonant, 125
semivowel, 125
sonorant, 125
syllabic, 220–21, 302, 312
types of, 124–43
voiced, 218
voiceless, 218
vowels *versus,* 73–74, 109
Constricted sounds, 73

Contact assimilation, 203, 204
Contiguous assimilation, 203
Continuant consonants, 124
Contrastive stress, 251, 255
Cooing, 238, 274
Coronal, 349
Coronal division of tongue, 111
Creole, 154, 171
Creolist Hypothesis, 171
Cricothyroid muscle, 32
Cross-sectional mastery level charts, 250
Cross-sectional sound mastery study, 275–76
Cuban American English, 178–79
Cul-de-sac, 117
Culture, 167

D
Deaffrication, 266
Denasalization, 266
Dental, 113, 349
Dentalization, 215
exercises for, 384
Derhotacization, 223, 267
Devoicing, 218
exercises for, 385–86
partial, 385–86
Diacritics, 52, 58, 212–30
case study on, 229–30
clinical application for, 218
defined, 201, 232–33
dentalization, 215
exercises for, 384–94
lateralization, 216–17
palatalization, 215–16
for suprasegmentals, 226–30
syllabic, 221
used with consonants, 214–23
used with vowels, 223–26, 390–91
velarization, 216
voice symbols, 218–23
Dialects, 92, 149–96
African American Vernacular English (AAVE), 151, 168–73
case study on, 149, 165
change in, 153–55
defined, 150
defining boundaries of, 154–55
ethnic, 154
exercises for, 395–99
foreign, 173–92, 397–99
popular *versus* professional usage, 150–52
rap and, 172
regional, 97, 154, 155–65
social and ethnic, 166–73
variations of, 94, 95, 153–55
vernacular, 152
Diaphragm, 25, 26, 28
Digastric muscles, 31
Digraph, 61
Diphthongization, 100

Larynx (*cont.*)
  intrinsic muscles of, 32, 33
  posterior view of, 30
Lateral approximants, 123
Lateralization, 216–17
  exercises for, 384
Lateral s-productions, 137
Laughing, 238, 274
Lax vowels, 79, 81
Lenis consonants, 116
Letters, sounds *versus*, 318–23
Limited English proficient students, 173, 196
  clinical application for, 173
  language spoken by, 175
Linear phonologies, 270, 277
Lingua-alveolar, 110
Lingual, 110
Linguistic phase, of phonological development,
  241
Linguistics
  case study on, 11
  defined, 7
Lips, 3, 11, 22, 39
  retraction, 77
  rounding, 77, 97, 119
  spreading, 77
  unrounding, 77
Liquids, 145, 267
Long vowels, 80
Loudness, 5, 16
Low vowels, 75
Lungs, 26, 27
  volume of, 28

M
Machine-gun rhythm, 212
Major class features
  consonantal, 258
  sonorant, 258
  vocalic, 258
Malocclusions, 40, 41
Mandible, 3, 22, 39, 40
Manner of articulation, 115–24, 258–59
  continuant, 258
  delayed release, 258
  phonetic description of, 123
  tense, 258–59
Matrix, 292
  for recording consonants, 292
  for recording vowels, 292
  for syllable initiating and terminating
    consonants, 305
Maxilla, 40
Mechanical resonator, 41
Mediodorsal, 111
Mediodorsal division of tongue, 111
Mediopalatal, 113
Mediopharynx, 36. *See also* Oropharynx
Melody, 206
  speech, 208

Mergers, 159–61, 193–94
Midland dialects, 165
Mid vowels, 75, 82
Minimal pairs, 8
Misarticulations, 217
Monophthongization, 100
Monophthongs, 84
  diphthongs *versus,* 84
  vowels, 100
Multiple interdentality, 215
Muscles
  abdominal, 28
  cricothyroid, 32
  digastric, 31
  extrinsic, 31
  geniohyoid, 31
  infrahyoid, 31
  intercostal, 26
  intrinsic, 31, 32
  mylohyoid, 31
  omohyoid, 31
  orbicularis oris, 39
  sternohyoid, 31
  stylohyoid, 31
  suprahyoid, 31
  thoracic, 25, 28
  thryohyoid, 31
Mylohyoid muscles, 31

N
Narrow transcription, 52
  clinical application of, 53
Nasal cavities, 36
Nasal emission, 38
Nasality
  exercises for, 391–94
  symbols, 225–26
Nasalization, 100
Nasal productions, 117, 248
  characteristics of, 118–21, 144
  clinical application for, 118
  exercises for, 364–72
Nasal sounds, 37
Nasopharynx, 35
Natural frequency, 41
Natural phonology, 262–68, 276–77
  assimilation processes, 267–68
  phonological development and, 263
  phonological processes, 263
  substitution processes, 264–67
  syllable structure changes, 263–64
Natural processes, 263
Nicaraguan American English, 180
No Child Left Behind Act (NCLB), 196
Nonaspiration, exercises for, 386–87
Noncontiguous assimilation, 203
Noncontinuant consonants, 124
Nonlabialization
  of consonants, 221–22
  exercises for, 389–90

Nonlinear phonologies, 270, 277
feature geometry of, 272
phonological development and, 271–74
Nonlinear theories, 268–74
Nonnasality, exercises for, 391–94
Nonnasal sounds, 37
Nonphonemic diphthongs, 86
Non-pulmonic consonants, 57
Non-pulmonic sounds, 56
Nonreduplicated babbling, 239
Nonresonant consonants, 125
Northern Cities vowel shift, 156–58
Northern dialects, 164
exercises for, 395–96
Notation, phonetic, 52
Notation system, phonetic transcription as, 51–52
accuracy of, 51
communication and, 52
documentation, 51–52
Nucleus, 73

O
Obstruent consonants, 125
Occlusion, 40
Offglide, 85
onglide *versus,* 85
Omohyoid muscles, 31
Onglide, 85
offglide *versus,* 85
Onglides, 97, 98
Onset, 302
Open sounds, 73
Open syllables, 303
closed syllables *versus,* 303
Open vowels, 80, 82
Oral cavity, 36
structures of, 115
Orbicularis oris muscle, 39
Oropharynx, 36
Orthographic letter system, 68
Orthography, 60
system, 68
Overlaid functions, 24

P
Palatal, 110
Palatalization, 215–16
exercises for, 384
Partial assimilation, 205
Partial devoicing, exercises for, 385–86
Partial voicing, exercises for, 385–86
Passive articulators, 113–15, 144
alveolar, 113
dental, 113
glottal, 113
labial, 113
mediopalatal, 113
oral cavity structures, 115
phonetic description of, 114
postpalatal, 113

prepalatal, 113
velar, 113
Peak, 302
Perception
clinical application of, 7
of speech, 5
Perceptual biases, clinical application for, 64
Perceptual phonetics, 5. *See also* Auditory
phonetics
Perseverative assimilation, 203
Pharyngeal cavity, 35
Phonation, 22
dysarthria and, 36
Phonatory system, 22, 29–35
overview of, 23
Phone, 3
Phonemes, 8, 10–12, 12, 16
distribution of, 303–7
inventory of, 14
notation for, 53
Phonemic analysis, 281–312
phonemic inventory and contrasts, 291–301
Phonemic assimilation, 205
Phonemic contrasts, 292
Phonemic diphthongs, 86
Phonemic inventory, 291–301
Phonemic transcription, 52
Phonetically consistent forms, 242
Phonetic analysis, 281–312
Phonetic notation, 52
Phonetics
acoustic, 3, 5, 41–45
articulatory, 3, 72–104
auditory, 3, 5
defined, 2, 3
form, 13, 17
function, 13, 17
as perception of speech sounds, 3–7
perceptual, 5
phonology and, 13–15
physiological, 22–40
as production, 3–7
as transmission, 3–7
Phonetic Teachers' Association. *See* International
Phonetic Association (IPA)
Phonetic transcription, 50–69
in articulation test, 286–87
case study on, 50
defined, 52–53
for foreign language teachers, 51
guidelines, 65–66, 69
as notation system, 51–52
purpose of, 60–62
using, 62–66
Phonetic variability, 242
Phonological development, 236–77
case study on, 236, 249
defined, 246
distinctive features and, 256–68, 259–62
first fifty words, 241–45

Phonological development (*cont.*)
  natural phonology and, 262–68, 263
  nonlinear phonology and, 271–74
  nonlinear theories, 268–74
  prelinguistic stages, 237–41
  preschool child, 245–51
  school-age child, 252–56
  theories of, 256–74
Phonological disorders, 14, 290
  case study on, 281
Phonological idioms, 251
Phonological process, 263
  suppression, 269
Phonological variations. *See* Foreign dialects
Phonology, 246
  clinical application of, 9
  defined, 7–9
  form, 13, 17
  function, 13, 17
  linear, 270, 277
  natural, 262–68, 276–77
  nonlinear, 270, 277
  phonemes, 8
  phonetics and, 13–15
Phonotactic constraints, 303
Phonotactic processes, 154
Phonotactics, 9
Photo Articulation Test (PAT-3), 284
Phrasal stress, 209
Physiological phonetics, 22
  anatomical-physiological foundation of speech
    production, 22–24
  articulatory system, 39–40
  clinical application of, 25
  phonatory system, 29–35
  resonatory system, 35–38
  respiratory system, 25–29
Pidgin, 171
Pitch, 5, 16, 206, 207
Place, 272
Play, vocal, 238–39, 274–75
Plays (dramatic), pronunciation in, 65
Pleura, 26
Pleural linkage, 26
Postdorsal, 338
Postdorsal division of tongue, 111
Postpalatal, 113, 349
Predorsal, 111
Predorsal division of tongue, 111
Prelinguistic behavior, 237
Prelinguistic jargon, 241
Prelinguistic stages, 237–41
  canonical babbling, 239–40
  clinical application for, 239
  consonant-like sounds, 240
  cooing and laughing, 238
  jargon stage, 240
  prosodic feature development, 241
  reflexive crying and vegetative sounds, 238

  syllable shapes, 241
  vocal play, 238–39
  vowel-like sounds, 240
Prepalatal, 113, 349
Preschool children, 245–51
  prosodic feature development, 251
  segmental development, 246–51
Pressure
  alveolar, 27
  atmospheric, 27
Primary cardinal vowels, 82
Primary function, 24
Primary stress, 226
Processes
  assimilation, 267–68
  natural, 263
  phonological, 263
  phonotactic, 154
  substitution, 154, 264–67
Production, 11
  approach phase, 116
  characteristics, 3
  charting accuracy, 67
  of consonants, 108–45
  features, 74
  fricative, 121–22
  light and dark /l/, 142
  nasal, 118–21
  release phase, 116
  "s," 133
  "sh," 135
  speech, 21–47
  stop phase, 116
  stop-plosive, 117–18
  variations of "s," 4
  vowel, 93
Progressive assimilation, 203, 205
Pronunciation, 7
  of British English, 92
  received, 65
Prosodic feature development, 241, 245
  of preschool children, 251
  of school-age children, 255–56
Prosodic variability, 155
Protowords, 242
Puerto Rican American English, 179
Pulmonic consonants, 57
Pulmonic sounds, 56

Q
Quasi-words, 242
Quiet breathing, 33

R
Race, 167
Rap, dialect shift and, 172
R-coloring, 93
  central vowels with, 96
Received pronunciation, 65

Spanish American English, 174–78, 397–98
Spectrography, 43
Speech
    aberrant, 135–36
    breathing, 24
    case study on, 200
    in context, 200–212
    defined, 2
    in diacritics, 212–30
    mechanism, 22
    melody, 208, 231
    perception of, 5
    sound source for, 33
    spontaneous, 66, 222, 289–91
Speech disorders, fricatives and, 119
Speech-language pathologists, 62
Speech production
    anatomical-physiological foundation of, 22–24
    case study on, 21
    overview of, 21–47
Speech sounds, 2, 73
    development, 247
    function, 7
    perception of, 3–7
Spelling, problems, 61. *See also* Orthography
Spoken syllabification, guidelines for, 302
Spontaneous speech, 222
    case study on, 290
    citation-form articulation test *versus,* 66
    exercises for, 400–401
    sampling, 289–91, 311–12
Spreading, 202
S-productions
    case study on, 133, 222
    clinical application of, 133
    lateral, 137
    types of, 133
Stage accent, 65
Standard English
    Formal, 152
    Informal, 152
    vernacular English *versus,* 152–53
Sternohyoid muscle, 31
Stimulability testing, 288–89, 310–11
Stop phase, 116
Stopping, 265–66
    age of suppression of, 266
Stop-plosive productions, 116, 126–27, 248
    aspiration and nonaspiration of, 219
    characteristics of, 117–18, 144
    exercises for, 338–41
    unreleased, 220
Stops, unreleased, 220
Stress, 209, 211, 232
    contrastive, 251, 255
    phrasal, 209
    primary, 226
    secondary, 226–27
    word, 209, 210

Stressed syllables, unstressed *versus,* 324–29
Stress markers, 226–27
Structured Photographic Articulation Test II, 285
Stylohyoid muscles, 31
Subglottal, 28
Subglottal air pressure, 34
Substitution processes, 154, 264–67
    affrication, 266
    alveolarization, 265
    case study on, 266
    deaffrication, 266
    denasalization, 266
    derhotacization, 267
    fronting, 265
    gliding, 267
    labialization, 265
    stopping, 265–66
    vowelization, 267
Suprahyoid muscles, 31
Suprasegmentals, 59, 206–12
    diacritics for, 226–30
    duration symbols, 228–29
    features of, 201
    juncture symbols, 227–28
    stress markers, 226–27
    syllable boundaries, 229–30
Surface-level representation, 268
Swallowing
    dysphagia, 29
    function of, 37
Syllabic, 388–89
    consonants, 220–21, 302, 312
    sound, 125
Syllable-initiating segments, 312
Syllables, 73
    boundaries, 229–30
    categorization of, 312
    closed, 303
    coda, 302
    initiating segments, 302
    nucleus of, 73
    onset, 302
    open, 303
    reduplication, 242
    shapes, 241
    stressed *versus* unstressed, 324–29
    structure, 301–9
    structure changes, 263–64
    terminating sounds, 302
Syllable-terminating sounds, 312
Symbols
    diacritics, of International Phonetic Alphabet, 213
    duration, 228–29
    of International Phonetic Alphabet, 55–59, 64, 129
    juncture, 227–28
    nasality, 225–26
    phonetic, 54
    suprasegmentals, 59
    tones, 59

voice, 218–23
voiced, 213
voiceless, 213
word accents, 59
Systems
alphabetic, 54
analphabetic, 54
articulatory, 22, 23, 39–40
phonatory, 22, 23, 29–35
resonatory, 22, 23, 35–38
respiratory, 25–29
transcription, 54–59

T
Teeth, 4, 22, 39
function of, 40
Tempo, 211, 232
Tense vowels, 79, 81
Testing
articulation, 282–88
citation-form, 282
stimulability, 288–89
Thoracic cavity, 27
Thoracic muscles, 25, 28
Thoracic resistance, 28
Thyrohyoid muscles, 31
Thyroid cartilage, 32
Timbre, 34
Tone, 59, 206, 207, 231
Tone-unit, 251
Tongue, 3, 22, 39
advanced/retracted position, 224
apical division, 111
coronal division, 111
dimensions of, 76
divisions of, 112
height, 78
mediodorsal division, 111
placement for "s" and "sh," 113
postdorsal division, 111
predorsal division, 111
raised/lowered position, 223–24
Tongue position, 39, 75
for apico-alveolar and predorsal-alveolar, 132
for back vowels, 92
for central vowels, 95
for front vowels, 89
for interdental and apico-dental productions,
131
for /j/, 140
for /k/ and /g/, 128
for /r/, 141
for /t/ and /d/, 127
for /w/, 139
Total assimilation, 205, 231
Transcription
audio recordings, 60
broad, 53
broad *versus* narrow, 53

narrow, 52
phonemic, 52
phonetic, 50–69, 52, 53
of rhotic diphthongs, 99
systems, 54–59
video recordings, 60
Transcription workbook
answers for, 402–11
approximants, 364–72
articulation testing, 400–401
centering or rhotic diphthongs, 379–83
central vowels, 373–78
diacritics, 384–94
dialect, 395–99
diphthongs, 357–63
fricatives, 349–56
letters *versus* sounds, 318–23
nasals, 364–72
spontaneous speech, 400–401
stop-plosives, 338–41
stressed *versus* unstressed syllables, 324–29
vowels, 330–37, 342–48
Transfer, 167
Transmission properties, 3
Two-word stage, 242

U
Underlying representation, 269
United States
midland dialects, 165
northern dialects, 164
phonological geography of mainland, 163–65
southern dialects, 164
western dialects, 165
Unreleased stop-plosives, exercises for, 386–87
Unreleased stops, 220
Unrounded vowels, 77
Unstressed syllables, stressed *versus*, 324–29
Uvula, 39, 40

V
Variations
consonants cluster, 154
dialectal, 153–55
free, 12–13, 17
phonological (*See* Foreign dialects)
of r-productions, 161–62, 194
Variegated babbling. *See* Nonreduplicated babbling
Vegetative sounds, 238, 274
Velar, 113, 338
Velarization, 216
exercises for, 384
Velopharyngeal mechanism, 37, 38, 46
resonance and, 38
Velopharyngeal port, 37
Velum, 4, 22, 39, 40, 115
Vernacular Black English. *See* African American
Vernacular English (AAVE)
Vernacular dialects, 152

Vibration
  forced, 41
  free, 41
  vocal fold, 8, 24, 34–35, 46
Video recording, as transcription, 60
Vietnamese American English, 180–81, 398
  consonants of, 181
  vowels of, 181
Virgules, 53
Vital functions, 24
Vocal fold vibration, 8, 24, 46
  mechanism in, 34–35
Vocal play, 238–39, 274–75
Vocal tract, 35
  as resonator, 43
Voiceless approximants, 123
Voice symbols, 218–23
Voicing, 124
  changes in, 267
  exercises for, 385–86
  partial, 385–86
  phonetic description of, 124
Vowel articulation, dimensions of, 77–78, 101–2
Vowel distortions, case study on, 224
Vowelization, 267
Vowel-like sounds, 240
Vowels, 4, 57
  allophonic variations of, 100
  American English, 75–78
  area of, 76
  articulation of, 75
  back, 76, 90–92
  case study on, 84, 100–101
  categorization of, 82–84, 83
  central, 76, 93–96, 373–78
  clinical application for, 93, 98

close, 80, 82
consonants *versus*, 73–74, 109
diacritics used with, 223–26
exercises for, 330–37, 342–48, 390–91, 395
extreme positions, 82
front, 76, 87–89
of General American English, 79
high, 75
lax, 79, 81
long, 80
low, 75
mid, 75, 82
monophthong, 100
nasality symbols, 225–26
Northern vowel shifts, 156–59
open, 80, 82
primary cardinal, 82
production of, 44–45, 46–47, 72–104
quadrilateral, 77, 79, 83, 86
quality of, 37, 44
rounded, 77
secondary cardinal, 83
shift, 159
short, 80
Southern shifts, 156–59
of Spanish, 176
tense, 79, 81
therapy, 98
types of, 84–99
unrounded, 77

W

Waves, complex, 42
Western dialects, 165
Word accents, 59
Word stress, 209, 210